Relationship Rewired

A COUPLE SURVIVES THE
EFFECTS OF A BRAIN TUMOR

Dot,
A beautiful lady with a kind heart...
With gratitude and love,
Martee

Enjoy!
Joe

Relationship Rewired

A COUPLE SURVIVES THE
EFFECTS OF A BRAIN TUMOR

Martha M Dumas and Joseph S Dumas

Pompano Pubs
2014

For Nancy Tharler, LICSW
For taking the initiative to help us through one of the worst times of our life.
and
Margo Greenhow
For knowing when and how to reach out to a friend.

CONTENTS

ACKNOWLEDGEMENTS

The greatest gift one can give another is *giving*. We have been on the receiving end of that precious gift throughout the experiences associated with Martie's brain tumor. We are fortunate to have loving people in our lives who gave and gave and gave, and then gave some more. They play an important part in our story.

There was a generous preparing of cooked meals during the radiation treatments by Martie's friend, Margo Greenhow. How we looked forward to them on Friday of each week. Our heartfelt thanks to you, Margo. And to neighbors and friends, who provided meals that seemed to show up at our door just when we needed them.

Thanks to the many drivers who gave rides when Martie wasn't allowed to drive, or just to give Joe a break.

We are indebted to our son, Ken and his wife, Danielle, for the sleep-overs during the many weeks of grueling radiation. At the same time we couldn't have managed the radiation treatments in Boston without the generous help from special friends, Robert and Anna, and Beverly, dearest friends who opened their homes for us. Many thanks to Linda who drove Martie back and forth to the Brigham. And to additional friends who filled in the gaps.

Much gratitude goes to our son, Tim, who was living in Montana at the time of Martie's four weeks of hospitalization. He called every night to say, "goodnight, Mom." That was a treasure for her. In addition, Martie's friend, Martha from high school, and Carol from our Buffalo days, called to wish her well as each day ended. Martie looked forward to those calls every night.

Acknowledgements

Humble thanks go to Anna, Beverly, Margo, Billy and Barbara, Anne, and Donna, for staying with Martie during her early recovery at home when Joe returned to work. Martie relishes those times.

Friendship and thanks to Les and Eileen Gladu for their willingness to always listen without judging, and for being available in the way only next-door neighbors can.

Martie has a shopping bag that represents an abundance of *giving*. It was filled with cards, flowers, candies with her name imprinted, hundreds of emails, teddy bears, and games. There's a multitude of you, around the country. You know what you did. Nothing was too small. Every act of *giving* was gracefully received, and touched our lives.

To all the doctors, nurses, aids, rehabilitation specialists who worked with us at Cape Cod Hospital and at Spaulding Rehabilitation Hospital. And to the doctors, radiation therapists, social workers, nurses at Brigham & Women's Hospital. We are in awe of what you do. Special gratitude to our therapist. When we got derailed due to the trauma, you got us back on track.

To Nancy Tharler, LICSW, social worker for Dana-Farber, who divided her work with the Brigham, and made time for us while Martie was undergoing radiation treatments. We are impressed with your skills and kindness, and for helping us through a terrifying time.

Many, many people supported and encouraged us in the writing of this book. Thanks go to:

Martie's friend, Margo, who introduced her to Barbara Potzka. Barbara had the wisdom to notice Martie's re-telling of her 'story', and invited her to join a writing course, *Memories to Life Stories* at the Academy for Lifelong Learning held at the Cape Cod Community College.

Dorothy Swanback, coordinator of the course, *Memories to Life Stories*. Martie appreciates Dottie for her nurturing guidance and important suggestions as she wrote and read chapters from her book.

The students in the class, *Memories to Life Stories*, who encouraged and supported Martie over three years as she wrote chapter after chapter. She remembers hearing, "This book has to be published."

Martie's diligent and dedicated readers of drafts: Sue Andrew, Barbara Hayes, Susan Kaplan, Karen Kierstead, and Alice Barkin, who took the time to read every chapter as Martie wrote it. We are deeply indebted to you for your valuable comments. Your encouragement to Martie to keep writing always lifted her spirits, and helped her to keep going with her story. To Alice: Martie enjoyed special times with you as you both reviewed each chapter together over the phone.

Samantha White and Susan Andrew, both clinical social workers, who provided invaluable assistance with clinical ideas.

Janet Nichols, Mary Dumas, Beth Ellis, and Helen Klein, who read early chapters and provided the encouragement and support that Martie needed in the beginning of her writing.

Kay Kramer, Mary Nyman, and Linda Jackson, friends and writers, who spent many lunches strategizing about 'the book'.

The many friends and people who know Martie from the various activities she pursues. You know who you are. You are the ones who always ask, "How's the book?"

Anne LeClaire, notable author from Chatham, who graciously agreed to read our book and provide a quote for the back cover. It was at the Cape Cod Writer's Conference when Anne taught a course in *Memoir Writing* that Martie met Anne, and Susan Kaplan. Anne provided wisdom and encouragement to Martie for the first chapter. The publishing of our book brings the three of them together again. Our humble thanks to you.

Steven H. Manchester and Suzanne Strempek Shea, both published authors, offered hours of guidance and advice through many emails, as we worked to get our book published.

To Tempe Goodhue who meticulously read every word as she edited our manuscript. How you kept all our details in your head astounds us.

Paulette Richard-O'Rourke for her guidance and support of Martie throughout the writing and publishing of the book.

We are indebted to Susan Kaplan who partnered with us in publishing this book. She provided a great sounding board for many ideas, especially on the book title, creation of the book cover, and so much more.

Danielle Nordin helped us untangle the mysteries of MS Word© headers and footers.

We cannot leave out our special daughters-in law, Joanna Dumas and Danielle Dumas, both writers, themselves. Martie is grateful to you for your interest and encouragement at every step to continue writing.

Acknowledgements

To Martie's colleagues at Natick Holistic Therapies for their patience and concern of Martie during our trying times. Special thanks go to Sue and Nedra for covering Martie's clients all those months before she closed her practice.

To Martie's clients for their everlasting patience and understanding especially during the interruption of their treatment.

To Joe's colleagues at Bentley University for their support. Special thanks go to Lena Dmitrieva, who helped us navigate the maze at the Brigham, and for giving rides to Martie.

Again special thanks to our sons, Kenneth and Timothy. This was a tough ordeal for all of us as a family. We always know we can count on you to be there for us with your love and support.

AUTHORS' NOTE

Throughout this book we have written our own, separate sections describing how we experienced events between January 2007 and September 2012. Each section is formatted in different fonts.

Martie's looks like this.

Joe's looks like this.

We have changed the names of all of the medical personnel we mention: doctors, nurses, social workers, etc., to preserve their privacy. We have not changed the names of friends and family. We use their actual names, with their permission.

The events we describe are based on Martie's medical records, which we have obtained from the relevant hospitals, and our memories. The dialogue we quote is from our notes and our memories.

FOREWORD

Whoosh, I am propelled back to consciousness from the anesthesia. I turn my head and see Joe by my bed, just like I wanted. My face is moist from tears. "This. Is. So. Hard." He places his hand on my shoulder, a familiar gesture of comfort.

A wave of panic hits as I realize I'm in the ICU. What's happened? His thumb circles my hand as he assures me, "Nothing out of the ordinary, it's standard protocol for Cape Cod Hospital." I've come through major surgery. A tumor was removed from my brain. I feel a sense of relief the surgery is over, and that I am alive. I believed I would die, especially after that awful seizure in the ER a few days ago.

———

It's forty-eight hours after the surgery and I cannot move any muscles on the left side of my body: my arm, leg, or torso. None of those muscles respond to my **willing** them to move. That's how the brain works, doesn't it? We will our muscles to move, and through intricate channels of electrical impulses, messages are sent from the brain to those muscles of the limbs we want to move. But my muscles seem dead. Immovable. Half my body feels marooned. I close my eyes, feeling helpless. One half of me has life and movement, the other is dead weight.

My life is turned inside-out. Did I do something to cause the tumor? The paralysis? I'm a *goody-two-shoes* who does all the right things: nutritious diet, work-out in the gym, daily meditation, yoga classes. A week ago I was off Cape in my office assisting psychotherapy clients, then preparing to meet Joe for dinner. Now I am in a hospital bed partially paralyzed.

There's a tightness in my chest that's starting to consume me. I am scared.

This fear reminds me of a story of Buddhist monks whose monastery is located on the top of a mountain. One day the director needs to go down to the village for supplies. He instructs his monks to lock the door after he leaves, and **not** open it for anyone. He will return in a few days. Later that evening the monks hear a knock, which they ignore at first, but as the knocking becomes bolder, they open the door. Who is standing there? Fear. He strides in quickly before the monks can shut him out. The monks quiver at his sight and hide in a corner. In response to their quivering and shaking, Fear grows larger and larger. Fear grows so large he crowds the room. The monks feel helpless.

The following day the director returns and sees the situation. He takes one look at Fear looming over the monks and says, "Fear, come with me. Let us sit and have tea." As the director talks to Fear something mysterious happens. Fear begins to shrink. He becomes smaller and smaller as the Director talks to him. Eventually Fear slides under the door and disappears.

I will have tea with *my* fear. I bring two cups. I push a cup toward Fear and pour the tea. He appears uncomfortable as his over-sized bulk hangs off the chair. I watch him shrink smaller when I ask, *"How will I find myself?"* Passing the cream I continue, *"Will I be whole?"* He shrinks down a bit more. I take a sip of my tea and feel encouraged to ask, *"Will I be loved?"* He's now the size of a small child. Boldly, I question him, *"Will I walk again?"* Fear has become a puddle under the chair.

Finally, I put my tea cup down and ask, *"Will you listen to my story?"*

Each day you define
more and more
who you are becoming
and how you want
your life to be.

—Hallmark

WAKE UP!

I see three firemen at the foot of my bed. What are *they* doing here! Am I dreaming?

My head falls back on the pillow as I search for sleep, but it eludes me. I don't know what time it is. Probably the middle of the night—when time is suspended and everything in life seem grossly out of place. You know what I mean. The time when feelings become dark and sometimes perverse. When the day's events are relived, and get exaggerated and out of focus. Doubts pound heavy, fears scream louder, thoughts go wild, and anxiety springs into action. It's the time when bad dreams occur—even nightmares. It's also the time when medical surprises and compromises to the human body occur. That's the time—the middle of the night—when I wake feeling disoriented and far away, like something out of the ordinary has happened. I remember a remnant of a conversation. I don't understand what prompted Joe to announce, "I'm going to call 911."

Oh. *That's* why they're here.

———

Why do I call 911 within about two minutes of getting whopped on the head by Martie's arm? I wish I could tell you it was after a logical analysis of the situation. But it didn't happen that way.

After the hit woke me, I see it is 2:30 a.m. I walk around the bed to Martie's side. She seems to be awake but is not moving. I stroke her bare arm and say, "How you doing?" She responds with an "OK" that feels more like, "It's not OK." When you have been married to someone for

43 years, you know when you are not making an emotional connection. I wasn't getting through.

It's at that moment my unconscious puts together the pattern of events that occurred over the previous few days. It pops into my head that there's something neurological going on. A startling insight! Perhaps because I had been asleep, my rational left brain is at rest allowing my intuitive right brain to see the pattern. I have no other explanation.

Then my left brain takes over. Having been trained as a scientist, I decide to test the insight. "I'm going to call 911."

Silence. "That's the emergency number," she says in a flat, emotionless tone. I expect something like, "Do you think you should?" or "What if it's only an allergy?" or "Yes, do that."

There *is* something seriously wrong.

I pick up the phone handset and move into the hall. I hesitate. What will I say? What if the dispatcher cross-examines me about the need for an ambulance? Can I convince the firefighters to come? There is no time to rehearse. I dial. (The following conversation is from my memory. I have no doubt that if we had a transcript, the dispatcher followed proper procedure.)

"Hello, emergency dispatcher."

"My wife needs help."

"Can you give me your phone number?"

I give the number.

"And your name?"

I give my name.

"Where are you calling from?"

I give the address.

"You are calling because?"

"There's something wrong with my wife. She's very distant. It's not like her." If the dispatcher asks for more symptoms, I don't have any.

"What is her age?"

"61."

"Someone will be there shortly."

"Thank you." The cross-examination I anticipated never occurs.

———

One of the firemen walks over to the side of my bed and I realize there are not three firemen but two. In my hazy state, I mistook Joe for the third one.

"Can you sit up?," he asks. I struggle to move and he assists me by moving my legs over the side of the bed. I sit upright. "Where did the blood on your pajamas come from?" I look down at my pajama top and notice the blood stains.

"I must have bitten my tongue again, like I did earlier this afternoon."

After that things happen fast. "Get the stretcher!" the fireman orders his partner, who flies down the stairs. Now the fireman grabs me under my arms and helps me up.

"Get on the other side of her," he calls to Joe. With Joe and the fireman on either side of me, we slowly and tentatively go down the stairs. When I reach the bottom of the stairs, I stand next to Joe and watch while the other fireman rearranges my living room furniture so he can prepare the stretcher for me. How can there be a stretcher in my living room? This is an eerie scene. My living room? A stretcher? Out of the corner of my eye I see an ambulance in the driveway. The lights are flashing, pulsing rapidly in such a way that I think I see snow. But it is not snow. It is the strobe effect from the flashing red and blue lights that creates the illusion of snow. There has been no snow yet this season—it is January 17, 2007.

———

As I walk down the stairs from the second floor holding onto one side of Martie, the EMT holding the other, I look down into the living room and see a very large gurney. "This is surreal. This can't be happening."

———

My mind starts to wake up to the events around me. I have no shoes or slippers on. I'm in my pajamas. Where's my coat? I can't go out in the cold like this. Where are they taking me? Can Joe come with me? Will I be all right? What's happening? I have so many questions I am beginning to scare myself. In addition,

I'm too weak or groggy to begin to figure out much less take any control of this situation. I feel myself go into a state of bewilderment—call it shock, if you like—because that's how I feel—in shock. If I don't go into shock I will start to feel, and this bundle of feel is too scary now. It is pummeling against a solid wall I call bewilderment. One feeling begins to ooze its way out, the dominant one—*terror!*

I must calm myself and let this bewildered state infuse my mind; otherwise I will not be able to get through whatever lies ahead. Let these firemen do their job and take care of me. I remind myself that these young men are trained professionals who know what they are doing and I, in my foggy state, promise myself I will let go of my need to control and will trust them. In one swift movement the two firemen bundle me up in a blanket and swing me onto the stretcher. They wrap me snugly so I feel warm—even my feet.

"We are headed to Cape Cod Hospital emergency room," they tell Joe. "You can meet us there. But *don't* try to keep up with us."

They strap me tightly in the stretcher. We proceed with a bounce out the front door and over the grass to the back of the open ambulance. One smooth movement propels me up and into the ambulance where I meet a third EMT and view a set of monitors. I start to relax and doze again. The last thing I hear before we leave the driveway is a loud thud, the impact of the ambulance doors as they are shut tight.

As I look through the window of the ambulance and see Martie propped up in the gurney while they hook her up to the monitoring equipment, I think, "They're taking her away. Will I see her again? Will she know me?"

In the ambulance, I wake up and drift in and out—not really in and out of consciousness, I'm in a sort of a dream-like state. I look around at the EMT watching the monitors. He turns toward me.

"Do you feel comfortable, are you warm enough?"

"Yes." I am reassured he's there. I feel relieved and safe now. Maybe someone will find out what is wrong with me.

I have not been right for quite some time. But I haven't been able to pin down just what is wrong. I don't even look myself. I see that in the mirror. I look pale. Even had a facial to see if that fashionable teen-Gothic white would disappear. It didn't. When I established a new primary care doctor on the Cape and told him I was very fatigued, in fact, unusually fatigued, he repeated back to me my stressful schedule—working off Cape with my psychotherapy practice and the hard traveling back and forth. He ran blood tests, all values normal. I know I could have persisted with him, but I was afraid. Yes, afraid he would find something.

What came to mind was a conversation I had some months ago with my Aunt Ann, my father's youngest sister, who told me her story of feeling fatigued and "oh so tired, like I've never felt before." Her symptoms mirrored my tiredness, and were the result of an aggressive cancer. Her story scared me. Even though I knew down deep that something was wrong, I was afraid to pursue it. And then again, I rationalized, I had no other symptoms. My blood levels were normal.

So I agreed with my doctor that my tiredness really was due to my work schedule, which I had to admit was grueling. It went something like this. On Tuesday morning Joe and I left our home to go off Cape to our respective jobs— he to Bentley College and me to my psychotherapy practice in Natick. We had lived in Natick for 30 years raising our two sons, and moved to the Cape two years ago, in 2005. In moving to the Cape, we fulfilled a long-held dream. We were happy with ourselves. We made it happen.

A colleague convinced me to commute from the Cape and continue my practice in Natick. I liked the idea because I was very proud of my practice. I grew it from nothing in 1999 and hated the idea of closing it and saying good-bye to all my clients. Joe enjoyed his work in the usability engineering field and had many colleagues in the Boston area. Bentley was a good fit for him. He was teaching, mentoring, and consulting. Also, we were not old enough, nor were we ready, to retire. Driving off Cape like this allowed us to live our dream and not dip into our retirement savings. It worked for us.

Our friends perceived this arrangement as hard and tiring, and it was. But for us it was part of our journey and an adventure. We met at the Red Roof Inn on Tuesday evenings—arriving in separate cars. We couldn't travel in one car because of our different schedules. Joe took care of the check-in, and I the check-out.

What do you suppose the management staff thought! We had them guessing for a long time. We drove home on Wednesday evenings. And on Thursdays we were very tired. We had been following that schedule for two years.

———

Back in the ambulance I drift off to sleep but have a sense of being shifted around. I sense darkness like we are not outside anymore. I feel like I am riding in a long, dark corridor. I guess the ambulance has come in through a garage. The EMTs manage to get me out of the ambulance. We roll along through the back entrance to the ER.

I am awake now as we enter the emergency room. The lights are very bright. The stretcher upon which I am securely strapped is being rolled down the hall. Cape Cod Hospital is small but growing. It bears no likeness to the fictitious urban teaching hospital of *ER*, the TV series, where there is a constant stream of people pouring in the ER doors, and staff running every which way to confront the next crisis and participate in the next drama.

Instead, at 3:30 a.m. I see a large area with desks, nurses, aides, and people who appear to be doctors. Who are they all? What are they doing? It looks like they are hanging around waiting for somebody or for something to happen. On the other side I see small cubicles with beds where patients and their families wait with anxious looks. All are awaiting answers about what has frightened *them* in the middle of the night.

The EMTs are guiding me into one of the cubbies to settle me into an available bed. As they begin the transfer from stretcher to bed, I hear the nurse say, "On my count..." At the same moment, I feel the need to stretch my left leg. That's when all hell breaks loose. Everything in my body begins to shake—all at once, and I mean shake uncontrollably. I can't stop it. Nothing like this has ever happened to me. I can't feel my body. I can do anything to stop it. I'm terrified. What is happening? Somebody do something! Somebody help me! I am out of it...out of my body...don't know where I...seem to be in space. What am I to do? I try to call out for help, but my throat closes up. I try telling them what is happening. I can't even move my head. I don't even know who's with me. I feel all alone. Will I ever see anyone I love again? Where is Joe? I want to tell him I love him. What about my sons, Ken and Tim? There's no time to tell them...they're not here...I believe I am dying. Everything goes dark.

I guess I created a little drama of my own.

To my surprise, after the seizure I am paralyzed on my left side—from my left shoulder all the way down to my left foot.

———

I am surprised when the emergency room attendant calls my name. I have only been waiting about half an hour. During that time I breathe and try to keep from thinking because there is nothing positive to think about.

"Your wife is in room 13."

"How appropriate."

I am self-conscious as I walk through the emergency room. No one seems to notice me. Some nurses and doctors are walking with purpose, others typing at computers. I see the patient rooms along the far wall and walk to #13.

I look in to see a nurse busy with wires. Martie sees me and bursts out crying. "I thought I would never see you again...had this awful seizure... thought I was dying...I was shaking...I can't move my left leg or arm."

My mind goes blank. I feel the adrenalin spreading through my body. My hands shake. I move toward the bed and grab her hand, her left one to calm us both. No response. I bend down and hug her as best I can. More tears. My legs begin to vibrate.

I manage to get out, "What happened?"

Martie talks about moving from the stretcher to a bed and having a seizure and after that not being able to move. They did a CT scan and she is waiting for the results.

"Do they know what's causing all this?"

"I don't know. Nothing seems to make sense."

I am guessing that she had a stroke. What else could it be?

I look up at the monitor above her head. It's a Hewlett-Packard monitor. By chance I had worked on its design in my earlier days as a human factors consultant. It shows very abnormal readings. Her blood pressure is 151 over 50. Her pulse is racing. Her breathing is shallow.

The numbers don't lie, and they are not good. I keep the monitor readings to myself so as not to upset Martie even more. Later I realized that this is the first instance of my caretaking of her. I have to focus on her needs at this moment and put my panic away, where it will not be a threat.

The ER doctor walks in.

"The CT scan shows a brain tumor, probably a meningioma," he says. I hear the "-oma" part but not the rest of the word. This is the first indication of what the problem is. "Meningiomas are usually benign," he adds. That's a relief.

He reports he has called the neurosurgeon, who will be in around 6:30 a.m. to talk with us. The neurosurgeon has prescribed an antiseizure medication to start right away. We have three hours to make sense out of this.

When Joe is finally allowed into the room, I am overjoyed to see him and tell him so, and of my very deep feelings for him. And I am crying. He, in turn, is happy and full of relief to see me. I tell him of the terrible sensations while undergoing that awful seizure. He says the nurse reported to him that "Your wife had the seizure during the transfer from the stretcher to the bed, and I needed to tear off her pajamas to quickly hook up the IV and heart and oxygen monitors." Joe is helping me remember these details, and informs me my cubicle number is 13. He also looks at my readings on the monitors. He doesn't say anything, but I can tell he is alarmed.

Shortly thereafter the attending ER doctor talks with Joe and me. "The CT scan shows a tumor located on one of the outside layers of your brain." A brain tumor! Instant, paralyzing fear. Will I die from this? But then I hear, "It is benign." I exhale a breath I didn't know I was holding. Oh, I am so relieved. Are they sure?

It is the size of a plum! Do you know how big a plum is? (To this day I cannot eat one.) This tumor is resting on my right motor cortex, which is why I am paralyzed on my left side. This also explains why I experienced weakness and some loss of control when I tried to put on my jeans after biting my tongue earlier in the day. It is confirmed now that the two episodes I experienced yesterday and during the night were seizures.

It is about 4:30 a.m. and the attending ER doctor gives me antiseizure medication through the IV, along with a relaxant. In the meantime, Joe and I talk and process what has just happened.

And talk we do. Joe keeps me talking so I won't fall apart. He is very good at that. He reminisces about the early days of our marriage and the struggles we endured. He talks about "shuffling off to Buffalo" with our three-month-old infant son, Ken, in the backseat of our red Volkswagen Beetle. He brings these times up to remind me—and, I am sure, himself—that whatever we're facing here, we'll get through it and find our way. As we always have.

We also look back and start to piece together some of my most recent symptoms, which at the time seemed meaningless. The weekend before my seizures I experienced a strange stabbing pain in my right cheek. It came and went intermittently, and it hurt. It hurt so badly I had to place my hand on my cheek every time I felt the pain. I took Ibuprofen but it didn't touch the pain. I did not call my doctor because it was Saturday; if the pain persisted I will call him on Monday. Thoughts of going to the ER were dashed when I pictured myself explaining a pain in my cheekbone when otherwise I felt fine.

Then there was the smashed glass on the kitchen floor when we had neighbors over to watch the Patriot's playoff game. I put ice cubes in a glass, and in my mind's eye I believed I placed the glass on the counter. But the glass fell directly to the floor and smashed. My friends said I needed glasses. In my puzzled state, I countered with, "No, it was misperception." How did I know that?

I met with Joe on Tuesday, the day before my seizures, and, with a laugh, told him of the incident in my office where I spilled a cup of water all over my client, the office furniture, and myself. Another strange incident, and another misperception.

On Wednesday I did not feel well – but could not put words to my symptoms. I felt out of my body. I planned to meet my colleague, Sue, for an early breakfast before we meet our clients.

I'm not feeling any better after breakfast and feel as if I'm walking in slow motion as I enter my office building. My first client is a no-show. Always a disappointment. Today the feelings of disappointment seem distant. The second client is at home waiting for a plumber. She asks if we can do a phone session and I agree.

Later I place some phone calls, eat lunch, and listen to my inner self. I do not feel right. My stomach feels like someone has grabbed it and put it in a vise and twisted it to a torture level. I consider canceling the afternoon clients. I need to go home. But I *never* cancel clients when I am sick. I can always transcend any symptoms to be present for them and listen to what they need.

I ask my inner self, my angels, too: *what should I do?* I call my afternoon clients and reschedule them to the following week. Each one is supportive, giving back what I have taught them. After listening to their well-wishes and *it's good you're taking care of yourself, Martie,* I pack up my things. I call Joe and leave a message to tell him my plans and make the 90-mile ride home to the Cape and took a nap.

After waking from a nap, I noticed my tongue is ripped to shreds. Must have been my teeth. I felt fine otherwise, but that certainly was odd. Then I noticed I had trouble putting my left leg into my jeans. I had no control over my left leg; it wavered back and forth, but would not go into the pant leg. Finally with both hands I guide my leg into my jeans. I stand up, decide I feel fine, and walk down stairs and wait for Joe. I say to myself that the wobbly leg must have been an anomaly.

———

I was surprised when Martie left me a message that she had canceled her clients. The phrase she used was her "late clients." They were not actually that late but midafternoon. Normally, when she is not feeling well she toughs it out and keeps her appointments. It's more of a hassle to cancel and reschedule them. So she must be hurting. Lately she has been pale and she complains of pressure in her sinuses. While she has plant and animal allergies that might produce that symptom, this is January and we have no pets.

This winter has not been a good one for her health. She is tired most of the time. I have not seen her rosy cheeks for a while. On the other hand she has driven off Cape every week to see her clients and that has to take its toll. This is the second year we have been working several days a week a two hour drive away. On the nights we stay together at the Red Roof Inn, we do not sleep well. We often joke about it. We are not sure why we have

trouble sleeping, it's not particularly noisy and the beds are typical motel quality. Go figure. I will find out more when I get home tonight.

———

As we talk in the ER, we both realize that biting my tongue was my first seizure and had I not cancelled my afternoon clients I might have had that seizure on the road.

———

Time goes by and shift changes occur. It is looking like daybreak, and we find nurses from both shifts stopping by to talk. They realize we both have had a difficult night. They are reassuring and compassionate. They tell us about the neurosurgeon we will meet. His name is Dr. Anderson. The nurses speak highly of him—both personally and professionally. He has a good reputation as a skillful surgeon. These words are comforting, especially since this is the man who is will cut into my skull and probe with his hands and instruments around my brain!

It's 6:30 a.m. "Good morning, I'm Dr. Anderson." He exudes confidence as he shakes our hands. He has an air of authority but also a down-to-earth composure. His youth hits me immediately. He is younger than our sons, who are in their forties. But it is the young doctors who have had the teaching opportunities and are alert to new technologies and the best methods. He is a man of small build, average height at about 5 foot 9 inches, with short dark hair with strands falling forward in a natural way across his forehead. He has a ready smile and dark brown eyes that twinkle in synch with that smile. He wears rimless glasses. He has me at ease immediately.

Dr. Anderson appears to know about me and what occurred in the night. The first thing he says to me is that I am "going to be fine." He repeats this comforting phrase several times during our conversation. He confirms that I have a meningioma. He explains that "most meningiomas—95 percent—are benign. In many cases meningiomas grow slowly. Sometimes, depending on where it is located, a meningioma may reach a relatively large size before it causes symptoms. As they grow, meningiomas compress adjacent brain tissue." He looks right at me as he says this. He continues by saying, "Your tumor has pressed against the right side of your motor cortex."

Dr. Anderson pulls a cart with a computer on it, Joe and I can view the tumor on the CT scan. We are not familiar with reading these scans and are not sure what we are seeing. Later, Joe remembers seeing the tumor as a different color from the rest of the brain and pretty big. I have no memory of it. Dr. Anderson says, "Your meningioma is pretty large, but it's in a good place—on the top of your skull."

"Oh great!" I think.

"I know I will be able to get at it and remove it." Again he reassures me I am "going to be fine." He is confident it is benign as the vast majority of them are. His major concern is that I not have another seizure because that would complicate things. He verifies the correct dosage of the antiseizure medication.

Dr. Anderson says he plans to perform the surgery on Tuesday—five days from now. He bases this decision on the expectation that the swelling on my brain will soon decrease and the pressure on my motor cortex will lessen enough to allow normal movement to return to my left side. Then I'd go home. And wait for Tuesday. He asks me to perform tasks to determine my muscular strength. I fail them completely. I can't shrug my left shoulder or raise my left arm to push my left hand against him. I can't lift my left leg to push my left foot against him. After that evaluation, he decides I am to be admitted. I'll go to the recently opened Mugar Building and onto a floor that was opened the previous week. I'm relieved because I don't know how I could care for myself at home. I'd need assistance getting in and out of bed as well as help with just about everything else. Joe is relieved because amid all this chaos and questions, we now have a plan. As he puts it, "This is the beginning of a plan to deal with this."

Dr. Anderson leaves for surgery. Joe goes home. I go to Mugar 4.

———

I am in my room on Mugar 4. It's a beautiful private room with a large picture window. My view is of fields and the nighttime sky. There is a long window seat that can be used for a bed if someone cares to spend the night. The nurses and their staff all love this new wing. Each floor has advanced technological features for tracking patients.

Now that I have been admitted and am in my hospital bed, I'm feeling that sense of relief I felt in the ambulance. I'm being taken care of. I am safe. Thankfully, I am staying. Above my bed there is a sign warning all who come near: "CAUTION SEIZURE." There are special pads on the sides of the bed to protect me in case I have another one. No, I won't! There is much attention paid to me as I need assistance for most actions, especially getting in and out of bed. It takes two people all the time. I pay attention to learn the names of all the nurses and nursing aides, as well as the housekeeping staff. This keeps my mind occupied, plus people like it when I remember their names.

On the other hand, I am starting to get scared. I need to get back my state of bewilderment. The first time I became aware of it was back in my living room last night as I stood in my pajamas and bare feet watching the EMTs prepare a stretcher for me. It seems the bewilderment not only pushes the barrage of feelings back, it keeps things from being real and it helps me operate in a numbed fashion, as if things are an illusion or suspended. So far I think I have been moving along in a robotic manner, doing what I have been told and not really getting a chance to react or process any of what is or has happened. It is way too much to grasp. That's why I'm looking my comfort zone—my bewilderment.

I think about the idea of going home. I'm grateful I didn't. It would have thrown me right out of my comfort zone, and a heavy dose of reality would have come crashing down. Experiencing the familiarity of home would have broken through my protective state, and I would have had nothing to do but think about all that has happened and all that is to occur. Now I realize I am facing brain surgery, and I'm scared.

Things that have just occurred in my life—those seizures, the ambulance ride in the middle of the night, hospital admittance—are so out of the ordinary, so out of my day-to-day-experience that I can't catch my breath or wrap my arms around it. What's happening...to me...and to Joe...and to my life! One minute we were going along with our ordinary life, and the next thing—WHOOOSHH—it's out of our control It's like a slap upside the head. Only in this case it's a series of seizures brought on by a meningioma that's been growing inside my skull, for years probably, and is now pressing on my motor cortex. Presently, it—the tumor—wants OUT! And, frankly, with all the trouble it's been causing me, I want it out, too. I need my state of bewilderment back to protect me from thinking about the details of surgery. A group of doctors will actually go into my head...my skull...with a saw...oh my god! I can't go there.

———

I do some research on meningiomas. Here is my layman's explanation. The root of the word is the term "meninges," which are membranes that cover the brain and spinal cord. They help protect the central nervous system. The cerebrospinal fluid flows within the membranes, which are crisscrossed with veins that carry blood back to the heart.

Meningiomas form on the outside of the meninges—no one knows why. They are not inside the brain. As they grow, they push aside the brain, distorting it. They take a long time to grow, so most are not discovered until people are in their forties and fifties. Meningiomas are the most common type of brain tumor, accounting for 20 to 30 percent of them.

As far as I can tell, there are four strong correlations between meningiomas and other factors. First, they are twice as likely in women as men. Second, they are known to grow faster during pregnancy. Hence estrogen is assumed to be somehow related, at least to the rapidity of growth. Third, meningiomas occur more frequently in people of color than in Caucasians. Again, no one knows why. Martie is Caucasian.

The final correlation is with exposure to radiation. Scientists found that people exposed to radiation from the atomic bombs dropped on Hiroshima and Nagasaki had a higher incidence of meningiomas than would otherwise be expected, and the closer to the epicenter of the bomb, the larger the effect. If there is a known link to radiation exposure, say from radiation therapy, the tumors are called "radiation-induced meningiomas." Martie has not been exposed to above normal radiation.

Most tumors are discovered when they present themselves via symptoms. The pressure on the brain from the growing tumor can cause headaches, seizures, or other symptoms that depend on just where the tumor is pressing. In Martie's case, we now know that she had at least two seizures in the 12 hours before the big one in the ER. There may have been others we were not aware of. The left-side paralysis came from the pressure on her motor cortex on the right side of her brain, made worse from the swelling from the seizures. It is hard to believe that a tumor could get to be the size of a plum before it caused symptoms but it did. The most common location for meningiomas, like Martie's, is near the top of the brain. This location is actually a good one, if you have to have a tumor, because it is easier to remove surgically.

Complicating this picture is the fact that not all meningiomas are the same. Fortunately, only about 5 percent are malignant. Most, about 80 percent, are called "typical." They are slow growing and do not invade adjacent tissue or bone. They often are left alone if they are not causing symptoms. The rest, from 10 to 15 percent, are called "atypical." You can tell by that vague name that scientists don't know much about them. They grow faster than typical tumors, and they do invade adjacent bone and tissue. As we found out later, Martie's tumor was atypical. That is why it ate into her skull, and invaded and blocked the sagittal sinus, a major vein. Atypical tumors are more likely to recur than typical ones. That is why atypical tumors need to be treated more aggressively.

———

I am trying to get myself acclimated to the situation around me—in a hospital and facing surgery—brain surgery. The next thing I know I am being wheeled out of my hospital room and down to the Radiology Department for an MRI. I've never had an MRI. They ask if I am claustrophobic.

"I'm not sure."

I'm placed on a narrow bed with a sheet over my body and a plastic contraption over my face to keep my head in place. I *am* beginning to feel claustrophobic but say nothing. Head first, this narrow bed slowly moves me into a hollow tube—all the way in so my feet are almost in, too. Did I mention that the machine surrounding this tube is gigantic? Now I truly feel claustrophobic. I still say nothing. Instead, as the technicians begin the procedure, my body responds. My legs and lower body begin to squirm. Even my left leg is moving slightly. Very soon into the procedure, the technicians stop and say they will try again later. They agree that I'm claustrophobic. The technicians are compassionate. They make a recommendation to Dr. Anderson that I receive 10 milligrams of Valium the next time. Several hours later, with 10 milligrams of Valium in me, the MRI scan is performed successfully.

Later in the day—it's Friday now—Joe and I meet with Dr. Anderson. He wheels in a cart with a wireless computer. The Mugar Building is completely wireless. Dr. Anderson has trouble logging on at first and gets help from a staff member. It's his first attempt using the computers on this newly opened floor. Joe, who is in the computer field, comments about this, says, "It's a common problem people have everywhere in a new environment." Once Dr. Anderson gets the system up and running, he shows us a more detailed look at the tumor. It is not only resting on my motor cortex but also entwined in the major vein on the top of my brain—the sagittal sinus. I listen to all this information as if it were the weather report—like it is interesting news. I cannot respond.

Dr. Anderson begins to discuss the surgery. Oh my God. Is he really going to talk about this? He will make a horseshoe-shaped incision on the top on my head. Joe muses, "Just like the hood of a car, so you can look inside." What would I do without his humor? I discover I'm now on the surgery roster for Monday morning. The doctor is fearful that I may have more seizures. "The sooner the better," he says.

Whew! This is a ton of information to digest. I don't know if I am going to cry or scream. Joe helps me by distracting me. He tells me about the people he has begun to notify. He begins with our two sons, of course: Ken, who lives in Brookline, Massachusetts, with his wife, and Tim, who lives with his wife in Montana. Both sons are surprised and then filled with concern and finally relief after speaking with their dad. Joe has assured them both that I am in good hands. Joe also called my brother, who lives on the Cape, as well as my two sisters. He called his sisters and our next-door neighbors. Joe is a man of few words. How can he make these phone calls short?

Our sons are stunned, as is everyone else. Ken, in his usual coping mode, needs more and more information. He wants answers. For Tim, being so far away, it is difficult. He doesn't know what to do, whether to get on a plane. Joe and I lived away from our family for nine years; we understand what Tim may be experiencing. Joe advises Tim to wait.

———

Joe reports that a couple of my friends have called. I began to perk up now because there are many who need to be notified. I began my litany of, "Oh, but did you call…?" "You have to call…" I have a legion of friends. I pick up friends like little boys bring home puppies. I have friends from every activity I do, every job I have had, every school I have attended—even kindergarten, and I feel they all need to know. This activity keeps me from thinking about my fears and the seriousness of my surgery. My brother, Billy, is my first visitor. Yes, I cried, he cried, I was so happy to see him. I cry when I see every visitor.

But, wait! What about my clients and my private psychotherapy practice in Natick? Today is Friday. What do I do? I have a business off Cape. I share office space with several colleagues and have financial responsibilities. I have appointments with clients next Tuesday and Wednesday and in the weeks after that. None of my clients know what has happened to me and that they won't be seeing me for a while. I need to get some word out to them. How will I do that? They need to be informed, too.

I remember reading an article in the National Association of Social Workers newsletter—that's my profession's monthly newspaper—about a clinician who died and what happened to her practice. It was chaotic. The article suggested a plan be put in place for emergency events. Well, I am not planning on dying (now that I survived that scare with the seizure in the ER), but I need to get something in place, and quickly. I need clinicians to cover for me while I will not be available. My clients need clinicians to bridge this gap. And Joe is not the one to do it. He has enough on his hands, and clinically I can't put that kind of responsibility on him. And there is the confidentiality issue.

I devise a plan. I assign four of my colleagues to talk to my clients right away. I apportion out my clients among them. I write out a script for Joe to read to my colleagues over the phone. This script gives my clients information on the immediacy of my illness and my surgery. As part of this script I let them know that for an unknown period they can talk with and/or meet with the designated clinician. I am very specific that I am not available by phone.

I feel proud of myself for mastering this, for taking care of my clients at such a crucial and frightening time. It took my mind away from me. I also feel sad and disappointed that I could not talk with them myself and assure them that I will be OK.

Will I be OK? I don't know. What is going to happen after this brain surgery? Who knows these things? What happens when someone gets into your brain and starts cutting and maneuvering around? It's not the same as when the abdominal cavity is opened and the organs get jostled. In the case of the brain, the skull is cut with a special saw. I discovered that someone invented the saw specifically to STOP the second it hits soft tissue. How great is that! Still, this is a lot to swallow.

Everything else in my life seems to be in place—my family has been notified, some friends, too. My business and my clients will be taken care of. Now I need to prepare myself for surgery. I often support clients through situations such as surgery, chemotherapy, or childbirth. I think about what I say to help them and can use for myself, including visualizations that I will use during the weekend. Another important item includes involving people close to you—whom do I want to see when I wake up in the recovery room? That gets me thinking. Well, Joe, of course, then Ken and his wife, Danielle, my brother, Billy and his wife, Barbara. Yes, that'll do it. I would love to see Tim and his wife, Joanna, but that seems like too much to ask. They're too far away. Now all I need to do is wait for the surgery. I am ready—sort of.

———

My caretaking role continues with the phone calls. Over the next month I make several hundred. During the first few hours I call my sons, my sisters, and Martie's siblings. Then I spread out to additional relatives and many friends. Martie has a wide network of people with whom she keeps in regular contact. They need to be called before the operation. No one likes to think they are so far down the list that they aren't called soon after an emergency.

The calls during the first few days are the longest. You just can't call someone and say, "Martie is in the hospital with a brain tumor and is paralyzed. She will have brain surgery on Monday." It's too much of a shock to lay on people all at once. So I start with something like, "It's been quite a day."

I notice that once I start to tell the story, I can't stop, nor can I give a brief version. I need to include all the details. I also find myself telling

the story in my head while riding in the car going back and forth to the hospital and before I go to sleep and when I wake up.

The people I call seem to want details. Some express their amazement and sorrow. Others ask questions, many. I guess they need to calm their own anxiety.

A few people offer advice. I have a hard time dealing with people who want me to move Martie to a Boston hospital for the surgery. They are well meaning but can't accept our decision to stay at Cape Cod Hospital and with Dr. Anderson. Martie and I had discussed the pros and cons of a second opinion and moving. We felt comfortable with the doctor. I looked him up on the Internet. He is well educated and the doctors I talk with think highly of him.

We are less sure about the hospital. Cape Cod Hospital has a mixed reputation in the community among people who have been patients there. It's hard to make sense of the hospital ratings on the Internet, especially for an uncommon specialty like neurosurgery. But the ratings I can find for the hospital are quite good for many conditions. The kinds of medical problems that the Cape population tends to have, such as hip and knee replacement and stroke, are well treated there. Furthermore, the hospital has just opened a new wing and has a whole floor devoted to neurosurgery. Our assessment is that the hospital has had a spotty record in past years, but with the rise in the Cape population and rising income, it is improving, at least for many medical conditions.

We know that the Boston hospitals have great reputations, but which one would we choose? And which doctor? Will that doctor have the time to see us right away? Will the hospital's OR be available? Will Martie risk a seizure while being transferred? Can we even do that transfer with her paralysis?

We decided to stay at Cape Cod Hospital and put Martie's tumor in the hands of Dr. Anderson As I talk with friends and family on the phone, several don't agree. But I do not have the energy to debate the issue right now.

This caretaking is new. I'm not used to talking about emotional issues on the phone. It's not a guy thing. It actually helps that I have such a compulsion to repeat the details over and over.

It is during the weekend before the surgery that I hit on the idea of a group email. I have created distribution lists at work but never at home. As the list of people Martie wants me to keep in contact with grows, I do not see how I can make more phone calls, even keep up the ones I am making. Also, it looks like the recovery is going to take quite a while.

So I create a group with all of the addresses for the people I have been talking with on the phone and I begin to send out email updates. This was the first:

Subject: Martie today

Date: 1/20/2007 6:43 AM Eastern Standard Time

Dearest friends,

I am using email to keep you informed over the next few days. Email is sometimes an impersonal way to communicate. But each day I will look at your names and our connection. Thanks so much for your thoughts and prayers.

This is Saturday. Yesterday went well. Her left leg is still not coordinated. She needs help to walk. Her mood is good. Eating well.

The doctor came in and wheeled in a cart with a computer and we saw the results of the MRI. It showed the tumor. It's about the size of a plum. It may be touching a major blood vessel, which could mean that part of it can't be removed. The assumption is that the tumor is benign, 90–95% are. The surgery is still scheduled for Tuesday. They are getting her in as soon as they can because of the size of the tumor and its location. Further growth or another seizure could result in damage to her left leg because of the location of the tumor.

I have attached a Word file that describes what these tumors are all about.

Thanks for your concern and continue to keep us in your thoughts.

Joe

Writing about the events has a different impact on me than describing them over the phone. This first email doesn't say much about my feelings, but future ones do. I have no idea how the messages are being received because, unlike a phone call, there is no one on the other end to talk back.

But it gives me time to sit and think and the freedom to say what I want to these people, many of whom I care for deeply.

It's the night before the surgery and he's walking away from me. Kissing me good-bye and walking out the hospital room door. A familiar pattern for us. One that has defined our relationship. I hate to see him go. I miss him. We've been married 43 years and enjoy being together. We have been apart a lot before but not like this.

Joe has been in the consulting field for over 20 years, and consulting work means travel. A few years ago, his consulting firm won a big contract with the New York Stock Exchange. For a six-year period he flew down to New York on Monday morning and returned on Thursday, or sometimes Friday, evening. They were long weeks, but I was working at a private clinic and the boys had begun to fashion their own lives with jobs and a separate address from home. Yes, we missed each other, but we were both busy with our careers, and I also was active with volunteering, yoga, piano lessons, etc. So, our times together at home became precious. But this separation is very different. It's as though I won the contract this time. I expect that I will explore the ramifications of all these feeling during my recovery. Can't go there now.

If I feel alone, he must feel the same. But what else is he feeling? This "thing" that is going on in our lives—I don't know what name to give it—may change our lives profoundly. How scary. How will it change us as a couple? There are many questions, worries, and unknowns with this thing. It is still so new. We are each making our own way in this new medical "travesty." Is that what I'll name it? Too negative. Maybe I'll just call it "Martie's brain tumor." It's short. It's clear. And, right now, it's meaningful.

I reflect back to our conversation in the ER when Joe reminded me that we will get through this because we always have. I look at myself now—paralyzed on one side of my body, even the left side of my mouth—my smile is crooked. I can do nothing on my own. I can't even will my limbs to move—and believe me, I've been trying. My body feels useless. I feel discouraged. I can't walk, I need to be transported everywhere in a wheelchair. Two people need to help me get out of bed, go to the john, take a shower, lift the wraps off my food so I can eat, even lift me up in my bed when my body slides down. This is quite a state for a woman like me, who has always been quite independent. I'm completely dependent on other people to help me with every little thing. What will the brain surgery do? Will my condition get worse?

I don't want to dwell on that. Although I am dependent on people right now, I am also determined. I believe what Joe has said: "We will get through this." I will get through this. Somewhere deep down inside the kernel of who Martie is, I *know* I will get through this. My determination will serve me now.

I talk with the nurses about the impending surgery, and they are encouraging that the outcome will be a good one. They remind me that Dr. Anderson is an excellent surgeon. He has ordered a sleep aid for me and I take it without hesitation. My surgery is scheduled for tomorrow—Monday at 6:30 a.m. It has only been five days since this journey began. A lot has happened. I have a premonition that there's a lot more to come.

———

Joe arrives at 6 a.m. Monday. I am happy to see him. He greets me affectionately. He is followed shortly by Dr. Anderson, who is already in his scrubs. I guess he means business. He enters with some unknown materials in his hands. They are identifiers for my head. When he is finished, Joe says there are blue markings on top of my hair, like what the electric and gas companies leave on people's lawn to identify their respective cables. We are both surprised that I still have hair on my head. I surmise it will be shaved in the OR. I fully expect to be bald after the surgery. Dr. Anderson reassures me, once again, that "you'll be OK." The nurse calls for the stretcher.

———

I don't sleep well the night before the surgery. I set the alarm for 5:15 a.m. I kept waking and looking at the clock to make sure I didn't miss the alarm. Each time I wake I run through the events of the past few days, from beginning to end, as if I am talking with someone on the phone. I have to repeat the whole story up to yesterday's preparations for surgery.

When the alarm rings, I decide not to eat anything and just get to the hospital. It being January, there is no hint of a sunrise. The night before I had followed Martie's instructions and called Ken and her brother Billy to let them know that Martie wanted them there with their wives when she woke up after the surgery. Ken and Danielle said they would be coming down in the morning to stay with me. I will call Billy when the doctor calls me to let him know when to meet us.

I am not sure that having five people in the recovery room is wise or even if the nurses will let us all be there. What if they say no? It will be my job to do the convincing. It is important to Martie. I am not sure why it is important, but she is wiser than me about these things.

I can't fail her again. When she and I were 21, Ken was born. I was working as a golf course groundskeeper, a summer job, at the time. I received a message late one morning that her water had broken, and she was taking a taxi to the hospital. I went home, cleaned up the towels, and changed my clothes. I found my way to the hospital and the waiting area for fathers. In those days, fathers were not allowed to see mothers until after the birth. I checked in and the nurse said that Martie was being prepared and that I should wait. There was no one else waiting. I waited all day. Supper time came and I asked if I should go to eat. They said I should. I went and came back and waited some more. I should have called Martie's or my mother, but I thought I would wait until I had some good news for them. Never once did the nurses seek me out with some status information. The hours dragged. Finally, I was told I could see her; it was about 3 a.m. She had endured about 15 hours of labor and Ken had arrived, a healthy boy. She kept asking for me during the labor but to no avail. That night was the one of the loneliest of my married life. I have always blamed myself for the separation. I should have been more aggressive. I believe that I could have at least got in to see her. I was a wimp! That wasn't going to happen again.

Martie's room is buzzing at 6 a.m. Nurses in and out. I hear phone calls from the nurses' station to the OR preparation room asking for instructions. Dr. Anderson arrives and seems wide awake and calm. He marks Martie's head with blue Xs, perhaps to guide the saw. His reassurance that Martie is going to be fine lowers my tension a bit. He leaves to get ready.

At about 6:30, two volunteers arrive wheeling the OR "taxi," patients ride free. I walk along the corridors with them to the prep room. It's an amazing sight to see all the activity, staff everywhere, beds along the walls, and wires, monitors, and equipment. Everyone has a sense-of-purpose face on. After parking the bed, the volunteers leave and the first of many staff approaches. It's always the same: a smile, a hello, and "your name and date of birth please." They hook up the monitors and insert a new, larger IV line, starting the saline drip. I am hoping that they will give Martie something to calm her. But they offer nothing.

In between the interruptions, I try to talk with her. It's not easy. I don't know quite what to say. We are both tense, and we both know that she is facing five-plus hours of surgery. What can I say? A guy like me just can't invent small talk on demand. Super Bowl talk seems a bit of a stretch. "It's going to be cold today," feels too impersonal. "I am scared shitless," would be honest, I guess, but it might be too upsetting for both of us.

The anesthesiologist approaches. I can tell right away who he is. No smile, no eye contact. He offers that he is covering for another anesthesiologist, no explanation why. I guess we get the pinch hitter. He keeps paging though a folder full of forms and notes. He asks about allergies and medications. He talks about his plan, which is quite general—more drugs at first, less later. He doesn't offer anything to calm Martie's tension—not his job, apparently. He seems annoyed that something is missing from the folder—the only emotion he shows. He leaves without a word of encouragement; he is the ultimate technician.

It's 7:30. Some patients are being wheeled through the large double doors. A nurse comes by with the Valium drip. I guess they don't want you to be drowsy while they ask all their questions. Maybe you give better answers when you are tense. I squeeze Martie's hand, give her a kiss, and tell her I will see her in recovery. She disappears through the doors. No windows here with which to see where they are taking her. I turn my brain off. It is my enemy at this moment.

———

I go home and have breakfast. Ken and Danielle arrive. We talk and do some cleaning up. Have lunch and wait for the phone.

About 1:30, Dr. Anderson calls, calm as ever. He says that everything went well. He is encouraged by the fact that Martie could move her leg and arm when he asked her to. It means the pathways are active. He does say that he had to put a piece of titanium mesh into her skull to replace the bone that the tumor had eaten away. (This is a clear sign that the tumor is atypical, but I didn't get the connection then). Also that the tumor has blocked a major blood vessel, her sagittal sinus vein, and that he decided not to try to remove all of it. But almost the entire tumor is gone, and the signs for a full recovery are positive. Hooray for that!

I call Billy to ask him and his wife Barbara to meet us in an hour. Then I call Tim, my sisters, and Martie's sisters. They are all relieved as am I. Off to the hospital.

We all meet outside of the intensive care unit. I call in on the phone and the nurse comes out. She seems to know who Martie wants there and asks us to wait a minute while she settles another patient. No resistance to having all five of us. I have to back off my readiness to do battle over Martie's request and the hospital's policy. I'll have to prove my manhood some other day.

The surgery takes five and one-half hours. When I wake I am in the ICU, not the recovery room, as I anticipated. I see Joe, my son Ken and his wife Danielle, my brother Billy and his wife Barbara—all the people I wanted to see the very first thing. So, you know I cried. Joe is holding my hand as I spoke my first words to all of them: "This is so hard, I didn't think it would be this hard!" and then I cried some more. They were comforting. I told all of them I was happy to see them. There are no phones allowed in the ICU for obvious reasons (patients are too busy healing), so Joe told me he had called Tim and told him that the surgery went well and that I am OK.

Joe informs me I have on a white turban bandage, just like you see in the movies. He also notices that natural coloring has returned to my face for the first time in months. I place my hand to feel the white turban and notice I still have most of my hair. It seems the surgical team shaved only the top area of my scalp, where the team needed to cut into my skull. I notice slight movement on my left side. I can move my left arm and left leg a little bit. I am filled with hope and encouragement. I am happy to be alive! As much as I like socializing, sleep overcomes me and I drift away.

A HORSESHOE-SHAPED INCISION

Back on the hospital floor, Mugar 4, I begin my recovery. There are 39 staples in my skull keeping the horseshoe-shaped incision knitted tightly together so it will heal. The incision is approximately 3 1/2 inches long and 3 inches wide—about the size of my hand. I also learn I have lost a portion of my skull. The tumor, as it began its rapid growth, pushed its way into my skull and destroyed the bone. That part of my skull was replaced during surgery with titanium steel mesh— imagine the technology!—and kept in place by special cement. When my fingers migrate to the top of my head, it feels strange. Not just because I feel my skin there—my bald spot—but because I feel small bumps and tiny indentations that weren't there before. I guess that's the cement and the titanium mesh underneath. It feels creepy.

I fall asleep easily the first night but every two hours someone comes in to check vital signs. In addition, I awake automatically between midnight and one o'clock. I wake up scared. What's just happened to me? Why am I alive? How did I get this tumor? Dr. Anderson has assured me it is benign. He also tells me there are pieces of the tumor still present by that major vein, and they may need to be removed through radiation. I fall asleep and wake again at five. Again I am scared, and I want to talk to Joe. It's too early. I don't want to wake him. I watch foolish things on TV and wait for 7 o'clock. Is that too early to call?

Seven o'clock comes—or is it quarter to?—and I call Joe and wake him. This is the beginning of a daily early morning ritual. I cry.

"How is it that I can breathe on my own?" I begin sobbing. "How can my heart beat the way it is supposed to?" I am frightened and don't know exactly why.

Joe always has a way with his words and is able to soothe me and bring to this situation some sense of normal, a showing of reality.

"The doctors have a plan." He answers in calm words. "Day by day, we will get through this together."

A calm wave begins to hover. When I look back on it, I don't know how *he* did it. I am sure he was scared, himself, and exhausted, too. Here he is being awakened early (for him) to a terrified and weeping wife, and yet he always comes through with his soothing and loving affect.

On Tuesday she is back at Mugar, in a different room from her weekend stay. On Tuesday night, Dr. Anderson comes in. He does his check of her mobility, asking her to move various body parts. She can't lift her left arm or move her hand or fingers or lift her leg or wiggle her toes. He's concerned because she has less mobility than before the surgery and less than the day before. She should have more. (She said later that it didn't seem any different to her because she couldn't feel any of those muscles either before or after surgery.)

Dr. Anderson suspects brain swelling and, perhaps, bleeding, neither of which is good. He orders steroids, the miracle drug that promotes healing, reduces swelling and bleeding. I watch as the nurse brings in a big needle and injects the steroid into the IV line. We are all hoping for a miracle, except for Martie, thank goodness, who seems unaware of how serious the situation is. If the swelling or bleeding does not stop, what then? More surgery? Spreading paralysis?

On Wednesday, there is no change except for the side effects of the steroids. Martie is up in more than one sense. Her mood is positive, she talks more than usual, and she can't sleep. Right after the surgery, sleep came easily. Now that benefit is lost.

On Thursday, I go to see her after lunch and sit down beside her.

"Watch this," she says, looking down at her left hand. After a pause, she begins to wiggle her thumb like she was thumbing for a ride. We both smile and giggle. That movement is the first sign that the steroids are working. The beginning of recovery. The steroid injections continue for a few more days. Our first but not last encounter with that miracle drug.

———

In one of his visits, Dr. Anderson talks about my paralysis. "Back in the 1970s people who suffered paralysis after neurosurgery were sent home without any further rehabilitation. If they recovered use of their muscles on their own, they were considered lucky." I listen thoughtfully. What is he trying to say? "But over the years, research has shown we can retrain the brain." Part of the plan for me is to go to a rehabilitation hospital as soon as I recover from the surgery, and when there is an opening.

This is a shock. I guess I thought there was a pill, like a steroid or something, to get my muscles going again. But rehab! Isn't that a place for old ladies in their eighties who break their hips, and maybe die? Or, after motor vehicle accidents, for folks who are paralyzed and never get their muscles moving again? Should I be nervous here? I remind myself that Dr. Anderson has guided me carefully, and he has been right so far. The surgical outcome has been successful in a number of ways. I can speak. I can recognize Joe. I know who my family members are, and my friends, as well as all the medical folks. I can process my thoughts. I have a long-term and short-term memory, of sorts. The right side of my body is working. I guess the left side is calling out for rehab.

———

Just about every morning during Martie's hospitalization and rehab she calls around 7 a.m. Sometimes it is closer to 6:30. I look forward to them. They are our time for reflecting on and digesting what is happening. The events are so traumatic that there is little time to think about or feel what they mean. I make it through the day by putting one foot in front of the other and moving forward. Even driving alone in the car, I try not to think about the meaning of what is happening. I have enough stress for now.

During the calls, we talk about our feelings a bit. Martie has more access to hers, so she often starts off crying. I know from our years together that her tears are a good sign. They help her release the emotional tension. For my part, I need to listen. Martie needs to be heard. I reflect back her feelings and try to provide some perspective—telling her that she should cry, be scared, and feel alone. It's not that I am her therapist. Just giving her space to let some of the frightening thoughts and feelings out.

I can't let myself feel too intensely. It's not that I am without feelings. I just need to keep the flame on simmer. By listening and talking about what is happening, I am helping Martie deal with her trauma. It helps me some. But I am holding off my internal reflection until some indefinite time in the future.

———

A new doctor appears. She walks in early one morning while Joe is visiting. Her name is Dr. Lincoln and she, too, looks quite young. As she introduces herself and hands us her card, I wonder why I need a radiation oncologist. She goes on to explain that I had an "atypical" (it's the first time I've heard that word) meningioma. She emphasizes the pieces of the tumor left reside on a critical section of my brain.

"There are two schools of thought here on the best way to handle these leftover materials," she begins. "One is to radiate the pieces that are left. Two is to let them be and check them periodically with MRIs."

Joe and I look at each other, astonished. "Go on," says Joe.

"Your case will be the subject at the Tumor Conference Bureau in Boston in the coming weeks. At that time we'll have a better idea how to handle your situation, and if radiation is necessary." She leaves the room saying, "My office will be calling you for an appointment."

Why a radiation oncologist? Dr. Anderson did mention the possibility of radiation for the pieces of tumor that could not be removed surgically. But I thought that radiation would be optional. I don't want anything to do with it. Still, I can't help but feel important because my case will be the focus of attention at a Tumor Conference!

———

Remember the white turban bandage? The one that was put in place after the surgery to cover the 39 staples. I decide it needs a snazzier look. White can be so boring, especially in a hospital. I send Joe home with instructions to find some of my scarves and three of my best costume jewelry pins.

When Joe returns, he ties one of the scarves around the white turban and pins it in place with all three pins. Yes, all of them! Tears well up as he does this. He is tender and clumsy at the same time. The white turban falls into my eyes and he spends time fussing with it. He works to get the turban bandage back on my head, and then manipulates the scarf. Joe can be all thumbs, but he manages to get everything in place: the white turban, the fashionable scarf, the pins. He so wants me to look pretty. That's why my tears.

Everyone who comes into the room comments on this new style, from the docs to the folks who sweep the floors. I have started a new fashion trend!

———

I miss my sons. A lot. I miss Ken and I miss Tim. Ken lives two hours away, in Brookline. He calls, but I'd just love to see him. If he came, he could stay with Joe and help him around the house and keep him company.

Kenneth Andrew is our oldest son. He was born in June 1965 a year after we married and two days after Joe obtained his degree from Boston College. Life became hectic as this beautiful, tiny, golden-haired, blue-eyed boy entered our lives, and we began our parenting apprenticeship. In September, we prepared to leave our first nest. Joe was accepted at graduate school in Buffalo, New York, where he planned to earn a PhD in cognitive psychology.

We traveled many times back and forth between Boston and Buffalo in our new red Volkswagen Beetle with Kenneth sleeping in the back seat in a carriage bed. We were the first in our families to move far away from home. It was a stressful time in our lives—Joe worked hard at his studies, and I had a part-time evening job at a local hospital to help with the finances. Kenneth grew fast, doing all the normal baby things. Meanwhile, the world around us was changing. The Beatles made their debut in the States. Also, there was much chaos, particularly the antiestablishment student uprisings at universities, such as sit-ins and demonstrations.

By the age of seven, Ken had many interests: photography, filmmaking, and science fiction. *Star Trek* became a favorite. He and his friends formed a *Star Trek* club in our garage. Over the years he became a collector —a serious collector, and managed to accumulate a generous down payment on his first condominium when he sold pieces of his collection. At one time we had a *Star Trek* pinball machine in our garage. We were proud of him. And he loved boasting to us that his collection really was "worth doing all those years!"

Ken's dream was to make and direct movies. He attended Syracuse University and while there made some unusual and creative movies. By graduation he realized that the unstructured life of a director was not for him. Instead he took his education and creativity and channeled it into mapmaking—cartography— and now is the primary mapmaker for an agency that services the Department of Transportation in Massachusetts. He is responsible for the state road maps, Massachusetts Bay Transportation Authority (MBTA) maps, park-and-ride maps, bike maps—whatever the Commonwealth requires.

He met his wife, Danielle, through a mutual friend. David was persistent and they were stubborn and resistant claiming, "but I'm OK in my life right now."

Their agreement to exchange emails almost ended when Danielle saw Ken's email address, "kosh,". To Danielle it meant Orthodox Jewish. (Imagine an Irish boy with a French name being Jewish!) David nudged some more. Eventually Danielle responded. What followed were many hours on the telephone. Ken and Danielle met. They fell in love. David was happy. Ken and Danielle were happy— and are now happily married and living in Brookline with their two cats.

Tim lives far away in Bozeman, Montana. Tim was born in 1968 in Buffalo, New York, two days after the Reverend Martin Luther King Jr. was assassinated. I was typing dissertations for PhD students at the time to earn extra money. Three weeks before Tim's due date my water broke, and someone was left with a partially typed dissertation.

Tim, born Timothy, was nameless for 24 hours because, throughout my pregnancy, Joe and I could not agree on a name. Finally Joe's mother suggested Timothy, and we loved it. We decided not to give him a middle name. My mother warned me I would regret it. She was right. Timmy always asked, "Why didn't I get a middle name?"

In both our families the tradition had been to name sons after fathers or grandfathers. Joe and I had strong feelings against this tradition. By giving our sons nonfamily names we were flexing our independence. We were defiant, in our small way.

Tim's formative years coincided with the escalation of the Vietnam War, the growing antiwar sentiment, and its many protests. While I was in the hospital recovering from his birth, demonstrations and rioting erupted outside the building over the King assassination.

We were overjoyed to welcome another blue-eyed son into our world. As a baby, Timmy had little hair—his head was covered with golden peach fuzz. Ken was almost three years old. Joe and I were ready to handle another child. But Tim had his own ideas. He did things and got into things and thought of things that Ken never dreamed of. Our former parental apprenticeship was no longer relevant. We began learning from another book, a different teacher—Timmy. We learned a lot from him, and a lot about ourselves.

From a very early age Tim loved sports and was always eager to toss a ball. I remember Tim as a youngster playing sports in the back yard, especially baseball, his love. I said "no" to organized school hockey and football because I was fearful of injuries. I remember the days he and a friend would sit watching a baseball or football game—but mostly baseball. They sat side-by-side on our couch in front of the TV with the volume on low, performing the play-by-play and color commentary into a tape recorder mimicking the announcers today.

Tim couldn't wait to play for Little League in Natick. As soon as he was old enough—age eight—we signed him up for the farm team. I can still see him beaming with pride when he wore his team's baseball cap and red shirt, complete with a number on the back. Thus began his baseball career.

He had dreams of playing for the big leagues—like most of the other boys. Year after year he played. We went to the games and watched him with his friends throw and fumble and sometimes make connections with the ball. While attending Tim's games I learned the rules of this most-loved pastime.

In high school, Tim played in the Babe Ruth League. That's when the most amazing thing happened. After all these years of watching Timmy and his friends fumble, fall, strike out, and miss fly balls, they were doing it. From the stands we heard the thwack as the bat made a mean connection with the ball. Out in the field their mitts were held high and in the right position to catch a fly ball. They were running fast and putting numbers onto the scoreboard greater than zero. It was fun to watch them. It was becoming evident that Timmy could pitch. This happened in his sophomore and junior years. I know I'm his mother, but he was good. He had all the moves down exactly as I saw them on TV.

Tim took his love for sports into a career. He chose to advance his studies at Connecticut School for Broadcasting. From there he got his feet wet at a couple of radio stations before falling into newspapers. At one weekly newspaper he called up the editor and talked him into starting a sports page. And it became successful! He eventually became a sports reporter.

While working in production at one of the radio stations, a young female reporter asked him to show her how to skate backwards and, as he tells it, "the rest is history!" He married Joanna on Halloween night. Their marriage was the first time Tim did something before his older brother, Ken. Tim and Joanna moved to Bozeman, Montana, where he is a sports writer for the *Bozeman Chronicle*. They are waiting to adopt a little girl from China. It is a long process, and we are all waiting patiently for her arrival.

Longing for my sons stirs another, deeper memory of mine—that of my mother. I wonder about the feelings she must have experienced 35 years ago when she was diagnosed with colon cancer. At that time she was living in Auburndale—a village of Newton, Massachusetts, the town where I grew up. And I, her eldest daughter, was living with Joe and our two boys in Michigan. I felt devastated at this news—cancer! My mother had just turned 50. Imagine turning 50 and finding yourself in a hospital with colon cancer. How could this have happened? And I couldn't get home to be with her—too many circumstances were out of my control at the time. I desperately wanted to be with her during the initial surgeries and as she received devastating news. I begin to think about what she must have experienced as I sit in my hospital bed and reflect on my own devastating situation. However, I think I am fortunate that my tumor is benign; unlike hers.

I realize how lonely, scared, and forgotten she must have felt. My feelings of guilt return. The guilt of not being there when her trauma first hit resurfaces and hits hard. I wasn't there with her during her struggle and her lonesome times— some of the things I am feeling now. This convergence of feelings—the old ones of guilt and the current ones of fear and loneliness—are smashing together on all sides like the waves of a nor'easter. I feel unsettled and I don't know what to do.

I decide to take some action—do something that my mother would have wanted to do back then but could not because it was impossible for her at the time—fly me home to be with her. I decide to fly Tim and Joanna from Montana to the Cape. I want so much to see Tim. And I believe he needs to see me, too, see how I am doing—that I really am doing OK.

Volunteers are a big part of hospital care. I see them daily; they transport me to tests in the main hospital and they deliver my mail. Twice a day I receive heaps and heaps of cards along with flowers and plants. They enjoy delivering them and often announce that I receive the most. I love the "flowers" that are edible, the ones I receive from my brother, Billy. I nibble on it. I share it with the staff, along with the cookies, specialized M&Ms, chocolates, etc.

This outpouring of love is astonishing. I do not expect the gifts, the cards, the phone calls, the visitors. I start to hear from friends from everywhere—the ones I have scooped up from every corner of my life. Naturally they were all shocked, scared even, when Joe contacted them. Now they are here, or on the phone, or there is daily evidence of them in the mail. My sisters come to visit, my brother, too; Joe's sisters come with our nieces...my neighbors...some of my colleagues. I cry when I see each of them or hear their voices on the phone. They are equally happy to see me—see me alive or hear that I am alive, that is. Those make for joyous moments, loving moments.

I feel special, like a rock star or a queen. I have never experienced such attention, such caring, and I never realized how important I am to so many people. I am humbled. It is remarkable and, at the same time, overwhelming. I don't have the language to express it adequately. The best way I can think of to express this rush of love toward me is this: If there is a place, a feeling, a sensation, a space in the universe called heaven, this has to be what it's like!

One friend from high school, Martha, has made a healing shawl. It is crocheted beautifully with silky yarn in light turquoise shaded colors that give off an iridescent look. It's finished with a double-knotted fringe on each end. The nursing staff admires it and loves—is compelled even—to touch it. Everyone who comes into the room is drawn to it. The healing shawl goes everywhere with me—to MRIs, CT scans, blood tests—and the nursing aides always ensure it covers me at bedtime.

Cape Cod juts out into the Atlantic Ocean like a flexed arm, and is separated at the shoulder from the rest of Massachusetts by the Cape Cod Canal. There are two bridges crossing the canal – the Bourne and the Sagamore. Whenever someone comes to the Cape to visit, we Cape Codders use the phrase they came "over the bridge".

Two colleagues from my psychotherapy practice come over the bridge to visit. One walks in with the biggest dish garden I have ever seen. It is so big that she makes her entrance into my room wheeling it on an office chair. Edie is a gardener, and she designed this dish garden especially to help me heal. It is a beauty, with flowing greens that include pothos, a peace lily that is blooming, and a trailing philodendron, among others. While taking the time to visit, she does my nails, and we spend a lot of time just talking. Tender moments.

My friend and colleague, Sue, also visits and brings the best lunch. Because she wasn't sure what I would like, she delivers a potpourri from the best sandwich place in her hometown. I, who have been ravenous at each meal, eat them all. She also made "Martie's Comeback Tunes," a CD with songs she specifically chose as uplifting music to help me heal.

Sue, like Edie, is one of my colleagues monitoring and covering a good number of my clients. We take the time to discuss them, especially in terms of what's happened to me. Most of my clients are still reverberating from the suddenness of my catastrophe. We talk about how it is affecting them. Sue says most of the therapy sessions are taken up with questions about how I'm doing. We also talk about her children, my healing, and what my recovery plan is beginning to look like. It looks like it's going to be a long time before I get to go home.

After Sue leaves I play the CD. I do feel like a rock star with my own CD! The songs she has chosen include: *"The Theme from Rocky," "Eye of the Tiger," "Lean on Me," "You've Got a Friend," "I Am Woman,"* and *"I Can See Clearly Now."* The careful and loving thoughts that Sue put into my CD flood my soul. Tears again.

Later that night as I fall asleep I think of ways I can send the love back. One set of folks I think of first are the firemen/EMTs of Yarmouth Port who responded so quickly to our emergency that night and were very helpful to Joe and me. What can I do for them? I will make them supper. That's something I am sure they will enjoy. Several menus float in my head before I settle on the best one: roll-up lasagna with sweet sausage and my killer brownies for dessert. I play with these recipes in my head as I fall asleep.

During the second week after the operation, the full extent of my new role begins to take shape. I teach and consult at Bentley University during

the day three days a week, and also teach an evening course in the Master's degree program once a week.. Most of the year, I work two days on campus and one at home. During semesters when I teach, I have to stay near the campus an extra night.

I postponed my first class, which had been scheduled to begin on the evening of the operation. A week later, I have to leave for the two work days and the extra night for teaching. It's a welcome distraction to get back to work. My colleagues are very supportive. In fact, the first flower arrangement that arrived after the operation was from them. As I arrive on campus, some of them need updates. Others have not heard the whole story. I go through the details. Again, there is the compulsion to tell it from beginning to end. I never become bored, even if some of them may.

With Martie in the hospital, the household chores fall to me. I take her dirty clothes home every few days and wash them along with mine. In between phone calls, I clean the house, sort of, and pay the bills. I eat out or with Martie.

It is the beginning of a reversal of roles. I have spent my life being a provider, and it has been very important for me to be a good provider. In high school and college I had a friend, and our families knew each other well. My friend had five siblings, and his house was a bit chaotic. His mother was always screaming at them, and his father was never home. When I was about 15, his father moved to California with a girlfriend and left his business to his abandoned wife. When I told my mother the news, her comment was, "Too bad; he was a good provider." I was not sure what my mother had in mind, but I took her comment to mean that a man's role in the family was as a provider first, and that that role was even more important than his consistent presence.

Having a man who was a good provider was central to Mom's well-being. She was one of 11 children growing up in a lower-working-class section of Chelsea, Massachusetts. Her father, Tom Higgins, was a printer. When she was about nine, in 1917, she had a tragic accident. She was dragged under a car for several hundred feet. The worst injuries were to her legs: the skin and muscles on them were scrapped off, leaving the bone exposed. The local doctors wanted to amputate one of her legs, but my grandmother refused and had her moved to Children's Hospital in Boston.

37

There the doctors used a new procedure to graft skin and muscle from her lower legs over her knees. It worked. She spent years in recovery. From her I learned persistence along with a fear that bad times were never far away. She said repeatedly that I was not going to be "spoiled," which meant that I would *not* talk back and that I would *not* get into trouble.

My father was a construction worker, his title was "heavy equipment operator." He operated a "steam" shovel, later powered by diesel fuel. He worked six days a week and had two weeks of vacation a year, only one of which could be in the summer. My mother made a good catch in Dad—someone with a steady job who didn't drink to excess, her definition of a good provider.

I believe that I continued the tradition of providing for my family. I was good at it. But being a caretaker is another matter. No training, no male role models, no time to learn.

———

Determination. I have discovered early on in this journey that my determination is driving my recovery. However, another piece of my personality has also sprung loose in helping the recovery: my laughter and sense of humor. I seem to find something funny to say, make a play on words, add a comedic quip, or make a wisecrack about whatever is happening to me or whatever I see. No sarcasm, please—just humor. I do this to bring a smile out of others. I enjoy making people laugh. It is part of making a connection with them. And people like that. They, in turn, have a warmer feeling toward me, and they remember who I am.

When I worked in the business world, I wore many hats: research analyst, demographer, tech support analyst, data center manager, and financial analyst. In all those positions, I learned to frequent the "F word." Had to. Everyone used it—all the time—for everything. When I transitioned to my new career as a psychotherapist, I needed to tone it down and not use that word...as much. Sometimes in a session it was warranted and I did use it—but judiciously. One only has to look at me, see my sweet-looking face, to presume (wrongly) that I would never, ever, utter *that* word. No one would ever believe that that the F word could spring forth from this mouth. I would use the word, of course, to not only shock people but also to make them smile.

Before my recent surgery, one of my every-day phrases, especially in business, was, "Well, it's not brain surgery!" Now that I have actually undergone brain surgery, I am proclaiming out loud—in the hospital, for everyone to hear, and to all my visitors—"Well, I didn't just have brain surgery. I had *fucking* brain surgery!" Most people laugh, a few are embarrassed. For themselves. For me. I'm not sure. I find out from my friend, Anna, that her husband was shocked because he never believed I could say such a thing. No one told me to stop. And I didn't. I guess I have a case of disinhibition. The nurses find it hilarious.

I ask Joe to bring my camera to the hospital. I take pictures of everybody, and I mean everybody—Dr. Anderson, the nursing staff, meal delivery folks, and the young men and women sweeping the floors. When I get a group together, like the nurses and their aides, instead of asking them to say cheese, I query, "What else would you like to say?"

You guessed it. "FUCK," they scream.

Toward the end of the first week after the surgery I feel better each day. I notice continued improvement in my left hand and left leg. Dr. Anderson visits me daily to check on my motor activity. He also peeks under my fashionable turban to inspect the healing progress. It is going well from his point of view. I am feeling hopeful for the first time.

———

Lying in my bed waiting for the winter sun to rise. The field outside my window is beginning to lose its darkness and the light is shyly peeking its way through as if testing to see if it is safe to come on ahead. It looks like it will be another cold day. I hear we are in the throes of a frigid period—unseasonable for the Cape. I am happy to be ensconced in a warm bed and in a warm room with lots of good and capable people taking care of me.

Cape Cod Hospital, today, is different from its community hospital days of 30 to 40 years ago. Since the late 1970s there has been a steady increase in the population rolls, and the medical profession has kept pace in order to deliver the needed medical care. Today the hospital's Cardiac Group of Physicians is one of the top rated in the country. Since my brain surgery, I have learned that Neurosurgeons of Cape Cod shares top billing. This new building alone—the Mugar Building—is testament to the excellent professional medical care on the

Cape. The floor I am presently on was finished a week before I had my first seizure. Everything here is new. All the technology is state-of-the-art and competi-
tive with the Boston hospitals. I am lucky to be here.

We, on Cape Cod, are lucky to have David Mugar living here in the village of
Cotuit. He is a local philanthropist who pledged $5 million, then another $5 million for this new hospital addition. The second $5 million came with a challenge
to inspire other donors to match his initial donation—all for the development of
this wing. The wing is named after his parents, Marian G. and Stephen P. Mugar.
What an honorable testament to one's parents. The building, when complete, will
be 102,000 square feet and will include four inpatient floors that will house 120
private rooms. The completed floors now have rooms with a bath, a staff work
area, and a separate area for families. Long couches open into a bed to accommodate family members who may choose to stay the night. Each room has natural
wood accents and makes use of natural light through supersized picture windows.

Artwork is everywhere, in my room and in the hallways. Cape artists introduce themselves and unveil their artistry. I find it extraordinary that the planning
folks had the vision and foresight to include our local Cape painters in the final
details for this new wing. During the many times I am transported to tests, I enjoy
viewing the art—the views of dunes, the sea, children picking shells. As I am
wheeled through the connecting corridor to the previously existing hospital (the
main hospital), I notice another art medium—stained-glass windows—rows of
them high up on the walls. The main hospital houses the Radiology Department,
and I am a frequent traveler for CT scans and MRIs (no frequent traveler points
though).

It's during these trips that I get my chance to see these delicate, hand-blown
windows of French and German design. The designs are fluid with no discernible
shape, leaving the viewers to ponder and decide on her own what feeling the glass
is projecting. I also note that the windows, which fall in a series of rectangles and
then small thin vertical shapes on the side, have the effect of a three-dimensional
surface. The shapes and colors play into landscape views in the windows. And,
as the light changes from the daylight into the evening, so do the images. Such
is the brilliance of this artistry, all of it arranged with the intention of soothing
and healing.

I contemplate all this as I try to get a grasp of what has happened to me the
past few days: the seizures, the 911 call, the ambulance ride in the middle of the

night, the paralysis, the surgery with my new titanium plate, the recurrence of the paralysis, and now my recovery. There's so much to take hold of and take in and digest. It's like biting off a large piece of what looks to be an expensive cut of medium-rare steak. My favorite. Instead, not only did I bite off too much, but the piece of steak is too tough to chew, and I cannot spit it out. I have to keep on chewing. I think I will be chewing on this for a long time.

I am comfortable in the hospital. I remember when I was in training to become a clinical social worker. During my first-year internship, I was a hospital social worker and learned about this comfort factor. Some patients get quite accustomed to being taken care of and all their needs being attended to—three squares a day, a roof over their heads, a nice warm bed to sleep in, people in different roles managing their safekeeping. When it comes time for discharge, anxiety and possibly resistance can arise in those patients. Well, that was 15 years ago when patients remained in the hospital for more than a night or two. I have been hospitalized a bit more than a week now with no signs of discharge. And, yes I am quite comfortable. I feel safe. I feel taken care of.

A ritual has evolved: before I go to sleep each night, three people very dear to me call for a few minutes just to say good-night: my son, Tim; my friend, Martha, from high school; and my friend, Carol, from our graduate school days in Buffalo. The calls are very touching, and I look forward to them every evening.

Another cold day coming. It is my usual 5 a.m. wake-up time and dark outside. Five a.m. is a busy time. That's when the phlebotomist arrives to withdraw my blood before I eat. After many mornings, and evenings, too, of this unpleasant routine, I finally ask why. My blood levels are low and the doctor is monitoring them. Hmmm. Is that why I am hungry all the time and practically inhale my food when it arrives? Joe remarks on how fast my food disappears from my tray. And I eat everything.

It will be another few days before the transfer to a rehab hospital. Neither of us knows what this means or what I will be doing there. I know the goal is to regain the strength in my left side and to retrain my brain.

Joe and I have our 7 a.m. phone call. Lately, we have been reminiscing about our early days together. We met in high school, both members of the Dramatics

Club. I joined to become part of a social circle—translation: to meet a guy. Joe joined to have something to put on his college application. We both became part of the senior play production, *Ten Little Indians*. Adapted from Agatha Christie's book, the plot involves 10 guests who are invited to an island for a weekend of festivities. One by one they turn up dead. Fred Narracott is the character who rows each guest to the island. Joe (a.k.a. Fred) had the first line in the play, announcing, "All the guests have arrived, sir!" I was the production manager in charge of stage props and ensuring actors were in the right spot at the right time. Sometimes I whispered their lines if they needed a nudge. I was also responsible for knowing where the gun—which did get shot—was located. Fortunately, it had blanks.

We began to get to know each other—flirting and having fun with the play. It premiered in December, just before the Christmas break. Also before the break was the much-anticipated Christmas Cotillion, a semiformal dance, held on Saturday, December 16, 1960. I still remember the date! And yes, Joe asked me to be his date. I was thrilled and out of my mind with excitement. We danced the night, talked a lot, and learned more about each other. I discovered that Joe was born six days before me, in Somerville, while I was born in nearby Chelsea. I think I was falling for him. I had such a good time. And, oh yes, he kissed me goodnight. It was the sweetest kiss.

Then we return to the topic of rehab and what that means for me, for us. Will I walk again? Will I be able to dance? Joe sounds pessimistic. I am not. I am determined. I will walk again. I see myself walking again in my house. Joe has not had me home for almost two weeks. He's doing laundry and cooking and shopping and cleaning. And he's alone. I know this is hard for him. I think a lot of him being alone and in his new role.

When I insisted Joe get in touch and keep in touch with all my friends, this was a new role for him. Most nights he sits at his computer and sends an email noting the status of my condition and the events of my day, and his day. As each day flips by, there are more and more people to add as "Recipient" on the email list. As he relates this to me, I sense that this is a valuable outlet for him. He is a first-rate writer. He gathers his thoughts and expresses them each night through email. My friends and family tell me that these emails are quite special and beautifully written, and that someday I should read them.

———

Dr. Anderson seems pleased as he enters my room with a bounce in his step. Joe is with me as he delivers the news that I will be transferred to RHCI on Friday. "RHCI" stands for Rehabilitation Hospital of the Cape and Islands. Dr. Anderson exudes optimism as he speaks of that hospital, confident that I will be walking and responsible for my daily care by the time I leave. He goes on to say I will be there about four weeks. Four weeks! Joe and I look at each other. It seems like forever—four more weeks. The doctor hands us a brochure. I do not read it right away. Joe leaves to do some errands.

Later in the day I finally, but reluctantly, pick up the brochure. I hold it in my lap and ponder all that has happened, still trying to make some sense of it, but I can't. I am here in a hospital. My friend, Martha, who works at a rehab facility, informs me that I'll be working in therapy three hours a day. I can't imagine that. How will I do that? I feel tears on my cheeks. I guess it's time to read. Either that or watch the Jewelry Channel. That's what I call the Home Shopping Channel.

I begin to read.

RHCI is also on the Cape. It is affiliated with Spaulding Rehabilitation Hospital in Boston, one of the nation's leading rehabilitation institutions; Massachusetts General Hospital; and Brigham and Women's Hospital.

It certainly has outstanding credentials.

RHCI is dedicated to excellence in providing specialized programs while providing reha-bilitation care. Their mission is to help individuals reach their full potential in function and independence following a disabling illness or injury, surgery, or chronic illness. As a rehabilita-tion hospital, RHCI provides more medical, nursing, and therapy services than are offered at nursing homes, such as round-the-clock physician coverage, an average of three hours of therapy a day, nurses with specialized training, and comprehensive neurological inpatient programs designed to help patients return to their homes and community.

I put the brochure down and cry softly. It is hard to take all this in.

———

I remember a time 20 years ago when I was hospitalized for abdominal sur-gery. I had asked my surgeon if Joe and I could have dinner together in the hospital. He agreed. I decide to repeat that experience here, especially since it is to be one of my last nights in the hospital. A male nurse on the 3 to 11 p.m. shift is pleased to put in the request to the kitchen for another meal, two chicken dinners. But no cocktails, please! Not with my medications. I do miss my martini and a glass of red wine, but there will be time for that later.

Joe and I enjoy our meal together. It is our first dinner since my ambulance ride in the middle of the night almost two weeks ago. The nurse props me up in a wheelchair and things are arranged so that it feels like we are at a table for two. It is romantic and warmhearted just being together like this. The mood hovers around me in such a way that I actually believe the clear night sky has conjured up some stars to join us, along with that sliver of a moon, which sheds its light our way. It's special to have Joe here eating with me instead of taking wraps off my food, watching me eat, and then going home.

Soon, I will be off to RHCI. (A few years later RHCI became Spaulding Rehab of Cape Cod).

———

Here is what I wrote in my email that night about our dinner:
On Saturday we had a romantic dinner. No candles. No martinis. No, not at Chillingsworth by the Sea. In two chairs beside her hospital bed. The décor was hospital white. The lighting florescent. The waitress wore a hairnet and gloves but was quite attentive. We had the house special—chicken, rice and carrots—nutritious if underspiced. Ever the debonair fellow, I cut up Martie's chicken for her. A special treat for desert—a dish of pears. Does life get any better than this?
After I composed this humorous picture of our dinner, some not-so-funny thoughts bubbled up: what if this was a prelude to all of our future dinners? Would I always be helping Martie get into a chair, opening the little packet with her tea bag, cutting her meat? Her paralysis had to get better—didn't it? After almost two weeks post-surgery, her left side was only a little better than before. How much more movement would rehab provide? How do you get un-paralyzed?

44

———

I awake the next morning and speculate about the mysteries that await me at this rehab hospital. It is my usual 5 a.m. wake-up time. The phlebotomist arrives. My blood is taken. Surprisingly, a nurse arrives. It is early to see any of the nursing staff. She informs me I will *not* go to rehab today. There is no bed available. I will go tomorrow. "For sure."

How does that saying go? "Just when you think you have things all worked out, they change!" Now I wait another day. That won't be so bad. I'm comfortable here. I'm warm. People are taking care of me. I'm sounding like those patients I learned about when I was in training as a hospital social worker.

Joe arrives shortly after breakfast. We mull over the latest digression from the plan. Up to the present we both have been clobbered by so many complicated out-of-our-control life events that this one item hits us hard. We talk and soothe each other.

A noisy stretcher comes barging into the room interrupting our conversation. It is rolling loud and fast on its wheels, and shoved by two laughing EMTs—a young man and a young woman. Neither one says hello or asks who I am. Joe runs out of the room to find a nurse. There are no nurses to be found! Where do they disappear to? When Joe returns to the room the EMTs are rearranging the furniture and moving the stretcher so it aligns with my bed. Everything is happening so fast I cannot get a word out of my mouth. Joe looks just as rattled. The stretcher is positioned alongside my hospital bed. As they bend to move me onto the stretcher, they announce they are taking me to Mayflower Place.

That's when Joe and I, in unison, yell, "Stop!"

"I'm not going to Mayflower, I'm scheduled to go to Spaulding."

They pause. One of the EMTs asks if I am so-and-so.

No. I give my name.

"Huh, we have the wrong room."

"You certainly do!" Whatever happened to checking name and date of birth? Isn't this supposed to be the routine? Talk about anxiety. Well, I have some now.

The nurse walks into the room looking puzzled. We tell her what she missed.

It's time again to think about readying myself for rehab tomorrow. I will need comfortable clothes—I am expected to be dressed every day so I can work their program. That word "work" is adding to the anxiety that was just stirred up with

45

those intrusive EMTs, and now I have a full roiling broth of it stirring around. How will I do what they ask of me? I guess that's why I'm going there—so I can wake up the muscles on the left side of my body. I look at my left side and ponder how this will all take place. I am amazed by the human body—that my left side can be so dormant now, and in a period of time—say two to three weeks—it will learn to move again. That must be the miracle of retraining the brain. On the other side of my anxiety, there is curiosity. I'm looking forward to participating in this program—this experiment, this routine. I want to be part of it and see how it all works.

I talk with Joe about the clothing I will need: socks, underwear, shoes. Three weeks before my seizures I had purchased new running/walking shoes made by Easy Spirit. How serendipitous! I wonder what kind of workout they will get at rehab. Joe's niece, along with my two sisters, seemed to know the type of clothing I would need. They bought me the prettiest outfits, in mix-and-match sets, all in soft cotton that feels good next to my skin. I like the idea of no longer wearing this boring hospital gown. I can't dance in this! I tell Joe about the clothes I want and where to find them. He leaves with his instructions.

I am taking pictures of everyone. It's my way of saying good-bye and thank you to all who have been caring for me. There are many folks: doctors, nurses, nursing aides, menu-hand-out people, meal deliverers, floor sweepers, volunteers—too many to count. I take many photos. Not of me but of them. I want a memento. Taking photos becomes an interesting task with only one side working. But I manage with my light-weight camera and a steady forehead and the group in front of me to pose quickly. And they do but with lots of giggles and do-over shots. Without any prompting, everybody wants to say FUCK, smiling and giggling the whole time.

It is mid-afternoon and the phone by my bed rings.

"Hi, Mom." It's my son, Ken, calling. "I'm calling to wish you luck at rehab. I know you will be fine and do well." Ken is positive and upbeat. His words sound like my own. How fortunate I am to hear him give back my own words. It's soothing. I feel his love. We have a nice chat as he tells me about his day, his work, and how his life is going. "I'll be checking in with Dad to see how you are progressing. "

"That's sound good, Ken. Bye for now. I love you."

Later the phone rings. It's time for my evening calls.

"Hi, Tim, how are you?"

"Good. How are you doing, Mom? Dad tells me you're really going to rehab this time. Tomorrow, is it? Are you nervous?"

"A little, I don't know what to expect."

"Yeah, the old unknown. I remember feeling relieved when you got out of surgery, and now you are going to rehab. You are brave, Mom."

I'm touched. I cry softly. Again, I feel fortunate—my son's words from his heart.

"We're making plans to fly to Boston and visit."

"Oh, I'm happy you're coming. I look forward to hugging you." Things are falling into place. They will stay in Brookline with Ken and Danielle, and travel back and forth to the Cape to be with Joe and to visit with me.

"Well, good-night, Mom. I love you. Good luck tomorrow."

The next time the phone rings, I know it will be my friend Martha.

"Hi, Martie, how are you?"

"A little nervous about rehab tomorrow and all the work expected of me."

"I hear your concern, but I have confidence in you. I've known you since high school and what you're capable of accomplishing. This is just another puzzle piece, another thread in your tapestry of life. You can do it."

"Thanks. Your words are special and they mean a lot to me."

"Good-night, Martie. I'll talk to you when you're in rehab, too."

The final call is from Carol.

"Hi Martie. Want to get to you before you left the hospital. How is it going?"

"Scary, going off to the unknown, not sure my body will cooperate."

"You gave us quite a scare with those seizures and then the surgery, and you came through it so well. Rehab will help you walk again."

"Yeah, scared me, too."

"Can't help thinking back to other difficulties you, and Joe, have been through in your marriage, and you've come through them. Also, makes me think back to what all four of us endured in getting through graduate school. We did it together."

"Boy, those were some days, weren't they? We were poor and struggling and just starting out in our lives."

"I have no doubt you will regain your muscle strength and be walking in no time. Talk to you tomorrow night at rehab."

As I fall asleep I feel the love of so many. I'm especially touched by the words from both of my sons. I feel wrapped in their love. What a privilege. And my dear friends. I am touched by their love and deep belief in me and in my recovery. I am a blessed woman.

———

It's Saturday, February 3, transfer day. I'm leaving this hospital I have called home for more than two weeks. I wake, blink away fragments of early-morning dreams, and contemplate my day. It's 5 a.m. and I notice a funny twinge in my lower abdomen. It is the first pain I have had, of any sort, since the intermittent stabbing pain in my right cheek the weekend before my first seizure. Brain surgery and all I have been through so far, and no pain. Until now. What's going on? Probably nothing.

The nursing staff informs me the phone system at Spaulding is similar to the one at the hospital. Also, my time checking in will be consumed with an abundance of paperwork: name and date of birth I'm sure. Because it's Saturday I wonder how much will I do, how full is the staff is on the weekend, will I have a roommate, will the meals be as good as here, and...and...and. I will call Joe once I am settled.

A nurse arrives with intimidating equipment—small cutters, tweezers, latex gloves, and a bottle of isopropyl—all resting on a tray on wheels that she drags behind her. There is an ominous look to this setup. What's going to happen? I feel relieved when she says she is here to remove the staples from my scalp. More twinges?

I sit on the edge of the bed as she picks up the tweezers and small scissors. She counts as she pulls. "One, 2, 3..." I hear the ping, ping, ping as she drops the staples into the tray.

"Ouch!" I exclaim. But she continues on, not stopping in her movements and ignoring my outcry.

Now she is up to "8, 9..."

"Oooh," I grimace and I try not to yell. But then, "Ouch, that hurts," I say as she continues counting. I can tell this is a task she is used to performing—not stopping in the middle of my cries or even when she feels a tug, pull, or snag in my skin. "Ouch, that's another one." She goes on with her counting, and I hear ping, ping, ping.

"Twenty-three, 24," she whispers under her breath.

"Owwwch," I say, followed by, "Sorry." What am I sorry for? She's the one hurting me. "Eeeesh." I try to be still as she counts and pulls and tugs. More ping, ping, ping.

"Almost done," she says, "32, 33, 34."

When she gets to 36, I let out a loud, "OUCH, what are you doing to me?"

She ignores me and I hear 39 and one last ping. "We are done!" She inspects the top of my head carefully. She cleanses the bald area with the isopropyl, especially where the stapes were just removed. It stings but only a trifle. "And you, my dear, have a nicely shaped horseshoe incision!" With that said she takes her tools of torture and leaves.

What a relief. I wish she had more to say. Like about how brave I am.

The nursing staff, the folks who clean my room, and the menu and meal deliverers are all in on the fun I'm having with my horseshoe-shaped incision. I'm sporting it now and proud of it. It's the day before the Super Bowl. This year in New England we can't cheer for our beloved Patriots. They were eliminated a few weeks ago. It was the same weekend Joe and I had that neighborhood party. The party when I shattered the glass—my first misperception problem.

I tell the staff, "Since I can't cheer for Tom Brady and the Patriots, I will root for Peyton Manning and the Baltimore Colts. After all I have their logo—the horseshoe—imprinted on my scalp! And Peyton better win MVP because I worked hard to get this logo put up here!" Everyone laughs. Next season, my loyalties will return to the Pats.

When the EMTs arrive they are quieter, smoother, and more professional than the laughing two who barged into my room yesterday. They check the room number, ask my name and date of birth. We finally are off to Spaulding, about 10 miles away. My lower abdomen is becoming more cranky. I wonder what's happening.

The furniture is rearranged deftly to accommodate their stretcher's alignment with my hospital bed. I'm transferred to the ambulance stretcher in one fluid movement. I have no coat or shoes, just like when I left my home over two weeks ago. The EMTs wrap me snugly for the ambulance ride.

As I am wheeled out of my room, the morning shift nurse informs me that because there was a one-day delay in my transfer, the antibiotic I had been receiving on a daily basis ever since I was hospitalized had been stopped a day early. I received the antibiotic because I was bedridden and thus prone to a UTI—a urinary tract infection, also known as a bladder infection. A UTI can be uncomfortable and painful. I am beginning to make the connection to the growing pain in my abdomen.

When the stretcher comes to a halt in front of the nursing desk the nurses and nursing aides from other shifts have messages of "being well" and "good luck." But the last was the greatest by far: "As you make your way through rehab, Martie, you must not only work hard, but have a fucking good time!" I laugh and feel a different twinge. The twinge of sadness about saying good-bye to the caring, compassionate, and professional folks on Mugar 4. My heartfelt thanks to all of them.

THE LONG WAY HOME

The reverse stretcher ride goes through the Mugar corridor. I view the paintings by the Cape artists and the beautiful stained-glass windows one last time. After the long narrow tunnel, the stretcher empties out into the sunlight. I am lifted into the ambulance for the 10-mile ride to Sandwich. It feels strange not to be going home. But, how can I? I can't walk, wash, or dress myself. No monitors this time. Two talkative paramedics tell me that Spaulding is a great place for rehab and that the food is very delicious. I should ask for the tomato basil soup.

I have a mix of feelings. I am in my own tunnel as I prepare for the next stage of recovery. I don't know where it will lead, or how long it is, or where the light at the end will be—if there is an end. When will I be able to be "me" in my own home, my own life with Joe? When, or will I, get my old life back? What about my private practices? Natick is surely out. Because of the seizures I won't be able to drive until July (six months, states the law), but what about my Yarmouth Port practice? I had so much marketing planned before the seizures.

Here I am talking like this, and I can't do so many things. Am I fooling myself into thinking I ever will walk again? And how long will it really take? I am a person who is not used to taking baby steps, although that is what I have frequently advised my clients to do. This is hard. This is incredibly and awfully hard. To come back from such a weak and debilitated state, and be strong and determined, and show a sense of humor through it all. There is the feeling of shame at being so dependent. The shame is a hard one to bear. I can't dwell on that one now. 'Nuff said on that topic.

There is something else though. The pain in my abdomen is more intense. I am convinced I have a UTI and am wondering...why? Why did they stop the medication when it is used to prevent infection? And who ordered that? I will suffer for this. I hope I can get some medication fast at Spaulding, and that the staff there will listen to me and not just see me as a poor half-paralyzed elderly (not that!) patient who doesn't know what she's talking about. I can still think and talk—and clearly. My speech has not been affected by the tumor, and I haven't had a stroke. But I know they won't listen. They will have their procedures: paper work first, then an order from the doctor, then the pharmacy, etc., etc., etc. As I said before, I will suffer for this delay...their mistake. Damn them.

We pull up at our destination. The Spaulding building is beautiful. I am admitted through the front door. There is a message here, different from a long tunnel, a garage, a back door. We are entering through the front door as if I am important. We go up the elevator to the second floor and stop at the main desk. I am directed to a beautiful, spacious, semi-private room. Do I have a roommate? The bed by the large window with a nice view is vacant—that must be mine. I like being near the window. The EMTs park the stretcher for a few minutes while the aides prepare the furniture to get me ready for the gurney-to-bed transfer.

I look to my left and see a woman who looks like a waif. Her face is round and puffy. She has steel gray hair with long bangs that fall in front of her eyes. The hair on the sides of her face is long and falls under her chin. It has a wavy look to it, but it needs a cut and shaping badly. The top of her head resembles those monks who sport a large bald circle with straight hair flowing around it, sort of like a halo. This is no halo. I look at her pretty blue eyes...and cry. That's me, in the mirror. I have not seen myself since the night of my seizure when Joe called 911. I'm horrified! Omigod-I-am-so-ugly! What has happened to me?

No recollection of the transfer to my new bed, my new home. I am busy working within myself so I will not have a sobbing panic attack. I'm trying to get a grasp of this new reality, of seeing this new self.

As it turns out, check-in is easy. No paperwork, just verification of name and date of birth. Spaulding has all my records from Cape Cod Hospital. Quickly though, I return to the present moment because the physical pain in my abdomen is now difficult to bear. I make my case with a nurse—I know the hierarchy—she is the one to inform. Off she goes.

After my check-in I call Joe, as we had planned. He will come with my clothes. There is a large whiteboard on the wall with my name on it welcoming me. It measures about five by four feet, and presently the only info on it is headings: GOALS, OCCUPATIONAL THERAPIST, PHYSICAL THERAPIST, SPEECH THERAPIST, RN NAME, RA NAME—the last two labels are for the shift nurse's name and the rehab assistant's name. With a board that size, it will get filled in later. Will I really need a speech therapist? Joe arrives and stays through supper. Because I am very uncomfortable, I eat little. I am still waiting for the doctor's approval for medication. The pain is worse.

When I am in pain time stretches. By now—early evening—I've been in pain a long time—a very long time, and I'm going to become a "high maintenance chick." That may be my introduction to the Spaulding staff. I am calling out for the nurse, the rehab assistant, anybody, for help, and asking, "What is taking so long?" There is no answer. I yell some more, "will somebody help me p-u-l-l-eeez?" If I could get out of bed, I could at least be pacing with the pain, but...I recall the brochure I read that Spaulding is a medical facility where a physician is always present. Well, "where is he?" I yell louder, as I writhe. Yes, I'm getting dramatic. Waiting for this doctor to give his approval is like being stalled in traffic on a two-lane highway at a construction site. I can see the traffic coming from the opposite direction, where I want to go, but my lane is stalled. I'm in a mid-sized car behind several SUVs and can't see the traffic cop up ahead. All he needs to do is wave his hand so we can all move forward. This is what I am waiting for, a wave of the hand.

Hours later, close to 1 a.m., the cop waves his hand, a physician is reached, an authorization given, the in-house pharmacy notified, and a nurse on the next shift administers the medication. It takes some time for my abdomen and my nerves to settle down. Eventually, I fall asleep.

Welcome to rehab, Martie.

———

The whiteboard hangs on the wall across from the foot of my bed where I can view its contents. Over the weekend it slowly comes to life as more and more information is added. I am told by my first rehab assistant, Dee Dee, that the bottom right-hand corner is important to check at all times. Along with the day's date it holds the names of the rehab assistant and nurse for the current shift. Because there are three eight-hour shifts each day, I need to be current with who is caring for me. My eyes travel up to the top right and see, for the first time, the name of the physician assigned to me—Dr. Davidson. Somehow I missed his name when I first arrived. He must be the "cop" who eventually gave a wave of his hand so I could get the medication I needed. I look forward to meeting him.

The other items that come to life on the whiteboard are coded statements that pique my curiosity. They appear to be about me and my condition, and maybe some are my goals. First I notice the words "left neglect." That's an interesting phrase. I wonder if that's for my left-sided paralysis. I am not neglecting my left side; it is with me all the time! There's another notation: "Support LLE when in bed or w/c pillows." These letters might mean I need pillows to help support my left side and my left lower extremity when I sit up in bed or in a wheelchair. I notice when I do sit up, I tend to lean to the left; sometimes I slide down. "Keep HOB (head of the bed?) elevated greater than or equal to 30 degrees <u>at all times</u>." That must mean I have to continue sleeping in a sitting position as I did at Cape Cod Hospital. There's no sleeping on my side, as I've been doing all my life. Sleeping on my back with this 30 degree elevation is difficult, but I will do it. I have an investment in helping decrease the swelling in my brain. Seizure guards are placed over the bed rails at night. These are for my protection in the event I have another seizure.

I like trying to figure out the coded statements—it makes use of the analytical side of my brain. I scan the whiteboard and notice "physical therapy" and more codes. Under the phrase "bed mobility," the HOB notation is repeated, along with an encircled *S*, which may mean supervised. There's "transfers" with double-headed arrows between the words "sit" and "stand." And another set of double-headed arrows surrounded by "B" and "W/C," followed by "SST." I'll bet that has something to do with a particular procedure for getting me out of bed, and another step for moving myself into a wheelchair, and all with supervision.

As I lie here in bed, I puzzle through these codes to get my brain involved and busy. To get out of bed, I must be supervised at all times. Specifically, I must be aware of my motions and my actions. That must be how the sit and stand works. I need to stand up before I sit down in the wheelchair. And then the reverse. I must sit and then stand before I transfer myself back to the bed, a chair, or wheelchair. I am sure it will take time, but it will happen.

The label Occupational Therapy, jumps out at me. What is that? I look down the whiteboard and see "grooming, bathing, dressing, toileting." And under toileting: "transfer, hygiene, clothes management." Different codes and more goals.

These activities appear to be straightforward: all tasks have an encircled *S* followed by other letters that stymie me. A label above these tasks says "Min A." Could this be minimal assist? I'll need lots of assistance in the beginning. Looking at all these words and abbreviations means I have lots of work ahead. But I'm looking forward to the challenge and ready to get started.

I think of myself in this dependent state. It's so different from who I was in the past, a can-do woman. I've always been able to do anything and everything—by myself. I'm also a go-to woman. When I received my undergraduate degree in economics and computer science at the age of 35, I became a career woman as well as a mother and wife. That was the personification of the "Woman of the '80s." I aspired to that role, and I was good at it. It was a challenge, but it gave me the energy and thrill to keep on. Where does that come from? I'm not sure if I learned it or if it came with me at birth—the way my DNA was arranged—or both. My paternal grandmother sailed to Boston from Ireland on her own when she was 19 years old. My father, the oldest of her nine children, owned his own business, helped his brothers with jobs and in other ways, and always did many things on his own. Here I am, once fiercely independent, now dependent on many people for everything! I am not, however, despondent about the situation. After all these years of doing it all by myself and trying to prove something—whatever it was—it feels OK to accept this help and love from other people. It feels soothing, like a warm bath. I like it.

More and more information appears on the whiteboard, and I realize it's the GPS to my new world in rehab. If I lose my way or need to know where I am going, or who is tending to me, I give the whiteboard a glance. It has all the current info and reference points I need.

———

Thoughts about my goals and current progress bring to mind other whiteboards in my business career. After receiving my undergraduate degree I worked as a research analyst at the Boston Edison Company (now NSTAR), a Boston-area electric utility. A promotion to demographer occurred a year later. In the late 1970s and early '80s, before whiteboards, many meetings were held discussing goals using cumbersome paper flip charts. While working for this regulated monopoly I became responsible, along with a team of other players, for developing a mathematical equation that would predict the migration of the population in and out of the greater Boston area. Our team worked toward a profit goal driven by the number of people in the Boston Edison territory. Various hypotheses about population trends were tossed around on these flip charts.

Three years later I joined a sales team at a computer software company. While there I traveled with sales reps to client companies and assisted these companies with their business strategies. Corporate goals were written on whiteboards. As a support analyst I helped to support these goals by creating solutions with computer applications.

The name of that company changed frequently. It was the 1980s—a volatile and dynamic time for the computer industry. Mergers and acquisitions of companies became the fashionable financial strategy of the day. For the next five years companies were bought and sold like buildings on a Monopoly game board. Each time a company was bought, three things happened: a name change, a reorganization, and layoffs. I was a victim of a layoff after working there only one year—last in, first out.

Suffering through that layoff was hard. My work, which I loved, was part of my identity, and that piece was ripped away—out of my control. I had a difficult time dealing with that. After many months searching, I was invited back to the same company, now under yet a different name (it had been bought again and reorganized, and there were layoffs). I was hired as the data manager. And there was more whiteboard activity. The data center was to close in two years and move to Pittsburgh. I had a job waiting there—in Pittsburgh—if I wanted it. I declined. I preferred to stay in the Boston area, and I did not want to disturb our sons' schooling. Joe was settling well into his career, and I knew the business climate would hold more opportunities for me.

There were specific goals and time lines and inventory disposal and financial guidelines to follow for the next two years, all scribbled and erased and scribbled again on whiteboards. It was a stimulating and interesting time for me. Plus, the experience not only proved invaluable, it beefed up my resume.

T.J.Maxx, an off-price retailer and at the time a fast-growing company, was the next stop after the data center closed. The time was 1985. They liked my diverse experience—computers and finance combined. Every major executive—and once hired, I met with all of them—had a whiteboard. My extensive experience landed me a position in the Finance Department that was tightly linked to the executive offices.

There were many strategic points, organization charts, operational policies, sales strategies, and profit forecasts on whiteboards that changed daily. And there was the annual budget, which was my major responsibility. I worked for T.J. Maxx for seven years, until 1992, when I discovered another passageway that took my life in a completely different direction.

———

I can afford time to reminisce because it is the weekend. My real work and those goals on the whiteboard will begin on Monday. Today I have time for visitors. And here they come, the ones I have been waiting for—my son, Tim, with his wife, Joanna, all the way from Montana. Pouring like rushing water, my love flows over them. I feel tears well up in my eyes as we both stretch out our arms for a hug.

"Hi Mom."

"I'm so glad to see you," I cry, and hug him hard. As he hugs me back, I am sobbing silently into his chest. My heart swells with happiness. He is here. Then I greet Joanna with a warm hug. We both shed tears as we hold each other. We share a close connection.

We have a great visit. Joe is here, too. Tim and Joanna flew in from Bozeman last evening. We talk a lot and laugh. For me it is comforting to have my eyes on them and to have them physically close.

It's Super Bowl Sunday and the game will soon begin; they are ready to leave. Tim and Joanna are staying with Ken and Danielle. Ken, who is not a sports fan, will be watching his first Super Bowl. It will be a family gathering but without me. I tell them I am rooting for the Colts, and Peyton Manning must win the

MVP award because "I worked damn hard to get this horseshoe-shaped incision imprinted on my head. It's not a tattoo. This is the real thing, 39 staples, and it is the Colts' logo." We all share a good laugh. They will return tomorrow. I look forward to many visits while there are here.

———

Mick Jagger. A rock star of my time. I love him, and the Rolling Stones. After all these years, Mick and most of his crew, are still going strong—like the pink Energizer Bunny. A few years back, I had the great good fortune to see Mick Jagger live. What a thrill! He began his concert with the very upbeat song, "Start Me Up!" From the first drum beat he began strutting across the stage. He pranced and danced, ran and hopped, even skipped across the stage. A broad smile spread across my face as I marveled at his energy and gazed at his craggy, lined face. He's like a trained athlete. He works the entire audience as he careens across the stage, microphone in one hand, the other on his hip. He sports that famous haughty but pouty look that today is iconic. Here comes what we've all been waiting for, he pushes out those famous luscious lips and teases us with his tongue—his other famous icon. His hips swivel out, the chin up, his head held high, and he bends forward to the audience—the screaming audience—and points his finger to us and yells "you" when the song calls for it. The screaming gets louder—and mine, too. The energy is electric. For 90 minutes he maintains this energy, song after song. And he's not even out of breath. What a workout! Mick must have lots of support to put on a production like that.

Ensconced in rehab, I will require lots of support, too. I'm looking for energy that, while not electric, needs to be sustaining. A new rhythm may occur once I get to walk again. And a new look will happen if I can manage to get a haircut. I'm not looking to put on a production like Mick Jagger. Instead what I must do is to get out of bed, on my own, stand up, move to a wheelchair, sit down in that wheelchair, and learn to manipulate it. Then, after learning to stand up, I will teach my body to move and position itself in front of a walker. I will learn to walk with this walker, progress to a cane, and ultimately, walk on my own. Wow! As I contemplate these individual sequential steps I stop and think: I too will be putting on a production. I too will be getting my own workout. And to do all that I will require my own support staff to "start me up!"

It's Monday morning and I'm aware of three more people on my support staff: the occupational therapist (OT), the physical therapist (PT), and the certified occupational therapy assistant (COTA), Steve. He seems to wear many hats. For now he brings around the daily schedule. He handwrites the three-hour schedule for each patient. The time is broken into segments of one, one-half, or two hours, depending on progress. For now, I have mostly half-hour segments with long rest periods in between.

Depending on the day, my OT will be either Tess or Dee Dee. These two young women help with my OT goals. While I was at Cape Cod Hospital, there was no dressing or dressing management because every day I wore a clean hospital johnny. Bathing and grooming were combined with the help of the nursing aide, who helped me clean up at the bathroom sink each morning and evening. I washed my face and brushed my teeth at the sink located within the bathroom. I could do only part of it with my right hand, and the nursing aide would help with the rest. Because I was seated in a wheelchair, I could not see myself in the mirror; it was above my head. Toileting was arduous. It took two people—usually two aides—to lift me from the bed to the wheelchair. Two people to stand me up and transfer me to a wheelchair, and one to push me in to the bathroom. Once there, the aide lifted me on to the toilet and left, giving me privacy. When I was finished, I pulled a cord that rang at a central desk, as well as outside my room. An aide returned to help me off the toilet and into the wheelchair, and to lift me back to my bed.

Tess is on duty today. She has a lovely smile. "Would you like to take a shower?"

"Is that possible?"

"Sure is." She is a young woman. Later I learn she is in her early twenties, a young mother with one child, and working at Spaulding with a vision toward nursing school. She tells me she loves her work. And it shows. Tess is patient and gentle as she works with me. She exudes a positive attitude and wastes no time in helping me up out of the bed. Briefly she shows me how to use my body, concentrating on my strong right side, and how to pivot myself so I can help her. With her assistance, I somehow get myself into the wheelchair, and we proceed to the bathroom.

The first thing I notice is the physical layout. The sink is not inside the bathroom. It's outside in my room for brushing teeth and washing up at night. It has a pull-around curtain for privacy. The bathroom, which has no tub, appears quite large to me, but it measures about 7 by 10 feet. It is large enough to hold a toilet on one end and a shower at the other. Without a bathtub, the space gives the illusion of being large. There is a drain in the floor where the shower is. The bathroom is fully tiled, and different tiles distinguish the floor, the walls, and ceiling. The shower has a special moveable chair, which faces shower controls like the ones found at home, and it has a hand-held shower nozzle instead of an overhead one.

I take my first shower supervised, as the whiteboard instructs, by Tess. I use the hand-held shower, which is awkward at first. I try not to squirt Tess. I wash my hair for the first time, but Tess has to rinse the soap from the back of my head. It's frustrating not to be able to rinse all of my hair. The water goes everywhere but the job gets done. We have to use several towels. I'm determined to get better at that. All in all, it feels good to take a shower.

Tess helps me get dressed, giving me tips and techniques along the way.

Her biggest is, "always dress your left side, the weak side, first. Then you have the strong side to help with the tugging and pulling." She even has tricks for the shoes and socks. For now, she has to tie my shoes; the fingers on my left hand are weak and lack coordination. But in time they will gain it. Tess says that practice sessions squeezing the special clay will help strengthen my fingers.

I make mental notes of Tess's tips and look forward to tomorrow's shower; I want to see how much more I can accomplish. Once I am in the wheelchair and fully dressed for the first time in a long while, I say to myself, "It feels good."…a little piece of normal coming back. This part of my OT rehab tires me out, and I return to bed for a little doze while waiting for my next appointment. I take a peek and see that it is physical therapy, in about an hour.

When I wake I am looking at Ann Marie, the physical therapist. Ann Marie is a slightly built woman, slender, and in her mid-to-late thirties. She stands about five foot nine inches tall with short, dark hair; a soft gentle voice; and an easy smile. Ann Marie has the physique of a runner. Perhaps she's active outdoors. In the beginning, my physical therapy goals are about moving my body up in the bed, managing the controls of the bed so the head of the bed is at a 90-degree angle, and using the strength and weight of my right side to hoist myself up and push my left side to the edge of the bed. Tess, my OT, helped me with these actions this morning, but with Ann Marie I learn more steps. Hence more work on my part (I didn't realize how much work Tess did for me this morning). Working with Ann Marie becomes tiring, and I haven't even got out of the bed yet!

I've moved my body to the edge of the bed and am ready for what Ann Marie calls, and the program on the whiteboard requires, the transfers. Here's where I get a chance to carry through on the code: sit-to-stand and stand-to-sit. I will try transfers in and out of bed. When I first stand up, Ann Marie has an aide on either side assisting me. This is not new. That's how I accomplished the transfers in the hospital, too. What is new is that the aides on either side of me are not doing the work, I am, and it is hard. They are by my side so I won't fall. I'm terrified of falling, even with all the support around me. The Woman of the '80s, who did everything, is now afraid to fall and to fail.

Leaning on a rehab aide on my right and Ann Marie on my left, I rise up slowly and carefully, with all the might I have in me. This is hard. I close my eyes and imagine standing. I'm still not up, but I am pushing and willing and pushing my body up, up, up. I'm working my body hard. I want it to be straight, and then I can stand. I manage to get my body up. But I fall, crash down into the bed. And I am tired. I fall back on the bed a few more times. I laugh. I am reminded of a toddler just learning to walk. She teeters, she sways to the left, then to the right, she holds her hands in little fists, and her arms up and out at her sides to counter her balance. She loses her balance and then, whoops-a-daisy, she falls down on her bottom. But up she gets, over and over, teetering and tottering, falling and swaying, and getting up again. I am the toddler.

When I can stand steady, Ann Marie puts a strap around my waist, while maintaining a grip on me in case I fall. Slowly I learn how to step, and pivot, to move my body I can grab on to the handles of the wheelchair, and sit down. Ah, success! I don't want to say it out loud, but I feel tired. That was a lot of work. First rehearsal for my new concert tour, done for today!

I wish I could explain what struggling to move using all the might I have in me feels like. It's like there's an empty space in my head. Something should be there, but it's not. I'm working against that nothing as if it is gravity. I am trying to put something back where it belongs. And if I work hard enough, there will be something there. That is, if I can get something up there in my brain to respond, like new pathways, new electrical impulses to fire, neurons or synapses, then I CAN DO IT! But it is a struggle. When I move my left-side limbs, it is as if there's nothing there with which to respond. That's the feeling, the obstacle I am working against. It is the best way I can describe the sensation when I try to move my limbs, when I try to…start me up.

"The Great Room." That name describes different types of rooms. In real estate brochures or ads it is used to depict a large family room or living room or even a game room. I've never seen one. Until now. That's what I call this large spacious room—the Great Room. As Ann Marie, my PT, wheels me to the room, I am astonished at its size. Cut a professional basketball court in half and that's the size. Without the basket and the balls, of course. The ceiling must be at least 15 feet high and has skylights. The natural light creates a peaceful sense. There are windows on one wall with the late-day sun pouring through. The February winter sun is low and bright, and shades are lowered to keep it from blinding us. What's that I spy over by the windows? Stairs—a make-shift set with three steps. Oh my! The daunting thought of climbing them catches my breath as I'm wheeled in.

There's equipment of all types—some familiar and some strange looking—resting along the walls and in use by several patients. I'm struck by a patient moving by me with his physical therapist. He's going very slowly, he's hardly moving but his eyes are darting all around as if he is confused and doesn't know where he is. He's enclosed in a strap-like container and hanging in it, from it, but at the same time he's trying to walk. I tear up. I want to know what happened to him. What's he trying to achieve in that contraption? Will he get better? Ann Marie whispers that he has had a stroke and that this harness is a new technique that helps a stroke victim find themselves in space—spatial relations. I cry some more because I feel lucky to have what I have. In comparison, I have lost so little. I can't walk either, but I know I will and on my own. In addition, I seem to have a sense of myself in space. I feel scared for him. But I need to concentrate on myself, my recovery—what I have.

Every corner, between the corners, and the middle of the room are all occupied with diverse types of therapy. The middle of the room is for groups. As people progress in their rehab, they come together and play with each other around a table. Maybe I'll get there in time. There's a rectangular mat in each corner—like a square trampoline, but it's solid with a little give. When I sit or lie on it, it provides me with comfort. That's where we begin.

Ann Marie starts the actual movement of my limbs, my left leg and my left arm. I'm excited. I'm finally beginning my training—as if for the Olympics! It feels weird at first because there is no sensation at all, just her movement of my leg and arm while I observe. It's like I am watching somebody else crank up a machine—a thing. A thing that has no feeling.

But I do have *feelings*. Feelings of loss and fear and anxiety. What will become of me? What will it look like walking again? How will my life change? What about me and Joe? And then there's my practice...my professional life? Seeing the man in his harness...I don't know...he represents the barrage of feelings my state of bewilderment is trying to keep back...protecting me from feelings. There's a flood of tears...a choked sob, ready to burst. I struggle to keep it in check...to shove it back into my state of bewilderment...back into a vault for now. No time for tears, only time to cope, time to heal, time to recover, time to retrain.

The Great Room becomes like a clubhouse for me. I remember when I was a kid I couldn't wait to go and meet my friends and play and trade cards and have secret passwords. Boy, am I old. Today kids have BlackBerry smartphones and Facebook and websites and iPhones. Whoever heard of clubhouses!

I am beginning to recognize and know the other patients. We nod to each other in the hall. Joe always says I have antennae coming out of me because I manage to find out who and what's going on in a crowd. This therapy room is no exception. People are patients here for many reasons. A look here, a piece of conversation there, and a shout of encouragement over in the corner. It doesn't take me long to learn people's names and what has occurred in their lives to bring us together in the Great Room.

Many are recovering from different types of strokes. Others have head trauma from falls. Still others are recovering from motor vehicle and motorcycle accidents. Then there's postsurgical problems like mine; people with dehydration, medication dosage problems, and some things I can't explain. It doesn't take long before I get to know everybody. It's fun to say hi and get on with my workout. And especially fun because I am beginning to feel. My muscles are "waking up," the phrase I use to refer to my muscles becoming activated. The medical term, or proper term, is "firing up." And I'm all for firing these muscles up and sending messages to my brain and then back again. I have a long way to go...much work to do in the Great Room...to get home.

I'm surfing through my sleep. I think it is early morning and time to think about this new day. I'm not willing to open my eyes yet. My body feels like it's made of lead and it cannot—it will not—move. I am tired. Exhausted is a better word. I have been in rehab only a few days, and I can't do this anymore. No, I'm not being a wimp. I truly know that my body doesn't have the strength to get up, take that shower, get dressed (even with assistance), and participate in any of the rehab activities today. My body simply can't do it. Not even the right side—the good side. How do I know this? Because my body is telling me, and I have a keen ear, if you will, when I listen to it.

I have always been sensitive to the cues from my body. Never spent much time on the couch, as in couch potato. Joe and I have always walked or biked. Recently, since 2003, I have become acquainted with strength training because of the effect it can have on my bones as I grow older. Joining a gym allowed me to try the treadmill, the elliptical, and other cardio workout machines. I loved the rowing machine at one health club. Exercise for my body has taught me to become in tune with it—the aches and pains, the twitches and the burns, the stretches and the tears, and so forth. In addition, for the past 10 years I've been a practitioner of yoga. I've taken two classes a week and practice at home. I enjoy it and get great benefit from it—the stretches, the postures, the deep belly breathing, and the relaxation. Over those 10 years I've become more and more in tune with my body and what it needs. I know how far I can push it with any particular yoga pose so it won't be painful. I became a Reiki healer also during that time.

Reiki is an ancient healing art form from the Japanese culture. It helps the body with stress reduction and pain relief. Reiki can work on many levels: physical, emotional, and spiritual. Becoming a Reiki practitioner allowed me to be in sync with my body. I often introduced Reiki to my psychotherapy clients. It sometimes helped them push through with their insights, and it always gave them an uplifting sense of self.

With all my training, my body became a teacher for me, and that's why today it says no. It needs to sleep. Tess, however, is having nothing to do with my body's message. I drag myself up, we get me into the bathroom. I shower and wash my hair, and she helps me get dressed. Tess comments several times about my lethargy, and the fact that I washed my hair faster yesterday. She notes that I can get neither my socks nor my shoes on today. I say nothing. Steve, the rehab assistant, comes by with the schedule.

"I'm really too tired today, Steve. I need to rest."

"We'll see about that." With a brusque manner, he leaves my room.

I fall back to sleep. I wake to see Ann Marie. Maybe they sent her because of our close relationship. We talk. She listens and I believe she hears me. She returns awhile later with the shift nurse, Kelly, along with Tess. It is obvious Ann Marie has spent time speaking with both of them. I feel she knows I don't have the energy to keep repeating my story. They leave my room again saying that they will call the cop, Dr. Davidson. He returns with the gang: Ann Marie, Tess, and Kelly. We have a little conference. I tell them all I am not malingering (I actually use that word). I explain I know my body and how it works and what it needs, and right now it needs sleep. I am not sure if it was the bacterial infection in my urinary tract, the transfer from the hospital, the continuing recovery from brain surgery, or the past few days of rehab work. Whatever the cause, my body is currently on strike!

"Give me this time and I guarantee you I will be ready tomorrow to do whatever you ask."

They ask more questions and discuss some options. They give in. What a relief! It probably wasn't easy for them to let me rest. I am here to work. They are taking a chance on me that I really need the rest. They leave and I go back to sleep for hours.

My body wakes me for lunch. Funny, as tired as I am I always wake for meals. I'm learning that's because my blood count is still low, and they're hoping that as my body continues to recover the count will rise. In the meantime I continue to eat everything in sight. After lunch I fall into a sound sleep. I wake around three o'clock to Ann Marie gently shaking my leg.

"How about we go to the therapy room for just a little while?" She says with a firm voice. I know this is a test of my willingness to work.

I agree. I use the controls in my bed to sit up. With the protocols I have learned and am beginning to master—the transfers, the sit-to-stand, the step to the wheelchair—we go to the Great Room. Once there Ann Marie helps me move onto the elevated mat and begins moving my left leg and left arm to send those messages roaring to my brain. My body is not tired now and it's ready to work. I'm retraining my brain again.

Our lifelong friends, Carol and Jim, live in the northern part of New Jersey. Carol calls me every evening to check in and see how my day went. We met Jim and Carol when we were in our early twenties. Both Jim and Joe were PhD candidates at the State University of New York at Buffalo (SUNY). Joe and Jim gravitated toward one another right away. Turns out, Jim and Joe were among the top PhD students of their graduating class. Throughout the intervening years—all 42 of them—we have remained friends. We have been in touch throughout our respective highs and lows, our scary times and our joyful times.

For Jim, living in northern New Jersey is the best thing that could have happened to him. He's in love with Broadway: shows, plays, musicals, operas, on Broadway and off. He gets a chance to see them all. I'm not kidding. When we visit, we see shows, singing the songs as we drive into and out of New York City. One of his recent favorites, and mine, is Mel Brooks' Broadway adaptation of his 1968 film, *The Producers*. In the show, Brooks makes fun of everyone—even Hitler. I was aghast at that one, at first. The show centers around two wise guys, one is a failed producer and the other is his accountant. Together they realize they can make more money by producing a sure-fire flop, *Springtime for Hitler*. It's hilarious watching them do just that. And, of course, it's a smash hit! As the play develops, the audience slowly sees that Brooks is poking fun at white folks, black folks, straight guys, gays, Catholics, Jews, young people, dumb blondes, and, my favorite, grannies.

I reference that musical because I am getting prepped to use a walker. I have always thought of a walker as the end of the line, when I am so old I cannot get around anymore. I can't use a walker at my young age of 63! I am a lady with style. I always dress nicely and with coordinating colors. Not that I am trying to impress anyone. I enjoy dressing for myself and looking nice. I love colors, fabrics, textures, design, putting colors together, shirts with slacks or a skirt and a jacket. Oh, a jacket. I have so many jackets my friends refer to me as the Jacket Queen. And then there's always a scarf, a beautiful silk scarf with many brilliant colors to coordinate an outfit. How will I do that, now? Drape it on the walker? I guess I could, but I'd have to be careful. It might drag and get run over by the walker's wheels. An old-looking, steel grey thingamajig in front of me is certainly going to ruin any look I am trying to achieve. Do I really have to do this?

Then again I need to switch my mind over to: I MUST do this. Looking nice be damned! Wearing fun colors and dressing with a flair aren't important now, are they? What is important is taking that first step, with that left foot, retrain that brain. Instead I ready myself, give myself a lift of spirits, and regain my sense of humor. I think back to an act in *The Producers*.

Sixteen dancing girls with squat-heeled tap shoes come high-stepping onto the stage. Each sports not only a skimpy sequined grey dress but also a grey wig adorned with curls to give the illusion that they are grannies. And if that isn't enough, what are they pushing in front of them? WALKERS! With taps on all four legs, no less. What a hoot! No split tennis balls on these legs and no wheels on their walkers. Not for these grannies. These walkers are their props.

And right now at rehab, in my room, I visualize those 16 dancing girls. I hear their toes and heels clicking as they chug along the stage. They clack their walkers down in front of them, making a heavy, loud tapping. The taps on the shoes and on the walkers provide a loud *click-chug*. The grannies use the walkers to pivot their bodies around and up into the air, and they twirl themselves around the walkers. They pick up the walkers and wave them over their heads as they twirl around again. I'll never be able to do that (wave the walker in the air, maybe), but visualizing them and hearing all the *click-chugging* in my mind causes me to smile as I venture out on my new walker for the very first time.

I stand beside the bed with Ann Marie. She has a quiet nature, such grace and confidence. Every time I work with her I feel more and more of her confidence as my own. After placing the strap around me, she places the walker in front of me and moves the furniture out of the way. I have good clearance now, nothing in my way. The walker feels good in front of me, not like the appendage I imagined. It's not heavy and I don't have to put all my weight on it. I can use it as a guide. All those OT exercises for my left arm and left hand are paying off. Slowly I push forward with my body, my left leg, and the walker. It almost feels natural. With sliced tennis balls on the rear legs and wheels in the front it's easy to glide along the floor. In no time my body, my left leg, and the walker become in synch—we are one! We leave my room, our destination is the therapy room. Ann Marie follows with the wheelchair right behind me for two reasons: if I fall and for when I get tired. I feel as if I can walk all the way—down the long corridor to the turn, and then down the next long corridor to the room. My body tires and I elect to sit down and rest a few minutes. But I'm up and walking again. This walking is freedom. I dismiss all the negative beliefs and feelings I previously held about the walker. The walker is helping me, and I now welcome it. No tap dancing yet.

As time goes on, Joe becomes part of my walking routine. He takes Ann Marie's place and he walks behind me with the wheelchair. He is quite insistent when it comes time to rest. He knows I will try to do too much. This week my brother Billy arrives in rehab (he has had bilateral knee replacement surgery). My therapy now encompasses walking to his wing for a visit. Day after day I continue on my journey and get stronger. I continue to think of those dancing girls though, and the energy they possess to dance the way they do night after night. What talent they have. And I continue to laugh at their curly grey hair and their swinging walkers laden with taps—*clickety-chug chug, clickety-chug chug!*

Watching Martie go through her rehab is eventful for two reasons: her progress and her attitude. Once she is over her infection, she has three exercise sessions a day. Her progress is the first encouraging sign for me since this adventure started. Visiting her once a day, I watch her be able to move herself in the bed; then sit on its side; then, with help, transfer to a wheelchair; and then transfer with no help. Once she is in the wheelchair they put a belt on her that I can use to hold onto her. With my support she can stand up and then take a few steps. A major achievement for her was being able to dress herself, especially putting on her socks and shoes. Such a simple task.

Within a few days she is walking down a hallway, about 20 yards. Then they moved her to a walker, which allows her to walk by herself without a push. Her walking is slow and she quickly tires, but the progress is consistently positive.

We since have learned that when the motor nerves have been damaged, nerve pathways that were less important become stronger and take over the function of the damaged ones. What an amazing feat this is! But this process of nerve strengthening only lasts a few weeks. Somehow the brain knows that it will get confused if too many nerves change. That process is why having rehabilitation right away is so important.

My impression is that almost no one likes to be in a rehab hospital. It's not only a lot of work but it seems to be an annoying stop between the acute care hospital and home. In the "old" days, you just came home after

a stay in the hospital. I watch other patients. They grumble and resist the work and ask constantly about when they will be leaving. Martie is just the opposite. She loves the process and the people. I don't understand how she does it. I couldn't. I'd have my head down and be ashamed that I couldn't walk by myself. And I wouldn't be going out of my way to interact with other patients. I would project their disabilities onto myself, making me feel older, slower, dying. Even though it would not be helpful to feel that way, that's how it would be for me.

Martie bonds with the rehab nurses and therapists, who love her positive attitude. They don't get too many cooperative patients. When we talk each morning on the phone, Martie goes over her progress and her schedule for the day. She enjoys learning how to dress herself and how to sequence her movements to make actions easier.

I'm encouraged and looking forward to having her home soon.

———

I miss Joe. Here, I am stuck. Literally stuck in this bed, and I miss him. He is here every day to see me and help me get through this ordeal and recapture my strength so I can put myself together again, so I can learn to walk. But I miss him. I wish he could stay the night, but there is no place at rehab to accommodate him—no cot, no pullout sofa that serves as a bed like there was back at Cape Cod Hospital. I wish he could sleep in the same bed with me, like at home. Sleeping with me in my fancy rehab bed would provoke quite a laugh. I have to sleep on my back with my upper body at a 30-degree angle. From an observer's perspective, it looks like I am sleeping in a recliner. I don't think Joe would be comfortable sleeping like that. Then there's the antiseizure pads. How would he manage those? There I go again, being practical in the middle of a yearning, an angst. But it would be wonderful to touch him, to know that he is here with me in the night when I wake.

I typically wake between midnight and 1 a.m. I remember waking early in the hospital, crying. Here at rehab, I'm not crying. Usually my body has slid toward the bottom of the bed, and the sheets are tangled, especially around the boots. The boots are great. They're put on my feet every night, along with everything else and hooked up to a small motor that keeps the blood flow circulating in my feet. Works quite well. But around midnight I need to get disentangled and get out of bed. The midnight nurses are attuned to my rhythm, and they know immediately what I want when I press the call button. I was tentative the first night until I realized that midnight to 1 a.m. is a slow period; paperwork is done, most patients are asleep, and they can—some are even eager to—tend to me.

"Hi honey, do you need to get refreshed?" is often how they greet me. Most nurses allow me to sit in the wheelchair while they freshen the sheets in my bed. Sometimes they bring me a cup of tea and crackers, and stay for a chat. I'm appreciative of their kindness. I have a bunch of CDs with me and they make sure the CD player works and that I have chosen my music before they shut off the lights. I return to sleep.

Until...approximately 5 a.m. Another familiar routine. The phlebotomist arrives to finger-stick me. My blood count is still low. I know because I ask, and I continue to feel tired. How is my body able to do all this rehabilitation work in this tired state? Don't know. Also, I continue to inhale my food. A couple of times a staff member from the dietary group comes by to check my weight. It's done with a scale built into the bed. Amazing! I don't want to know my weight.

I hear from Joe that he is quite busy; he's keeping our household together. He's paying bills, keeping up with the laundry (mine, as well as his own), vacuuming here and there, shopping for food, preparing meals for himself, and taking care of all those unforeseen things that crop up in a household. As a couple we have evolved into sharing those activities. In addition, he's making phone calls to some folks about my progress. In the evening he sits down at the computer and composes his nightly email and sends them to our friends and colleagues to give them an update.

Toward the end of my first week here, I continue to feel tired. The nurse on duty speaks to Dr. Davidson about it, and between them they believe I am feeling anxiety. They approach me one at a time about this. I emphatically state, "No, that's not how I express anxiety. I am just tired." Well, they continue talking to me about it, and I begin to doubt myself. Mainly because I have never been in this type of situation before—rehab, not being able to walk, etc.—and they are the experts (ha, ha). Eventually, I give in. What did I give in to? Xanax—an anti-anxiety medication. Because of my profession as a psychotherapist I am familiar with anti-anxiety meds. I am not sure I need Xanax but agree to give it a try. I take two to three doses during the day and one at night.

Then I speak up. "That's enough. I'm not taking this stuff anymore! I don't like what it does to me. It makes me feel jumpy."

"Perhaps you don't have enough in your system yet for it to work."

"No! I am not taking any more." It took another 24 hours for it to leave my system. I'm relieved. I was fooled again and wish I had listened to my body. I know when I am anxious and when I am tired. Live and learn. I'm in a vulnerable position. I am still recovering physically from surgery and my blood count is low. I am learning to move my limbs so I can walk again and using the strength I have to get in and out of bed. I don't have the time to experience any anxiety. When I experience anxiety I will know it! And, right now I know I am tired.

The bra is problematic. All prepubescent girls learn how to put on a bra the way their mothers taught them: either with the cups in the front or the cups in the back. To quote George Costanza of *Seinfeld* fame—"I know all about the cups!" My mother taught me to fasten my bra with the cups in the front. Over the years my fingers became deft in hooking my bra from behind, even a double-hook, in one smooth stroke. Now with the fingers on my left hand not yet coordinated and slowly moving but showing tremors, I am unable to do this. Tess, my OT, teaches me what she thinks is a simpler way. She places my bra on completely reversed: the cups are now upside down and behind me, with the hooks in front. My brain has been through a lot in the past few weeks and it is still reverberating from being manually pushed around in surgery. I'm having difficulty getting a grasp on this new method. I try and practice each day. The success-o-meter rings at the low end of the scale most of the time.

I manage to get my bra on each day. Some days the bra is on inside out. Another day only one hook is engaged. I will say, though, the cups are *always* in the front! One day, in my frustration, I just went braless—like we did in the late 1960s and '70s. The fingers on my left hand begin to get stronger and the improved coordination shows itself in the afternoon OT exercises. I added my own OT exercise in the morning. I started putting the bra on my way: beginning with the cups in the front. It was a challenge at first, to get those hooks engaged in the back, but I keep working the fingers on my left hand, and eventually...I can do it my way!

———

During one of my walking exercises with Ann Marie I spot a grand piano in the family room. It stirs my heart.

"I play the piano."

"You do? You'll have to play for us."

"I'd love to." Word about my piano playing makes its way through the nurses' chatter. I talk with Joe about bringing in my music. I dream about playing for them. I have been taking piano lessons, as an adult, for 15 years. I began with classical music, but my teacher, Mr. Ed, is a gifted musician and a composer, and he introduced me to different types of music. I began playing popular music as well as music from *the American Songbook*—music from the first half of the twentieth century, the music Frank Sinatra sang, and Tony Bennett and Mel Torme, and others of that era. I learned many left-hand arrangements: jazz 10th, walking bass, rolling 10th, 9th voicings, the stride, and Alberti bass. Over those years, I participated in 15 adult recitals. I was like a nervous bunny for each recital. I thought I would throw up before the first one. But I overcame my nervousness, somewhat, and began to enjoy performing. I look forward to touching the keys of the piano here in the family room.

The day comes and the accompaniment includes: my walker, Joe, and my music. I intend to sit down and play "Stardust"—the piece I played at my recital in 2004. I had been rehearsing the notes and chords in my head for days. I approach the piano, and Joe helps me move the walker to the side. I sit down on the piano bench. Joe puts my music in place. I play the first rolling chord for the introduction. It sounds OK despite my left little finger not being able to strike the first note. Then the first line of the song—the familiar refrain—and that works well. I look up at the music. I can read the music, but something strange happens. I cannot make the connection from my brain to my fingers. I can't put it all together. My heart sinks low with despair. It is the first time I realize there is another type of damage to my brain. Sure I couldn't walk a week ago and I am retraining my brain on that deficit. But this is different. It appears more on the neurological, or is it the cognitive level? I try a few more chords. They work, meaning they sound musical, but I can't get the song to reveal itself like it's meant to be played. I can't feel the music, or put it together. I stop. I manage a smile as Joe and I leave the room. I don't feel embarrassed or shamed. I'm mystified. I revert into bewilderment for protection. My brain needs more rest, and I need some comfort.

Do you believe in angels? I do. They are all here floating, wafting, and swirling around. They come in all sizes and shapes: tall, short, thick, and thin. And colors, too: white, black, tan, and yellow. They are the rehab assistants on my rehab team—very crucial people. These angels take on the human form of women and men, and are on-call every minute of each eight-hour-shift.

When a patient rings the call button, the first person to respond is the rehab assistant. If the need of a patient is a medical one, the rehab assistant will locate the nurse. But, for the most part, the problem is solved by the rehab assistant. They do the dirty work. They monitor, as well as deposit, a patient's urine and bowel movements. They clean up vomit when accidents happen. The rehab assistants are the ones who constantly help me in and out of bed, and into the bathroom. They work very hard. I find most of them to be caring, supportive, loving, and eager to help. In addition, they sport a smile along with a cheery and positive attitude. That's why I call them angels.

One particular lady—Rita—comes to mind. Rita checks in on the 3:30 p.m. shift. Rita is compassionate and supportive, and she knows my routine for the evening. I learn from the OT/PT folks that after my rehab workouts I will recover the strength in my back muscles, if I sit up in a chair, or the wheelchair, for half an hour—as opposed to lying in bed. I put this into practice and sit in a chair with a sturdy back after each meal, and for a longer period after supper. My goal is to make it to 6:30 p.m. That means I am sitting for an additional half-hour. A challenging feat, it is. But I notice, as tired as my back and side muscles become, sitting up is producing results, making them stronger. I feel the difference.

Rita pokes her head in my door every 10 minutes or so just to be sure I am not tiring too early. I am, but I don't admit it to her. I am determined to make the half-hour. Most nights I make it. Then Rita assists while I wash up for bedtime, helps me with a clean hospital gown, and settles me in my bed with all its bells and whistles—a.k.a. bed rails, 30-degree head elevation, antiseizure pads. I am ready to watch my favorite show, *Law and Order,* and wait for the good-night calls from my son, Tim, and my friends, Martha and Carol.

Ronald is another rehab assistant of note. A former truck driver, Ronald had to stop driving due to back problems that gave him excruciating pain. Mike prides himself on giving—of all things—the best back rub. And he is right. He does.

"People ask for me," he says with a huge smile! Like Rita, Ronald seems to anticipate what a patient needs; he prides himself on that, too. I note his disappointment when I don't request him. My reply: "I am sharing you with folks who need you more than me." He smiles.

Another rehab assistant comes to mind whose name I can't remember but whose actions I shall never forget. She answers my call bell when I need to use the bathroom. I sense something different as she hurriedly comes into my room. No greeting from her, not even a "hello" or introduction. She is not on my whiteboard and I have not seen her before. She lifts me out of bed without letting me do any of the work, places me in the wheelchair, and briskly wheels me into the bathroom. She lifts me onto the toilet, again without allowing me to help myself, and takes the wheelchair out of the bathroom, instead of leaving it for me to use when I am through. When she leaves the bathroom, she shuts the door so that the latch engages. I'm alone.

All the rehab assistants leave me alone in the bathroom. That's for my privacy, and I respect that. However, none of them has ever shut the door so that it engages the latch. Plus the rehab assistants always wait in my room, so they can hear me through the door when I need them.

When I finish, I pull the call bell. I wait. A few minutes pass, longer than I'm used to. I wait some more. Pulling the call bell again does not cause any new activity at the nurse's desk. That's the way it works. You pull it once. I hear nothing with the bathroom door securely closed. OK, now what? I look around the room. There is nothing within my reach that I can use to help get myself up. There isn't even anything I can throw against the door that would make noise. What I do see is the poster on the wall that says: "PATIENT IS NOT TO BE LEFT ALONE IN BATHROOM!" Ha, now what! With my soft voice (I say "soft" because that's the type of voice I've been graced with), I begin to yell, "Hello...hello...hello. Is anybody out there?" then louder and louder, "HELLO...HELLO!"

If the wheelchair had been left I could have managed to get myself up off the toilet, grab onto something in the bathroom, then step and pivot my way into it and wheel myself out the door. But no, she took it with her. I don't know what she was thinking. From my perspective, she was *not* thinking. I'm feeling helpless. "HELLO!" I scream louder, this time. "Anybody there?" I begin screeching those words over and over and over, and yanking on the call button cord again—mainly for something to do.

I am trying not to panic, but the longer I hear nothing outside and no one coming to open the door, the more frantic I get. Someone will come along eventually. Yes, that's true. But feeling as vulnerable as I am I can't wait any longer. And why should I? I've lost my sense of safety. I scream, "H E-E-L-L-L-L-P! H E-E-L-L-L-L-P M-E-E-E-E-E!" over and over and over. Finally, after I don't know how many minutes, somebody comes and opens the door. By this time I am in tears and shaking. She helps me to bed. It takes an hour or so to calm down.

I know the team was notified about this incident, and the rehab assistant was told to come by to apologize.

"I was assisting someone else down the hall," she says defensively.

She just doesn't get it. I never see her again. I call her the fallen angel.

Time alone. By myself. These days I don't have much time to think...or to feel. It's bedtime, the lights are out, all the staff are busy. I can breathe and feel. What is this *down* feeling that is seeping in? I get this way when feelings need to come out. One thing I know is that I am still feeling fatigued, and I want to know what is fueling that. Is it the low blood? They keep testing that daily. What's going on? I am working hard to try to walk, maintain my balance, wake up the left side of my body, and understand what the team is saying to me and what they want of me. Sometimes I don't understand, and my lack of comprehension concerns me. Is there something else going on? Do I have some cognitive issues or cognitive losses, deficits? That scares me.

What will I look like when I get out of here? I can barely walk. I'm doing all the exercises, and still I am quaking and shaky, and my left arm and those last two fingers—the ring and the pinky—show a tremor and can barely do anything. This rehab is hard, harder than I ever dreamed. How would I know? I've never been in rehab before. I never had a brain tumor before. Having said that, the horror of it all is pouring out of me and frightens me.

All these things have happened in a short time—barely three weeks yet—and are difficult to assimilate into my consciousness, my reality, my brain. And it's my brain that is the focal point, the organ that was injured. I thank my lucky stars that my tumor was benign, but the repercussions of it all are difficult to absorb. Seizures are the scariest thing in my world. It's the ultimate loss of control. Unlike bladder or bowel control, a seizure affects the whole body. I can feel it and not feel it at the same time. I feel suspended in space. I lose track of time and I don't know when it will stop—if ever. Terrifying.

How freaky is it to have a new piece in my skull? Knowing that part of my skull was destroyed by the tumor. I shudder. I know at some point I'll joke about it. But not now. Not tonight. The saw that cut into my head...I can't think now. I am trying to heal.

Working hard on getting out of bed, standing, pivoting into the wheelchair, braking, strolling with a walker. Is this me? The new me? I don't know if I can accept that as the *new normal*. What's going to happen at home? How will I manage? I know I can depend on Joe. That will be great, and difficult, at the same time. I'm used to being independent; now I won't be.

And what about Joe? How is all this affecting him? He is on the sidelines watching, but much more than that, he must be experiencing his own feelings at seeing me debilitated and dependent, not the independent, spirited woman he has loved for over four decades. He must be scared. He must feel fragmented. He must feel frightened. This is all new for him, too. So far he has said little about any of his feelings.

His role may change in our relationship, perhaps a role reversal in our marriage. I worry about not only my physical deficits but also my neurological deficits—the ones that surprised me at the piano in the family room the other day—and the cognitive deficits that are emerging, and the ones I don't know that may pop up later. Will he be able to handle them? Will he still love me? What about my sons, Ken and Tim? They've always seen me as the strong mother, now I feel small and vulnerable. What are they thinking and feeling? They must be scared, too. All these worries... these many concerns...what will happen? What lies ahead?

———

Valentine's Day. A happy day for lovers. A happy day for some people, not me. Over the years Valentine's Day has taken on a not-so-good aura, and I have come to despise the day. Take your red hearts, your stupid little cupids with arrows of love, those boxes of chocolates, the candy hearts with the oh-so-cute sayings because...it is not my kind of day.

In the early years of our marriage Joe was resistant to hearts, cupids with arrows, and chocolates—all things that would have made me smile. I was disappointed at that and felt unloved. As years went by, our two boys suffered chicken pox and mumps, one after the other, and I was a housebound mom taking care of two sick toddlers—around Valentine's Day. A few years after that, while living in Michigan and away from my family, I was notified that my mother was diagnosed with colon cancer—around Valentine's Day. Many years later, when the boys were in their early twenties, we learned the reason for Joe's troubling disposition, the beast he had been wrestling with for months—depression—the day before Valentine's Day. And several years after that, Joe's mom, who became very close to me when I lost my mother, died on Valentine's Day.

Here at rehab, two days before Valentine's Day, there is a cutesy blond occupational therapist who is rounding up a bunch of us to make valentines. Make valentines! Is she kidding! She's not. She's gathering us up with our wheelchairs and walkers. She's serious. She in her early thirties, has a low, seductive, and sweet voice, and she wants us to make a Valentine's card for our spouse or whomever our caretaker is. Do people our age, my age, really subject themselves to this? Where is Ann Marie? Where is Steve? Hello? This must be a conspiracy. I'm in my wheelchair and can't move quickly. I try to escape but Miss Blond Cutesy has one of her minions push me back to the table. I guess I'll be held captive for the 45 minutes it takes to make a silly valentine.

OK, I know, I know. My rebellious adolescent has emerged, and she doesn't want to make a valentine. I stuffed her down inside me. With my grown-up voice politely, but softly, I tell the adolescent that she can do this, even if she doesn't like Valentine's Day.

———

Two days later, on Valentine's Day, I receive an unexpected call from Joe early in the morning. I am puzzled, then worried. What has happened? My first thoughts go toward our sons and their families. I wonder if they are OK. Billy is down the hall from me, so I know he is in good hands. Are my sisters and their families all right? It's amazing the thoughts that can whip through my mind, and how, in an instant, I can pick up the hint of something different in Joe's voice. In his soft, steady voice Joe informs me, "Your father died—early this morning." I think to myself *Valentine's Day!*

My emotions are mixed: grief, sadness, anger, frustration, relief, disbelief. My father had been ill. He was suffering from chronic obstructive pulmonary disease (COPD) and seemed to be managing quite well the last time I saw him, which was at Christmas. He began to fail in January, right around the time I became hospitalized.

About a year ago it became clear to my sisters, Regina and Marian, who live closer to him than either Billy or I, that he needed long-term care—today's new term for a nursing home. They took on that responsibility, and the two of them worked hard to ensure he had a comfortable and supportive place to live. The relationship between my father and me, as well as the relationship my brother and sisters had with him, has been a complicated one. He lived for 93 years. Next month, March, he would have been 94.

Wow, this is an enormous chunk of news to chew on. What is my father doing—dying now when Billy and I are in the middle of rehab recovering from serious procedures? We cannot get to the services. Leave it to him to do this. This is not new. This is not the first time in my life that my father has "pulled the rug out from under me." But it will be the last!

The first thing I want to do is talk to Billy. After breakfast he calls me on the hospital phone. We need to get together. Since I am more mobile than he (he is not able to get out of bed yet), we will meet later in the afternoon, when my PT routine brings me with my walker and my wheelchair behind me down to his room.

When we meet we sob together and share our grief, our anger, our frustration. We can't believe that he died now, when neither of us can get to the services. We talk and strategize about renting a wheelchair car for the three-hour ride to get out to Athol where the wake and funeral will be on Friday night and Saturday morning, respectively.

What we don't know is that, at the same time, our respective spouses are talking to each other, strategizing how they'll tell us, "You are in no condition to go!" As time goes on, and Billy and I talk it through and realize: We Can't Go, as compelling as it seems. I mean, how can we not show up at our own father's funeral? We cannot go. Physically Billy is just beginning to get up on crutches, and I can barely use a walker, and I need a wheelchair behind me. We are both vulnerable physically, as well as emotionally. And we are each responding to our own traumas and still recovering from surgeries. It is too soon for either of us to be venturing out anywhere.

I think of the emotional aspect of this, and all the people who will be at the services. Billy and I are two among dozens of cousins, and many of them will be there. Thinking of some or all of these people who could be there makes me dizzy. I cannot go into the funeral home and see any of them—with or without a walker. They would all crowd around and ask questions and want to know what happened! I just know I can't handle that stimulation. I fall back into bed. No, I cannot go. Fuck!

Later when I talk to Joe about my decision, he is visibly relieved. He informs me our son, Ken, and his wife, Danielle, will represent us at the funeral. I feel a swell of pride at the idea.

The idea of missing my father's wake and funeral feels strange. How can I not say my final good-byes to him? It has been a long and hard and sad journey between the two of us, and now there will be...nothing? There will be no formal ending? I am a believer in funerals. The rituals provide healing and help in accepting death.

My relationship with my father has been tumultuous. I have been angry with him for many years because he turned his back on me and my siblings when he remarried after my mother died. His second wife took priority over us, and he pushed us away.

I find it sad that I will miss standing with my sisters beside his casket accepting loving embraces and condolences from my aunts, uncles, cousins, and friends. I will miss the rituals around the funeral, the eulogy (my sister, Regina, will deliver it), and the burial. Because he was in the Navy during World War II, representatives from the Navy will be present and taps will be played. There will be the folding of the flag. That ceremony, with the flag, is an honorable and momentous ritual I will miss the most. Perhaps that is part of my anger—not being there.

I speak to Regina and Marian. We share our grief and we share words of comfort. Our conversation includes the conflicting feelings we had with our father over the years. If I were not in rehab, I would be there helping Billy with the wake and funeral decisions. Being the oldest it would have fallen to me to make some of those decisions. Right now all those decisions and details feel very overwhelming to me. I express gratitude to Regina that she and Marian are there to do what is necessary, and feel confident they will take charge of them. And there are many to handle. I know they will manage the events; our father will have a beautiful and healing service.

All this to grapple with—and on Valentine's Day!

———

I hate Valentine's Day. When Martie and I were first married at 20 years old, I began to learn how different the worlds of men and women are. I knew about birthday and Christmas cards, but Halloween? Easter? Isn't Valentine's Day for people who are courting? Why would I be asking my wife if she would be my valentine? Do I have to prove my love again and again? I didn't get it. I was grumpy about the card thing and sometimes forgot. I could see that Martie was hurt but I just figured she would get over it in a few years. What was I thinking? I gradually came to the solution that getting a card was easier than doing battle again. I now buy a blank card and put my own words on it.

When I was in graduate school, I started getting tension headaches in the back of my neck. Every three to four weeks one would arrive in the early morning. They lasted for a day, and nothing helped except going to bed and waiting it out. It was a stressful time. I had to write and finish my dissertation to qualify for a PhD, and I had a very tough faculty advisor. He was young and trying to prove how smart he was to his colleagues. I wrote a 40-page proposal for my dissertation. His first reaction was, "Boy, you are a shitty writer. Rewrite it so I can tell what you are trying to say." Great for my self-confidence.

I am not sure if the headaches were the start of my depression, but I do know that as the frequency of the headaches diminished through my twenties, depression took hold. I didn't realize it then, but as I look back, I can see how it blossomed during my days at the university, after getting my degree. My mother suffered from depression throughout much of her adult live. It would get bad, and she would go to a psychiatrist who would give her pills that made her feel unpleasant. So she would stop taking them and restart the cycle. My mom's depression wasn't so bad that it disrupted the family. She had periods when she seemed always to have a headache and she would get irritable and angry at her lot in life. She was distant emotionally during those times, but she always got up and went to work and took care of my sisters and me.

My first job after graduate school was a real downer for me. I was an assistant professor in the Psychology Department at Oakland University, in Rochester Michigan. It was without a PhD program and without modern lab facilities. For eight years my goal had been to get my degree. I hadn't thought about whether I really wanted to be an academic.

I enjoyed being in the classroom and using my computer skills to help the other faculty members with their research. But I had no one to talk with who knew cognitive psychology. I was isolated intellectually, and I figured out that I had almost no chance to move to a more prestigious university. I conducted some basic research studies that were published in good journals and snagged a small grant for a summer. The publications gave me enough ammunition for a shot at tenure, which I was granted after five years. But all tenure meant was that I could stay at Oakland forever. A grim prospect.

The social environment at Oakland was toxic. I was the son of a construction worker and a factory worker. Most of the other faculty had parents who had been professors or real doctors. They assumed they belonged in academia, albeit at a second or third tier university. I felt lost. I was more comfortable with the students than with the faculty. I knew I was as smart as the faculty, but I found most of them pretentious and hypocritical. If I stayed in academia, I could move only laterally or down, such as to a community college. I would have to publish many papers or books to move up, but with no graduate students or facilities and no time for research, that was unlikely.

So I sat for hours in my office looking at the wall wondering what I had become. I was distant at home with Martie and the guys. I wanted something different but didn't know what. So I read books, taught my classes, and avoided my feelings as much as I could.

Just before my last year at Oakland, my best friend in the Psychology Department was denied tenure. That sad event propelled me to action; I started looking for a new career path. Later that year I resigned my position and took a job near Boston working for a federal government transportation research facility. That position allowed us to move back home and within a year buy our first house. But I didn't leave the depression in Michigan.

There have been several book authors who have tried to describe what it feels like to be clinically depressed. They all admit that words can't express it. It's not just a mental state, it's a physical one. It affects your whole body. For me, it felt like a shade was being pulled down that blocked any positive feelings. The darkness is ever present and colors everything. I could be standing in the doorway of a colleague's office having a perfectly normal conversation. At the same time, I would feel a punch in the stomach and a voice in my head would say, "You're failing at your job. Your colleague knows it. You're just pretending and it shows."

As I later moved up in my career, the depression followed me. I was still able to work hard and long hours in spite of what I was feeling. During my early forties I wrote a book on software design. While I was writing it, I had long periods of doubt about its acceptance. The voice would tell me that it would be panned and I would be accused of not having any creativity. I spent endless nights writing with my IBM PC with two floppy disks hoping to convince the voice that I had something useful to say. In spite of the depression, I was ambitious. I was determined to be a good provider. The battle continued.

The book was published, and my career flourished. I moved up in the consulting firm I then worked for. My boss, a newly chosen president of the company, asked me to take over the running of the local Boston office, and I was soon a vice president. I published a second book with a colleague that became recognized as a leader in its field. Better consulting contracts followed. Becoming a VP was scary for the son of a construction worker. My inner voice told me I was way out of my league and heading for a downfall. Staring at the wall didn't help anymore. I began to wake up every week night about 3 a.m., thinking about the previous day's events and what I anticipated for the next day. I was anxious most of the time, and there was a gnawing feeling in the pit of my stomach. I began to drink more, especially when I travelled, which became more frequent as my reputation as a consultant grew. To an outside observer my life was envious; to my inner voice I was a fraud.

The consulting firm did most of its work with the federal government and the Department of Defense. My work was with profit-making high-tech firms, such as Digital, Lotus, Microsoft, Hewlett-Packard, and IBM. The company had a chance to be part of a team bidding on an Air Force proposal for a very large contract. It would provide work for at least five people for as long as five years. My boss asked me to lead the proposal effort. I agreed but said that I would not lead the project if we won the contract because I was pursuing commercial work with high-tech industry leaders. I was fully billable, meaning I had plenty of contract work to do and the work benefited the company. There was no reason why I had to work for the Air Force.

We won the contract, and my boss asked me to lead the project. It was unfair but he had no one else at the time and life isn't fair. So I took on a project with an impossible schedule, no staff, and no experience with such a large DoD effort. It was hell for me for several months. My self-esteem hit a new low. I felt isolated, ignored, and, for the first time in a while, incompetent.

Late one afternoon, I was asked to make a presentation to an Air Force general and his staff about the project. During it, I was put on the spot about my company's work, which I defended as best I could but probably not very well. I don't remember anything I said but I know I was intensely angry. After I drove home that evening I was preparing dinner when I burst out crying. I couldn't stop. The tears and sobs kept coming. I had never cried this hard as an adult. It went on and on. I was angry at having to work on a project for which I was a bad fit while missing out on exciting projects I could be getting. I sensed that I had been depressed for a long time, and that I was not a good husband or father. I was a wimp and, if I couldn't change, I would lose Martie. I could think of nothing positive. After about 20 minutes, Martie came home. I continued sobbing. I couldn't explain why. I didn't want to admit that I might drive Martie away or that I was a bad father. But I couldn't stop crying. It was upsetting to us both.

We decided that I needed to get help. I called my primary care doctor and burst out crying on the phone with him. He prescribed Xanax and referred me to a psychiatrist. I did stop crying and the next day saw the psychiatrist. I soon found out he was incompetent but I did get on an antidepressant. Six months later, feeling better I stopped taking the pills, which lead to a relapse worse than the original depression. I was plagued with thoughts of suicide and finally agreed to be hospitalized. The day I was admitted was Valentine's Day.

It was embarrassing to be in a psych ward but it was the best thing I ever did. Eventually, I found a good psychiatrist, a psychotherapist, and a group therapist. Instead of backing away, Martie rallied to my support. She called the president of the company and told him to call me. "What should I say?" he asked. "Tell him you love him," was her reply. She called several of my friends and asked them to visit me in the hospital. Most didn't know what to say but that wasn't important. Being there was.

The hospitalization was a turning point in my life. Martie and I started talking more openly about our feelings, and she was reassuring about my fathering. I could not have crawled out of that hole of depression alone. It's the relationships that matter. Ours took a turn for the better. Martie's resilience was amazing.

After 10 years of one-on-one psychotherapy with a great therapist and 13 years of group therapy, I believe I made it back to a place that most people consider normal. I still take antidepressants. Under the supervision of my psychiatrist I have tried eliminating the pills. Every time I do, I relapse into depression after four months. It's like clockwork. I've given up trying to make sense of what my body does to my mind. As long as I take the pills, I'm not depressed. I've accepted the bargain. And I will always hate Valentine's Day.

Emotionally, I lost my father a long time ago, not long after my mother died. I thought I had dealt with the anger, but it's erupting again. What was he doing dying now, in the middle of all the difficulties I am going through? I can chalk it up to one of those mysteries of life. Like those family secrets buried in Ireland, there will be no answer. Or, maybe it's because I was not there to say a final good-bye to him when he was dying. And now I won't be able to do that at any of the services.

Ireland. It's where it all started—my blood, my DNA, my ancestry. Three of my four grandparents were born in Ireland. I only knew one of them, Emma, my paternal grandmother. The info I have about my grandmother is sparse and lean. I learned about it over the years—a piece here and a scrap there. There was little information coming from the family because she didn't share any with her children. The following notes are from what little I heard over the years.

When Emma's mother had remarried and begun her new family, Emma, as a teenager, felt out of place. At the same time her peers were leaving for America. Her brother, John, had sailed to America a few years before and could arrange passage for her if she desired. In 1906, at the age of 18 and with her mother's blessing, she crossed the Atlantic—alone. The voyage was difficult for her. She was overcome with seasickness the entire time. She eventually landed in Boston to settle in a new land and start a new life. How courageous is that!

To know my grandmother was to behold mirth. She had a Mona-Lisa smile, a twinkle in her eyes, and always a story to tell. Once we grandchildren got older we realized her stories were just that—stories. Like the one where she had a job in the circus riding bareback on a horse. Then there was the story of her beginnings. She said she grew up in the Mountrath section of Dublin, but whenever we cousins went to Ireland, we discovered that Mountrath was 60 miles southwest of Dublin. With the sparse info she had provided in her tales, none of us could find her listed in the ancient texts in the Irish National Archives. The year I visited Ireland, I spent an entire day pouring through those texts. The first thing I noticed was that her name, Emma, was hard to find—there were so few listed. I even went so far as to look in volumes five years before and five years after my grandmother said she was born—November 1, 1888. By the day's end I cried tears of frustration.

I believe my grandmother did not want to be found or her past to be known. She left Ireland for reasons none of us will ever know. When she left, she never looked back. There are many secrets buried there. In discussions with my uncles and aunts—her sons and daughters—they said she never talked to them about Ireland. Not a word. One time, when her children became adults, they approached Emma about a trip to Ireland. She wasn't interested. When her own mother died my grandmother was pregnant with her fifth child and clearly not able to return for the funeral. Like me, she missed the funeral of a parent.

I am the oldest of four children. My sister, Regina, is next at three years younger than me, then my brother, Billy, at six years younger, followed by, Marian, who is 10 years younger. With Ireland as our roots, Catholicism permeated our family. The families of our grandmother were all close. We grew up in the '50s, a time when fathers worked and most were unavailable. My father William, called Billy by his siblings and Bill by my mother, had his own business and worked 24/7 (before the phrase was coined). As kids we rarely saw him. Hence he was unavailable. My father was a good man, a gentle man, a man who worked hard to provide for his family. A man who loved us. To me his quietness was made him somewhat of an enigma. My mother, Martha, married him in 1942—she was a war bride. I didn't know much about her home life but guessed it was chaotic. She wanted something different—something better for her family. She was very loving—a kind woman, a strong woman, a wise woman. Her family was the most important thing to her, and she wanted the best for us. She created a loving family environment and a household where we would all eat supper together. Often that meant waiting for our father to come home. And typically it was after seven o'clock in the evening. But I got my homework finished! Both our mother and father would tuck me in at night with hugs and kisses, and my father would say, "good-night, sleep tight, holler when the bugs bite!" That would make me giggle.

When my mother died in 1974, I was devastated. For the four of us kids, it was our first acquaintance with grief, and it was horrible. She died before her time at the age of 53. I didn't know what to do, how to deal with that catastrophe. I felt abandoned. I've grappled with her early death for many, many years and still do.

While I was dealing with my grief, I tried to become acquainted with my father—form a relationship with him. It was like he didn't know how. My siblings and I liked him. We had family dinners with him and he laughed a lot. He got to know his grandchildren, who were quite small. He had five at the time, the youngest born three weeks after my mother's death. He took us to lunch. We knew he was lonely and wondered if he would come to live with one of us. Then he began dating. He complained about loneliness. I wanted him to be happy. All I wanted was for him to notice me. I wanted to be with him, to share our lives. Isn't that the way it's supposed to be with families? He's my father, after all. That's what our big Irish family taught me. And that's what my mother had believed.

When he remarried, we were thrilled for him. We met the woman he was to marry and liked her. We looked forward to including her in our circle. We were going to acquire a step-brother—Richard had married Patti, and Regina grew up playing with Patti. Richard and Patti have three children. This was going to be so great! Our family was growing.

Dark clouds began to emerge that first Christmas, 13 weeks after the wedding. My father told me I had to call before I visited. It was a strange request because I had always called. Now when I or my sisters called, we were told not to come for various reasons. That not-to-come response became a regular theme, a broken record. My father continued to make many, many choices over the 26 years of his marriage that hurt me—hurt all of us. In essence, he excluded me from his life. He chose his new wife and her family over me. I knew he was listening to his wife, but that didn't lessen the pain. He moved out to western Massachusetts, over 100 miles away. Unavailable, again. Throughout the years of his marriage I never ceased trying to be part of his life. Why? Because he was my father, I was his oldest daughter. He abandoned me to be with *his wife* and *her family*. I now had been abandoned by both my parents, although only one of them by choice.

One time my siblings and I "kidnapped" him. It happened a few years after he moved to western Massachusetts. We four wanted to take him for a birthday lunch, we wanted to talk to him alone. His wife was recovering from a major operation and unable to go out. Arrangements were made with our stepbrother, Richard, who lived three doors down from his mother, and was very eager to help us in this ruse. He agreed to take over for my father and spend the time with his mother, thereby leaving my father free to have lunch with us. We figured it this way: if we could talk to him alone, he could explain what was going on and let us into his life. Well, explain he did. He yelled at us for not inviting his wife (who was bedridden) and he cried during the meal. It was awful. Afterwards, the four of us were in Billy's car, talking, crying, and feeling like we were all five years old. I don't know why, but we kept trying to see him, to get him in our lives. We lost most of the time.

One event clearly defines the relationship my father had with me. It happened years ago during a family wake. The funeral home was filled with uncles, aunts, and many cousins. I walked in with Joe and looked around the room to orient myself and see who was there. I spied my father on the other side of the room. At the same time it seemed like he spotted me. I saw his face light up, his eyes seemed to brighten. He leaped out of his chair, left his wife, and hurried over to me. Due to our strained relationship, and because I was in a state of shock at this new behavior, I did not move across the room to meet him halfway. I waited, in anticipation, for his greeting. He came closer and closer. I began to look forward to his hug and hello. I even had my hand halfway up in the form of a greeting. As he came within a half a foot of where I was standing, he hooked a right. With a hearty laugh and a wide smile he said, "Hello, Father, I'm awfully glad to see you," using both his hands to embrace the priest sitting not far from where I stood. I was stunned. I felt sucker-punched. He had done it again. As I turned around to get my balance, I noticed my sister, Marian, standing behind me with tears streaming down her face. She felt the same punch. I hugged her. No need for words.

My father has outlived two wives. Two years ago, in 2005, his second wife died. After she died, I discovered she had a gambling problem—she spent money every week of their marriage playing the lottery. It explained some things, especially their moving seven times in 26 years. But it did not explain everything. Her demise placed our father into our lives again. We had lots of questions, but he wasn't answering. My siblings were quite eager to be with him. I was not. I was reluctant, quite cold to the idea of seeing him. It took me time to sort out my feelings, my anger, before I could call him and arrange a visit.

As I prepared to visit, many emotions swirled and romped around my mind. I played and replayed several conversations. Most of them began with, "Dad, why did you...?" "Dad, how could...?" "After all these years..." "Twenty-six years is a long time to keep yourself from me!"

Two conversations kept reverberating in my mind. The first was when I screamed at him a few years ago yelling, "What about us..., your family?" Joe and our boys were struck with fear. They had never heard me yell with such rage, and at my father. Second, as the children in the next generation began getting married, there were conflicts and anger and hurt over his unwillingness to attend those weddings. He's their grandfather! Again I shared my angry words with him. Those tapes were playing in my head as I pulled into his driveway.

Of all the homes he had lived in for the past 26 years, I had yet to be in this one. It was a tiny two-bedroom home, in an over-55 complex. His front door was open (his front door is never open) and I could see an old man, bent over and hovering inside. He was waiting for me, as if he was looking forward to seeing me. I got out of the car to meet him at the door. He gave me a hug and cried and said, "I love you, I am so glad you came." Well there are no words to describe my feelings. All my rehearsed phrases flew away, like a bunch of angry crows. Here was love, like I never expected, that I had been yearning for.

The last time I saw my father was the week before Christmas. I traveled to Athol with Billy to celebrate Christmas with him and give him his presents. He was happy to see us, seemed healthy, no oxygen needed that day. My next planned trip had been for January 22. But that day abruptly became the day of my brain surgery.

Sometimes I wonder about it all. I guess he loved me in his own way. I'll never know for sure.

———

When Martie's sister, Regina, called on Valentine's Day with the news that their father had died, I felt the familiar anger I've had toward him for years. "Just like Bill Hayes," I thought, "to make it impossible for his children to get together for his funeral." That was the feeling. And I knew that the death would upset Martie at a time when she was very vulnerable.

For me, Bill represented some of the worst characteristics of the Irish Catholic father, especially his meekness in dealing with the women in his life. Like many males of his generation, his first wife, Martha, ran the house when the children were growing up. He was the provider, which is the role assigned to men. He worked six days a week, which is to his credit. But at home he was emotionally distant. More distant than my own father had ever been.

When Martha died at 53, the whole family was devastated. The children were all married, and they rallied around their father and gathered together several times a year. They hoped that Bill would find a new female friend. On several occasions, he introduced us to his latest candidate. When his new wife-to-be entered the picture, she was just the latest in a line of candidates. They continued to date and his children and I were happy for them. If Bill was happy, that was enough.

Bill decided to get married. That's when the friction began. His wife was a bit difficult to deal with: controlling, opinionated, and showing no affection for Bill's children. Still, Bill seemed happy, and that was most important. She would be Bill's problem, not his children's. Wrong!

The Christmas after the wedding, she began to insert herself into Bill's family's lives. She announced that she would not allow the children or grandchildren to visit for Christmas. Her reason? She had heart problems and couldn't handle the stress. She also began to monitor Bill's phone conversations. When Martie called to talk with him, she would stand beside him and comment. In short, she became a bitch.

They owned two houses when they married. They sold both and moved into a small house in Newton, close to his first wife's original house. We figured they made a good financial deal. But they soon moved west to Athol, Massachusetts, and then made other moves. The rationale was to be closer to her son, Richard, who lived nearby. But this meant long rides for his children to visit. Bill seemed not to care. He liked the house. When Martie and I visited, the agenda was always the same: a short discussion followed by a snack or lunch. His wife dominated the conversation, usually with her rants about her doctors or about critics of the Catholic Church. The Pope was her favorite. She never left Bill's side, making it impossible for Martie to talk with him alone. You could not talk to her, you listened.

They stopped coming to family gatherings, even grandchildren's weddings. When our son Tim married, he refused to send them an invitation because over the years Tim had watched Martie's agony at the emotional distance of her father. Bill and his wife continued to move to new houses. After she died, we learned that she spent $200 or so a week on lottery tickets. Their car floor was littered with used lottery tickets. That's why they had to move so much, to capture the real estate gain to pay off their debts.

My view of all this was that Bill was an adult and was responsible for his own relationship with his children. He was their father and they loved him in spite of his limitations. I can't tell you how many times Martie and I talked about this. How could she get closer to him? Should she tell him that she felt abandoned? Weeks would go by between calls, always initiated by Martie. After the calls, more tears. I admire what she did with the little she got from her father. She would say, "I know that's all I can get from him." She would not abandon him as I would have. I never tried to get in between their relationship. I always supported what Martie did. But I also made my position clear that he would get no break or affection from me.

I think that part of my anger with Bill was my own fear that I might become as weak as he was; that I would be wimpy when it comes to my relationship with my sons; that I would let Martie run my life. He represented the worst that I might become. My anger was very personal.

With this brief history, you can understand how I felt at the news of his death and my fear about its impact on Martie. I called her early that morning and told her the news. She was upset. I knew going to the funeral would put her in a bind. So I talked with Barbara, Billy's wife, beforehand, and we agreed that there was no way Billy and Martie would be going to that funeral.

When I visited that day, I was relieved to hear that Martie and Billy had already talked and agreed that they would not go. Martie seemed more upset with Billy's quandary about not being able to manage the funeral arrangements. I could understand his feelings. He had been a great funeral director in his earlier years, and I think he had imagined that he could somehow get closer to his father in death and, by running the funeral the way he planned, to somehow make a kind of settlement with his dad. Now that would be impossible. Just one of the many sad events in the life of that family.

I was grateful that Marian and Regina were handling the arrangements. I hoped that somehow the fact that the four siblings had to be separated during this difficult time might bring them closer together.

———

What! Are you kidding me? What do you mean, go home. I'm not ready yet. Look at me, I'm just barely gliding around with my walker! How can I go home? There's so much more for me to accomplish. Isn't there?"

That is my alarmed response to my team when they approach me with the news. "I thought I would to be here for two to three weeks!" I counter. "Or, at least one more week. I don't feel ready!"

Calmly and with soothing words they declare I am making such exceptional progress—with all my therapies—they have confidence I can transfer my new skills to home. I'm still not convinced. I wonder if they are pushing me out because of insurance. They answer with an emphatic no. I have more days of insurance coverage left. The case manager, Nora, reiterates that the team believes

I have "excelled" and am making "great progress." Wow! What an activity to be good at.

"She excels in gliding her walker around the halls of rehab." And, "She makes great progress in pushing herself in the wheelchair." But, "she still cannot get to and from the bathroom by herself." (My words, not the team's.) When will that one happen? Huh? Can I really go home before that transfer? The team assures me it's only a matter of time before I will do that. In fact, it could happen now. It's just for caution's sake that I am not allowed to do so. All I have to do is look at the signs posted in my room and in the bathroom, stating I am not to be "left alone."

There's one exercise I have not tried—the stairs. I remember those stairs. They looked very forbidding when I noticed them that first day. I'm going to get my chance. I am nervous though. Terrified is more like it. I must keep in mind that overcoming my terror and going up those stairs is my ticket to home. But, do I really want to go home? I have my doubts. I am comfortable here and am being taken care of quite well. Here comes the anxiety…what if something happens, like something bad—what will I do? What will Joe do? Can we both feel safe if I go home now, or in a few days? What if I fall, what if I have another seizure? Can I, can we, handle this? I am not ready.

What I need to do is a check on my goals. I refer to my GPS—the white-board—and scan it to check on my progress. As for dressing and clothes management, I take care of all that by myself—even the bra debacle is improving. I don't need any assistance. *Check.* Toileting and hygiene are the same, no assistance. *Check.* I still require help getting out of bed. But I have improved greatly with bed mobility, such that I can use my body to help me move in and out of bed. Once I am out of bed and standing, I can pivot my foot and leg and use my walker to get me to and from the bathroom. *Check. Check.* Two other goals accomplished. Bathing and grooming I had down pat last week. I take my shower and wash and dry my hair by myself. My rehab assistant doesn't get wet anymore. In fact she's hardly there, she has such confidence in me. She is just outside the door in the event I might need her. At nighttime, once I am helped out of bed, I can roll my wheelchair myself to the sink and wash up and prepare for bed myself. *Check. Check.*

Looking back to what I've accomplished, I have to admit that my OT and PT goals and accomplishments look impressive. I am walking along the corridors with my *Broadway* walker for a long, suitable distance that pleases Ann Marie. I am always accompanied—usually it is Joe or a PT assistant if Ann Marie has the day off. I continue to walk to the other wing of the hospital to visit with Billy. His progress continues, too. Someone always has the wheelchair behind me for rests, but I don't need to rest as often. I am able to self-propel my wheelchair to the Great Room by myself for OT play sessions in the afternoon with other patients. I've lost my resistant attitude for the Valentine play therapist and enjoy play time. *Check. Check.*

For PT today, Ann Marie and I travel down to the Great Room, me propelling myself in the wheelchair and Ann Marie walking beside me. We will meet my next challenge—stairs. I wheel myself over to the wall where the makeshift stairs are—three steps and a landing. I place the brakes on the wheelchair, stand up, and grab on to the walker that Ann Marie unfolds for me. I position myself so I can grab on to both stair railings.

"Remember," says Ann Marie, "the right, good foot goes up to heaven, and the bad foot goes down to hell."

"O-o-o K-a-a-y." I'm as nervous as a bevy of bees buzzing around hydrangeas. Ann Marie senses this and suggests in her soothing voice that I take a moment to stop, just relax and breathe. Tears well up. I know I am trying too hard (as usual). I stop. We breathe together. I begin again. I put my hands on the railing and place my right foot up on the first step. My weight goes down on that foot, and I bring myself up to the first step, which brings the left side of my body and my left foot up to join my right foot. I notice my left foot weaves a bit to the left and strikes the riser before it hits the step. I am now standing with both legs together side by side on the first step. Wow, I managed the first step! I repeat that all the way up: step two, step three, and onto the top landing. I am going up these stairs leading with my right foot, only just like the little toddler I spoke of back when I was learning to get out of bed. When a toddler begins to climb stairs she uses one leg leading to go up and one leading to go down, just like I am learning to do.

When I get to the landing, Ann Marie instructs me to turn around. I have railings on each side of me. Carefully I pivot. I begin my descent holding tightly to the railings. With my left leg and foot quivering, I place it down on the step. My whole body, as well as my left leg, is shaking. With all the rehab I have had on this leg, it feels surprisingly weak. Ann Marie is cautioning me to "take...your... time." I am scared I will fall. I gather my senses around me and proceed. With my left foot placed down on the top step, my right foot joins it easily. Then I proceed shakily to the second step. I place my left foot down again. I shake.

"One more step to go," encourages Ann Marie. I manage this last step, and both feet are now on the floor. Such a victory! My left leg is shaking and vibrating from the workout.

I'm worn out; my body is thoroughly tired. I look forward to returning to my room for a rest. Instinctively, Ann Marie knows this and opts to push my wheelchair back and helps me into bed. She speaks encouraging words to me. Again her confidence inspires me. With my eyes half-closed, she rubs my left foot and leg and says she looks forward to tomorrow, when she knows I will make even more progress.

———

I watch Martie go up the stairs in the therapy room. First she places the strong right leg on the first stair and lifts her weight with a grunt, like she is fighting gravity. She lifts her left leg, and it swings until the toe of her shoe hits the stair riser and bounces back before she can place her foot on the stair. She can't place her left foot directly on the stair. It looks like she has no control over the movement of her foot. She can raise her leg but not place her foot down. How will she ever get up the 12 stairs to our second floor? Is she really ready to come home?

I did some Internet research about rehabilitation after brain injury. My layman's understanding is that when an area of the brain that controls motor movement is injured, other circuits may become stronger to compensate. For any movement of the body, there are some nerve pathways from the brain to the spinal cord that are more important, the primary pathway, and some that are less important, the secondary pathways. After brain injury to a primary pathway, some secondary pathways may get stronger to compensate. Some movements that are impossible right after injury come back as these secondary pathways strengthen. That process is one of the reasons that rehab after injury is so important.

But there is an important limitation to this process: it lasts for only a few weeks after the injury. If it continued without a limit, the brain

would get confused about which pathways control which movements. So the rehab of motor movement is most important during those critical few weeks. If you don't use it right away, you lose it. If we had known about that process, Martie might have worked even harder to rehab her left side during those early weeks.

There is another aspect to movement that we gradually became aware of. It's called proprioception. When you pick up a pen from a table, you don't have to look at your arm. You look at the pen; if you do it often enough from the same position, you may even not have to look at the pen. The reason is that there is feedback from the movement of your muscles back to your brain. Your brain knows where your arm is and where it is moving. That same feedback allows you to walk without looking at your feet, and walk in a familiar place in the dark without seeing your feet.

As Martie was walking up the stairs at rehab, her brain didn't know where her left foot was, so it had to wait until her foot hit the stair riser before she could put it down on the step. She also had to look at her left foot as she walked to know where it was. She could not walk steadily without looking down. She had lost her proprioceptive feedback from her lower left leg and foot. Would it come back?

There's another member on my team I have yet to mention. She is a social worker and her name is Amanda. She hands me her card. I read the initials after her name—LICSW. They stand for Licensed Independent Clinical Social Worker. I am familiar with the initials because that's the same credentials after my name.

To become a social worker and earn those professional letters takes years of hard work. I began my graduate work at Simmons College School of Social Work, located in downtown Boston. I chose the full-time track and began in the fall of 1992. My foundation course work included human behavior and development, social policies, methods of practice, racism, statistics, and social research. The two-year course of study left scant room for electives, but I did manage to include alcoholism and family structure and dynamics. In tandem with my intensive course work, I completed a clinical internship each year.

My first internship was at a major hospital in Worcester, Massachusetts. Two days a week I assisted patients and their families on the medical/surgical floor. I discovered my strong suit was empathy, which helped patients and their families to trust me. My empathy was especially valuable when one of my patients died. The loss was difficult for me but devastating for the family. I became a major support for them during their time of grief.

On another case my empathy got me into trouble. A homeless woman I had discharged a few weeks earlier to a shelter in Connecticut managed to panhandle enough money to get a bus back to the hospital; she asked for me. The other social workers in the department were not happy. They discharged her back to her shelter right away because she had no medically justifiable reason to be in the hospital. My supervisor spoke to me about the incident. It was a learning episode for me. It was a lesson in boundaries—I needed to tighten mine. It was a lesson in personality disorders—this patient manipulated people: the shelter staff, the folks on the street who gave her the money, the Hospital Admissions Department, and the Social Work Department, especially me. And because I was there two days a week the other social workers were forced to deal with the consequences of the misalignment my boundaries and the backfiring of my empathy.

Three days a week a family service agency became home for my second-year internship. At this agency I discovered my passion for the one-on-one talking and listening sessions with individuals. I had a varied case load: a 9-year-old hyperactive child with attention deficit, a 13-year-old pregnant teen, a mom who struggled to work full time and understand her teenage daughters, a young adult with an alcoholic father, and an elderly woman who liked to come and talk. In addition, I co-led a teen group with another student. I have to say my favorite was the 9-year-old boy, even though he occasionally locked me out of the session room, typically when his mother forgot to give him his medication.

I received my master of social work (MSW) degree in May 1994. It was a hot, hot day but a special one. I had achieved a part of my dream: a master's degree in two years. I remember the excitement I felt as I prepared to walk across the stage. I was outfitted in a cap and gown, and the graduate hood for my school. When my name was called I held my head high, I smiled, my heart thumped. I did it. I was 50 years old and I was about to receive my master's degree. I was on the threshold of a new career. I felt pride in myself and in my work. Joe and our sons—Ken and Tim—were there extending congratulations. I could feel their pride in me.

Both sons were working and living at home at the time. They had seen me go to school, study, and take on those internships for the past two years. I often wonder what thoughts they had as they watched their middle-aged mother going off to school, taking on another career after they had left college.

I needed two more years of supervision before I could apply for the LICSW exam and become independent. I gained employment at a mental health hospital. It was my first job offer, and I considered it a plus. Working with people who are institutionalized was not available as a school internship, and this was an opportunity to gain it. In addition, supervision was available. I learned a great deal about the main debilitating mental health illnesses: schizophrenia, bipolar disorder, depression, anxiety disorders (the most prominent of which is post-traumatic stress disorder), and alcoholism and drug addiction. Equally important, I learned how to work with the systems these folks deal with: the state hospitals (most of which had closed), group homes (long waiting lists), shelters (most of which are full and have strict rules; no drugs or alcohol allowed, must be out of the shelter during the day, etc.), rehab facilities (for addictions), and length of stay restrictions (ruled by insurance companies).

While that job provided the supervisory requirement I needed, it was one of the worst experiences in my life. I place it second to my mother dying. Why? Because of the aforementioned systems. They put many walls in place that made it difficult for me, and the other social workers, to do our jobs. In addition, the hospital where I was employed gave scant support to social workers. It seemed as if wherever I turned, there was no support, no safety net, no comfort. I learned what it felt like to be a person with a mental illness and not have supports in place. It was frustrating and sad for them.

But my empathy for the patients remained. I discovered that I made an instant rapport with people diagnosed with schizophrenia or bipolar disorder. My empathy and my patience made it easy for them to talk with me. These folks taught me about life, especially about how to survive. One woman, who had an auditory hallucination all the time, taught me how to organize my patient load, even if she did boss the other patients around. In the afternoons I would gather all my patients to sign up on a whiteboard. She was always first. Then I called their names one by one to do their family and personal history. I used her idea for the two years I remained working at the hospital.

One of the most heartbreaking things I witnessed was a family whose 18-year-old son was experiencing his first psychotic break. He had been very involved in school activities and sports but became withdrawn over the summer, spending most of the time in his room with the shades drawn. When he joined the family for meals he hung his head and barely spoke. When his mother spoke to him she noticed a distant, far-away look in his eyes. She and her husband felt they were not reaching him when they spoke to him. Finally, after a visit to the family doctor, the family came to the hospital for an evaluation. The psychiatrist met with the family and the son. Many psychiatric tests were performed. I was in consultation with the heads of the departments of psychiatry, nursing, and social work. The eventual diagnosis: schizophrenia. While the testing was happening, I was comforting the parents, supporting them during this horrible time. I assisted in follow-up appointments and prepared education on schizophrenia and on the necessary medications.

I left the hospital after two years very knowledgeable in many areas: mental illness diagnoses, systems that are supposed to support people with a mental illness, and medications to help alleviate symptoms. I was ready to sit for the LICSW exam.

I passed on the first try, and immediately applied for the license from the Division of Professional Licensure Board of Social Workers. With license in hand, I claimed the initials—LICSW. Independence achieved. I worked two additional years in a private clinic for more experience before I opened my private practice in 1999, seeing clients one-on-one.

Now I find myself on the receiving end of professional sessions with Annette. I'm humbled. Annette is knowledgeable, kind, and supportive. I trust her. I sense her empathy. I like her personally as well as professionally.

"Amanda," I say one day after a meeting, "I'm the patient now, and I'm here to take in your helpful words." I continue to lean on her. She has much to teach me. When my father dies I ask to speak with her. We spend several sessions talking. She helps me sort out the tangles with regard to my father's relationship, as well as the strangeness of his untimely demise and my inability to attend his funeral. Emotions I thought were buried years ago surface, and Annette helps me with them. Now it's time for me to gather my thoughts and feelings around going home. Annette and I are working through those difficulties. And to my surprise there are many.

Just pack up. Joe will come and get me, and then we'll go home. That's what has happened in the past. That's what we rely on in life: what we've done before. Not this time. This time is different. Joe and I will be doing things differently, continuing our education in life. I have a feeling there are things I haven't even thought of yet, things that may erupt at home, not only physical things but emotional things, cognitive things. Gee, I am not sure I want to tackle those thoughts now. I put them off for later.

Bridget, my rehab assistant for the morning shift, asks if I want to visit the apartment.

"Apartment?" She answers by telling me it is a small set of rooms with two purposes, first for doctors who need to spend the night and, second, for patients like me who, when ready to go home, can venture in and get a sense of what it will feel like to be back home.

"I'd like to do that," I announce, projecting confidence in my voice.

Dee Dee and I enter the apartment. It's around 10 a.m., and there's no doctor here, so I don't feel like an intruder. The apartment feels big in contrast to my room. It consists of a living room with a couch, chair, TV, and for eating meals, a small table and chair. There is a tiny galley kitchen with stove, microwave, stackable washer and dryer, refrigerator, cabinets up and down. There is a bathroom with a shower, sink, and toilet. I stand there in the middle of the living room with my walker in front of me and I am totally overwhelmed. Who would think that being in this room, which is smaller than the large therapy room, could be so overwhelming? But it is. I look to my right and see the kitchen. I roll my walker over to the edge, afraid to move any further. I peer in. I have not seen my kitchen or any appliances in four weeks. Looking in takes my breath away. It tells me, actually screams to me, all the things I will need to do when I get home. All the things for which I feel I need more rehab. How can I go home now! How could I even plan a meal, never mind prepare one?

Dee Dee coaxes me over to the bathroom. She encourages me to step into the tub. It's impossible. I cannot raise my left leg high enough to get it over the rim of the tub! Dee Dee assures me that, with time, I will. These past two weeks I've taken a shower in a bathroom without a tub. How will I do that at home? The toilet seat is regular height. Dee Dee asks if I can lower myself on it. I can't. Panic.

"Dee Dee, I've had enough." No longer is there confidence in my voice. "I'd like to go back to my room, now."

"We can do that."

When I'm in my room where I feel comfortable and safe, Dee Dee senses my anxiety.

"You OK?"

"Yes, I'm going to rest now before my next OT."

"Call if you need me, I'll check on you later on."

As I lie down I close my eyes and do some deep breathing to reduce the panic. It helps. I continue until it's time for more work.

Later Annette and I talk about my reaction to the apartment visit, and she assures me it's normal. "Everyone has the same reaction as you." We discuss more points about going home. As we talk, my confidence returns. We review the discharge items for tomorrow's meeting with the case manager, Nora.

———

I receive word that I will be discharged to home Friday (two days away) and there are details to discuss. The next few days will be busy wrapping up my exercises and making plans. Joe has come in early to discuss them. My head is spinning, but I feel better knowing he is here and will be taking care of them, and me.

Nora, the case manager, meets with us. She talks about: what to expect, what not to expect, and what some of our needs will be at home. The Visiting Nurse Association (VNA) will check in first. We can expect to hear from them the day after I arrive home. They will call first to schedule the visit. Once the visiting nurse makes her assessment of our household situation, she will arrange the scheduling of the initial occupational therapy and physical therapy visits. There may be up to three visits a week for an undetermined time. Then there's Mr. Grab Bar, a business that provides all the new toys I will need: the raised toilet seat, shower chair, my own Broadway walker, a wheelchair, and a cane. Nora suggests we obtain the wheelchair and the cane from our local senior citizens center. Great. Now I qualify as a real senior citizen.

Nora gives Joe a business card for Mr. Grab Bar. "If you call him today, he'll install them for you right away. He's very quick and responsive. It's his business and that's all he does."

"How many steps to get into the house?" Nora asks.

"None. Oh, there is one from the garage."

Visions of yesterday's apartment visit flash in my mind. "It's going to be hard for me to get myself up that one step. Maybe we can get up with the wheelchair." I know my left side has minimal strength to lift my body up, even for that one step.

Nora turns toward Joe. "You can buy the grab bars in the hardware store and install them yourself."

"I can ask Buddy to help me. He's a neighbor who can do those kinds of things."

"So, that part is settled," she says, "Where is your master bedroom located, where will you sleep?"

"It's on the second floor," we both reply, "but we plan to sleep downstairs for a while."

Joe will be returning to his work at Bentley University once I'm home. He works there two days a week and will stay overnight at a local hotel. He has arranged with two of my friends—Anna and Beverly—to come down to the Cape for the next two weeks to stay with me overnight while he is away. When my friends are there, they will sleep in the guest room downstairs. Joe has set up a single bed in the room adjacent to the guest room, where I will sleep. I'll be next door and can call out to my friend if I need her.

All this attention is nice, but look what I have wrought. Well not me, but this brain tumor and the continuing road to recovery. I can't help feeling guilty about it, like I had something to do with the tumor and the resulting paralysis. I question what I'm feeling. Sadness, anger, and, yes, guilt that this has happened, and wonder as to where it will lead. What about our lives—Joe's and mine—together? What about my practice, my work that I love? Stop! I can't, I can't. If I give in to these feelings now, I will lose the strength, the determination, the momentum I have gained to continue on to heal, to recover. Back to bewilderment.

———

Today is the day before I go home. Joe came by this morning and took all my clothes and other things. We have a plan. Tomorrow he will come to Spaulding when I call him. There will be discharge papers, instructions, and so forth.

Probably lots of waiting around, but he wants to be here. We're both excited about my homecoming. It's been a long time. Things will be different. We haven't talked a lot about how it will be. I guess life will unfold and us with it. We will roll with it, as we have in the past. That's part of our plan, too. I am feeling very small, dependent, and vulnerable about it all, but happy we have a plan.

I am sitting in my wheelchair waiting for supper when I see Olive, the shift nurse, enter my room. I notice she is unencumbered. By that I mean there is no computer in front of her. Most of the nurses enter pushing a laptop computer on a rolling cart. It is almost as if the communication device they are pushing is a protective barrier. The computer contains info on all the patients, in particular medications, the required dosage, and time to be administered. Each computer is named after a town on the Cape—Hyannis, Bourne, Sandwich, Wellfleet, Yarmouth, even towns on the islands of Martha's Vineyard and Nantucket. It is unusual to see any nurse at this hour of the evening. Olive has fiery red hair, and today it is pinned up in the back and looks quite smart. It is Olive's typical fashion to emit a wise remark or a flip comment to make me laugh. But this evening I can tell by the expression on her face—a serious one—that she has something important to say. No jokes.

"Sweetie," she begins, "your discharge will be delayed a day. I am so sorry."

"Why?" I am astonished. I know it can't be because there is no bed like the last discharge delay, from the hospital to rehab. My home is ready for me. What could it possibly be?

"Your blood count is still low. You know we've been finger-sticking you every morning, your numbers aren't quite where we want them. We're going to give you a blood transfusion tonight. You'll receive two units after the evening meal."

Finally, they are taking some action. Maybe I won't be feeling fatigued anymore.

———

As the time for Martie to come home from rehab approaches, I get the house ready. With her coming home with a walker, sleeping upstairs is not going to work. We have a guest room downstairs with a queen-sized bed. But Martie says she is afraid of falling out. She is also worried about disturbing me if she has to get up during the night. It feels strange to have her express all those fears. She was never like that.

We decide that I'll sleep in the guest room and she'll sleep next door in her office. I ask a neighbor to help me move one of the twin beds from upstairs. I arrange a chair on one side of the bed with a mat on the floor in case she were to fall. The walker will be on the other side.

I really don't think that falling out of bed is likely, but for the past month Martie has had sides to her bed, often with pads in case she were to have a seizure. They make her feel safe and cozy.

With my neighbor, Buddy, we attach handholds by the step in the garage that leads into the kitchen. But Buddy and I are not confident about attaching the shower handholds, where to place them and how to make sure they're strong enough.

I have this fantasy about the TV show *This Old House*. I imagine Norm Abrams, the carpenter, saying to Bob Villa, the boss, "Well Bob, we started attaching the bars, but the tiles started falling off. Then we found that there were no studs in the wall and the house was unsafe. Looks like the owners will have to demolish it and build a new one."

At the rehab, they refer me to Mr. Grab Bar. What a guy! His real name is Mike MacDonald. He actually invented the bars that are easy to attach to bathroom walls and are strong enough to be safe. Watching him work is a joy. He knows exactly where the bars should go and has a device that finds the beginning and end of each stud behind the tile walls. He also likes to put on a show. He is proud of his skill, as he should be. He puts grab bars in both the downstairs and upstairs showers. They look like they have always been there. (The name of his business has been changed from Mr. Grab Bar to Get a Grip.)

With that taken care of, I go out to buy a few items: a special commode that is higher than the regular toilet seat and has a handle. A shower seat so Martie can sit while taking a shower. The walker will come home with her from rehab.

All of the equipment is paid for by our health insurance, except for the grab bars. Insurance will not pay for permanent fixtures to a house if the medical condition is temporary. The bean counters save some nickels. So I

pay Ronald for the bars and his labor. That's our only out-of-pocket expense for the past month's surgery and rehab. Thank goodness for insurance.

———

Once I get over my anger and initial disappointment about not going home tomorrow as planned, I call Joe.

"Hi," he says into the phone, sounding a bit puzzled. He just left me an hour ago. "Are you all right?"

"Yeah, I'm OK. But Olive, the nurse, just informed me I'm not going home tomorrow." I start to cry. The disappointment and the excitement and the planning all hit me at once.

"Gad. Not again, just like the hospital."

"You know those *stupid* finger sticks they've been doing for four *fucking* weeks to check my blood levels? Well they've finally decided to do something about it, and now, of all days, they're going give me a transfusion. What took them so long? Why not yesterday...or the day before...does anybody talk to each other around here?" Joe is silent on the other end of the phone as I move from sniffling tears to anger in one swift turn.

"It sucks," he says, "and it pisses me off, too. I want you home, it's been too long."

"I know, it's not like I can just get out of bed and leave here just because I'm mad."

"No, you can't, and you wouldn't get very far with that walker."

Now I am laughing and the anger is dissipating.

"What time will you get the *juice*?"

"Very funny. I'm not sure. They said 'after my evening meal' like we're aristocrats in England or something. I hope it's soon so I can get settled for the night."

"You sound better now. Will you be all right?"

"Yeah, I'm OK. Thanks."

I feel better after talking to Joe. I always do. What would I do without him. "When do you get the juice?" He has such a way with words, always making me smile. And it works. I relax. I'll await my good night calls, which are precious to me. Ah, here comes my evening meal.

I wait and wait and wait for my transfusion. Yes, my numbers are still low. I could tell because I am still eating everything, and very hastily, too. It is during the late-night shift that the units of B positive blood arrive. What a long wait! My one concern—no anxiety here—is that I will not be discharged tomorrow.

I'm awakened from a sound sleep. Well, as sound as one can get here in rehab. The night shift nurse introduces herself, along with a blood transfusion supervisor. Uh, oh, this is looking like a big deal—two nurses. They inform me they will ask my name and birthday several times during the transfusion of two units. The transfusion itself will take approximately two hours, and during that time the night shift nurse will take my blood pressure every 20 minutes. I can forget about getting a good night's sleep tonight.

In the beginning, the whole process fascinates me, and I decide to watch. It takes about 20 minutes for the two nurses to hook up their contraption to me, all the while asking me my name and date of birth. I watch as the blood begins to flow down the tube and into my veins. The red liquid, *the "juice,"* moves slowly, slowly up inside the transparent tube. As the blood begins to flow into me, instantly I notice a change in my body (I'm not kidding!). First, it feels cool, but soon after that I feel a great surge of energy. It reminds me of the Incredible Hulk, the comic book character. I feel as if I could jump out of the bed. Where is all this energy coming from? That is what I have been missing? How did I manage to do all the rehab work these past two weeks without it? No wonder I was tired all the time! That's why I've been inhaling my food. Now I'm beginning to feel much warmer. I never knew that blood in my veins could supply me with so much—warmth, nourishment, and energy. I sure wish I had this transfusion before I left Cape Cod Hospital!

They ask my name and birth date over and over and over throughout the wee hours of the morning. I can't really complain. I don't want to be the recipient of the wrong blood type or be alone if I have a bad reaction to the blood.

We do have fun with my blood type though. I keep saying, "just be positive," "B positive," "is there a little bee that is positive in here?" "I am being positive and I am being given B positive blood!" I had to have some fun every time I was awakened to have my blood pressure calibrated. Eventually I opt to have the blood pressure cuff remain wrapped on my arm for the remaining time. That cuts down on the number of wake-ups.

Why didn't I get this transfusion earlier? Who made the decision to wait this long? I know from what my body has been feeling—and it has been feeling tired and fatigued these past two weeks—that it could have benefited from the blood transfusion way back when. Geez Louise. And yes, fuck, too. What's wrong with these people? My next retort is: "It isn't brain surgery!" My blood count was low—for four weeks, for crying out loud. I just spent two exhausting weeks working to get my neurons in synch with my motor apparatus. I could have done a better job if my blood level was on par with the rest of my body. Where was the blood transfusion then, huh? Maybe I'd be in better physical shape to go home tomorrow if I had the transfusion sooner. What's going on here! I am in tears. But I don't want to travel down that road any more. Enough! Besides, I'm not a physician or a medical expert in hematology.

To think I arrived with a UTI and I am leaving with two pints of B positive blood. In between those events I regained a great deal of my life. The staff, my team, the rehab assistants, the nurses, the OTs, and the PTs—all of them—are phenomenal. I was treated with kindness, respect, and love every minute of my stay here. With their collective help I reached *all* my goals. I learned to dress myself, care for myself, learned to walk (albeit assisted, with a walker), and recovered the use my left arm and fingers, too. That sentence covers many acres of work.

It's close to 2 a.m. My body and I have been through a great deal tonight. I need to sleep. My music is on, and I fall asleep listening to my favorite soothing voice—Andrea Bocelli. With the blood transfusion I feel stronger. Tomorrow I'll be discharged—TO HOME.

Joe and I have plans. We will pick up the pieces of our lives that were smashed by the brain tumor, fit them together, and/or find new ones, as we begin our restoration. Finding out who we are *now* to ourselves and each other.

———

I'm riding home. Finally! I feel small in the car—invisible almost, and vulnerable. I have to lift my body up to see out the window. I never had to do that before, why now? I remember the last time I was driving on this highway. Now I am told I cannot drive for six months because of the seizures. Really, I don't ever want to drive again. Was it just 30 days ago—on January 16—when my body didn't feel quite right and I left my office in Natick early to come home? Today is February 17. So much has happened in the preceding month that it seems like years.

Joe and I drive along Route 6—the Mid-Cape Highway—toward our home, and I think of all the places we have lived. As we drive and I think of returning home, the beat of a song is penetrating my consciousness. My mind is full of songs, and these songs pop up and connect to phrases I hear or thoughts or occasions. I am going home and a beat reverberates. It goes "ba ba ba ba babba ba." Ah, now I've got it. It's a song sung by The Temptations, and it goes like this: "Poppa was a rolling stone. Wherever he laid his hat was his home." We have had several places in our 43-year marriage that we called "home."

We began in the city right after we married in 1964, in Allston, a section of Boston. It was the closest we could get to downtown Boston and still afford the rent. Joe and I grew up in the suburbs of Boston—about 12 miles outside. We wanted to make our mark. Like most young folks getting married at the time, we needed our independence and moved away from our parents. A small one-bedroom apartment was home for 15 months. We enjoyed setting up housekeeping for the first time as a couple. One year after we were married, Joe earned his undergraduate degree from Boston College—the first in his family to go to college. Two days after his graduation, Kenneth, our first child was born.

Three months later, we packed up and "shuffled off to Buffalo." Joe and I looked forward to that new adventure. We were excited about moving away, and beginning again and meeting new people from different parts of the country. Because we didn't know a lot about the city of Buffalo, our first apartment was located south of the city and the university. It was in a snow belt. When Joe began his teaching assistantship we knew we needed more income. With my medical secretarial experience, I landed a job typing doctor's radiology notes at the local hospital in the evenings. Working at night gave us an extra paycheck. Joe came home around suppertime after a full day of classes, teaching, and studying and would care for Kenneth. That's when I went to work at the hospital. As time went on, we both noticed there was a benefit to living closer to the university. Joe could walk to class, and I could have access to the car.

A few months later we placed an ad in the *Buffalo Evening News* under Flats Wanted—the term for apartments in Buffalo. Joe drew up the specifications for our needs: three bedrooms (we had come a long way from the tiny one-bedroom in Alston), and within walking distance of the university. A response came immediately from a couple in their late forties with two children—a daughter who eventually became our babysitter and an older son. We met and interviewed each other. It was a good fit. We moved in and stayed for the remaining three and one-half years until Joe finished his degree.

Our second son, Timmy, was born during the time we lived there, in 1968. We felt our family was now complete. Joe had one more year to finish his dissertation. While finishing, he began looking for a job to take us out of Buffalo. Would we go back home? Would the job market take us elsewhere?

"Ladies and gentlemen, please be sure your seat belt is fastened. We will be landing in a few minutes. Be sure all tray tables are placed back in position and your seats are in the upright position. The time here is exactly 2:45 p.m. Welcome to Detroit, Michigan." This was our new home for the next five years. I was a bit disappointed we didn't move eastward, but we went where the job was. Joe landed a teaching position at Oakland University in Rochester, Michigan—a small liberal arts college, part of the Michigan state university system. He taught psychology courses and conducted research. Again we felt excited about new beginnings. Joe had been a student for a long time—eight years—and this was a real job we said, jokingly. Through a university contact we were fortunate to rent a small three-bedroom ranch house with a large fenced-in back yard. Kenneth was now four and one-half and Timmy 17 months. Another new beginning. Another adventure.

After two years we needed to move. The folks we rented from returned from their sabbatical. Our next home was a rental also, through a bank. We lived in the bank-owned house, in Rochester, for three years. I was unhappy with this house. It was hard to hang my hat there. The house was located on a busy divided highway, and there were many other things, so I'll just add "etc., etc., etc." Joe conducted much research and published enough—he would not perish. He did receive tenure at the university, but something was missing for him. He needed to explore more options in his career. And we both wanted our boys to know their cousins, their family. We were ready to move East, closer to home.

Joe's mother began sending the Help Wanted section from *The Boston Globe* every week. It was fun looking for it in the mail. Joe also put out feelers, and after several months, something in the *Globe* caught his eye. Interviews were arranged in Cambridge. Joe got the job. We were going home! This was great news. At the same time we learned my mother's cancer had progressed. This was grave news. But she was happy we were all coming back home. It was 1974.

We lived with my parents for several weeks while we looked for a house, waited until we could close, and then moved into our first home—in Natick. We paid $37,500 for it. I was thrilled to hang my hat in this three-bedroom Cape, as were Joe and the boys. By this time Kenneth was nine years old and Timmy age six. We lived at that Natick address five years, but as the boys grew older we needed to expand. A beautiful, gracious-looking four-bedroom colonial was the next place we called home. As much as I loved our first house (we all did), I fell in love with the new one instantly—even before I walked inside. Twenty-five years we lived there. Highs and lows, sorrows, laughter, heartbreak, tears, but then joy and so much love happened in that house, that home.

As the boys grew older, traveled off to college and beyond to make their own homes, Joe and I followed through on a dream—living on Cape Cod. We had vacationed on the Cape for 20 years. A few medical scares for each of us (plus losing friends at young ages) convinced us to do it *now*—in 2004—rather than later at retirement age. We did. The Cape has been our home for two years. And we've not looked back. We're the two of us again—just as we began.

Like the first home we owned in Natick, the style of this house is a Cape. Not sure which type of Cape, but it has a low slung roof, a large picture window fitted with mullions in the living room, a brick front, a kitchen entryway, and an attached one-car garage. Without dormer windows, the house looks cozy and appears to be absent a second story. However, the second story becomes evident around the back, which has cedar shingles. In all there are four bedrooms.

———

We roll into the driveway and I see the familiar "Shorebirds" sign above our garage. My heart swells in my chest with joy. It feels good. I feel the beginning of a lump in my throat, and tears moisten my eyes. I remember how we contrived that name. Many homes on the Cape have signs on them—"Cape Escape," "A Slice of Life," "Dun Wandering," and so on. We wanted one, too, but what would it say? One cold April morning, Joe and I were walking on the beach, as we do frequently. We found ourselves walking nearer the shoreline because the sand is firmer, easier for walking. The tide was coming in and we were jumping back and forth, like dancers (but not as graceful), trying not to get our feet wet.

"You know," I said, "We are like those little shorebirds that skitter along the edges of the incoming tide and never get their feet wet." I laughed and continued, "Only they do a better job than us! Hey, how's that for a sign, 'Shorebirds'?"

"Do you think you'll need the wheelchair?" Joe breaks into my reverie.

"No," I state emphatically. I know he borrowed a wheelchair from the senior center. It is in the trunk of the car. I don't believe I need it. I know for sure it's not coming into the house.

Out of the corner of my eye I catch sight of the new grab bars on the sides of the door frames going into the house, and tears start again. The sight of these makes me feel ashamed, reminds me of my disability. Why should I feel ashamed? Not sure, but I do. I am guessing these are old feelings from my past. Part of my upbringing, where I am supposed to do everything for myself, not ask for, or get, help. Well, here I am with a wheelchair in my trunk and, any minute now, I'll have a walker in front of me, and I will need those grab bars to help me get into my house. Talk about help!

There are lots of feelings pushing through this morning, and I don't know how I'll stop them, or deal with them. I am going to take a deep breath and remind myself how fortunate I am. Some new concepts for me will be accepting that I need help, and that I need to ask for help and appreciate the help that is given me. Appreciating will be the easy part.

This is another beginning, the beginning of everything new in our lives—again. Another adventure but very unlike the new beginnings and adventures we've experienced together in the other houses. This is an inner adventure. It reminds me of a blank page and a puzzle at the same time. There's a heap of pieces in the corner. Some may fit and others may not. There are large chunks, moderate pieces, and tiny fragments. Some are old pieces from our past and a great number are newer pieces that will prove to be challenging to put, place, push, squeeze into place—for both of us—to create...what?

Joe gets the walker from the back seat and brings it around to my side of the car. He opens the door and assists me as I struggle with my body to get myself turned around, my feet on the ground, and my body up and out of the car. With his arm around my waist and my walker in front, we make our way to the kitchen entry door. This help from him feels new. Joe walks ahead and swings the door open. I see the grab bars on either side and think about the love and support of our neighbor, Buddy, who helped Joe install them. And that makes the tears that moistened my eyes awhile back pool again, and these tears are not going to hold. I place the walker up the one step, grab onto both bars, and with all my might, and with Joe's arm around my waist, I step up and enter my kitchen.

Now the tears are running freely. I'm in the kitchen, in my home. It's all familiar. My kitchen is arranged so that it is an open and central area with plenty of light. With the openness I can see into the dining room as well as the living room. It all looks beautiful, everything is in order. I'm happy to be home.

This is where my bewilderment was built one month ago, and this is where it starts to crumble. No longer is the bewilderment thick enough to hold back my feelings. As tears stream down my face, all the held back emotions are pouring out as my tears stream down my face: happiness, joy, grief, love, wonderment, fear. There are others I can't name. Mostly I am happy to be home...but...my father is being buried today and I am not there...and there are many pieces to pick up and put back together. So much work to do.

I look at Joe. "How will we do this?" I sob into his chest.

"One bit...one step...at a time."

PICKING UP THE PIECES

There's a lot going on. Much more than I can comprehend. To begin with, there are all these exercises, for my legs, my arms, my fingers. They're good for me, but I get weary of them, and from them. In the shower, I notice I feel steadier. The shower chair is my friend. I move easier in and out of the tub and am not as fearful about falling once I get my body settled into the chair. I don't have the words to explain it, but I have a feeling—a sense—my body wants to be standing upright when I shower and wash my hair, like I used to do.

I understand from all my years of yoga practice that my core—the middle section of my body—also benefits from these exercises. The leg strengthening from walking is building strength, not only in my legs but also in the middle/belly area of my body. Over the past several weeks the results of my hard work are converging in that one spot. My core. Soon, I will no longer need the shower chair.

The days go on, I feel the difference in my left leg and left arm; strength is returning, along with more movement and flexibility. Each week melds into the next, I notice myself naturally tending toward an upright position, not bent over when I first came home. Those are milestones, small ones but progress nonetheless. I feel it, and Joe notices it, as do my two visiting therapists.

Things are working out, going smoothly. I adhere to the rules I have been taught in rehab. I work my muscles as I follow the rules dictated by the Home Exercise Plan that has been fashioned for me. I am a person who follows rules. I don't know if I'm biologically wired to do so. Perhaps. Or maybe my upbringing taught me. Could be a bit of both.

A product of an Irish Catholic family who was scolded often to "do what you are told...or else," I often was on the receiving end of "or else." I was a happy little girl in my public school kindergarten, where the teacher looked like all the other adults I knew. By the time I made it to first grade, however, I was in a Catholic school with teachers who wore weird-looking clothing. They were very strict. I wanted to return to the public school.

Put a shy, quiet, girl like me into an environment of weird-looking creatures who doled out physical punishment on a whim, and the result is a girl who is afraid to speak. The molding began in first grade, with lessons motivated by terror. I hardly spoke in school. In that way, I thought, I wouldn't get hit, slapped, or threatened with having my tongue burned out of my mouth. Of course, then I was yelled at because I never raised my hand. And when I did speak, it was in a soft voice, and I was constantly told to Speak Up! During recess, however, I could talk up a storm with my friends. I couldn't win.

I'm winning now though. In my present circumstances, having learned to follow the rules is invaluable. It nourishes my determination to heal and walk again. Even if they are laborious or boring, the exercises help me as I retrain my brain. While I see progress, I do become tired. Not just from the exercises, but from what? Everything, it seems. I have a running list in my head from recovering from surgery to working my arm and leg muscles daily. The goal: to revive the neuronal memory so it can jump-start those muscles and remind them of what they used to do.

But I'm getting ahead of myself, as usual. I need to look back to see how far I have come, back to the first night, and day, of my return home.

———

It's a huge milestone to be home in familiar surroundings after being away for four weeks. My biggest obstacle is not the walker but me. I must remember to depend on, and to trust, the people around me. And the number one person I need to depend on, and trust completely, is Joe. Joe has been in my life a long time and I admit: I trust him, I always have. But now the tables have turned, the Monopoly card says, "Brain tumor **not** in your favor—take several steps back." I am brain-damaged and disabled. I am no longer the *independent go-to-gal*, the

113

I-can-do-anything woman. That part of me is gone, at least for now. And I feel stricken about that, feel some loss.

My internal dialogue protests and tells me: *it will come back.* I'm not convinced. Sure, I will learn to walk, in time; I'll lose the walker, then the cane. But things in my brain have changed, have changed me. Forever. How do I know that? I just do. I see it and feel it in the way I approach tasks and the way I look at things, at life. I will need to deal with these changes, whatever they are, as I progress in my recovery, as I heal. At least I am home in familiar surroundings with Joe, and with friends stopping by to help. I expect there will be some tough feelings to experience, feelings of loss, grief, frustration, helplessness. There I go again, getting ahead of myself. Why can't I let myself just *be*?

I help Joe with lunch, or maybe it works the other way round. The OTs' and PTs' words from rehab reverberate: "Be sure to get out in the kitchen and start cooking right away." And I do. At least I try. I find the walker cumbersome, and quickly learn to push it aside. I use the kitchen counter as leverage. My first success is boiling water for tea, but I need Joe's help in pouring the water into the mug. I can toast English muffins. Joe makes supper the first night, I'm grateful he can cook. My first home-cooked meal in a month.

Bedtime is different. We had not planned to sleep upstairs in our master bedroom. Joe will sleep in the guest room downstairs, and I will sleep next door on a single bed in my office. Why don't I sleep in the same bed with Joe after all my yearning for him while I was in the hospital and in rehab? Because after four weeks I became accustomed to the single bed and to sleeping alone. And then there is the boot I have to wear on my left foot, and I don't want to disturb him when I get up in the middle of the night, maneuvering the clunky walker.

When it's time for bed, Joe helps me get settled. My anxiety pops to the surface. I'm fearful of falling out of the bed. This single bed does not have rails on it, like the hospital bed. In my mind I will fall out, and am terrified. I need to feel safe and protected. Can Joe take care of me? Can I take care of me, like I'm supposed to do? These are two critical questions. I am not home 24 hours. It's too soon to know. Anxiety is pounding in my chest. I'm close to crying. I feel like a scared little kid and a frightened old woman at the same time—so vulnerable—over my fear of falling out of bed. Joe exudes calm and is resourceful. With the use of pillows, the walker, and tucking the blankets in tightly on one side, he ensures I will be safe. When I get myself into the bed and feel the tightness of the blankets and see the pieces of equipment and pillows around me—only then do I feel safe. The way Joe solves the bed problem relieves my fears. My fear was asking me, "Can he take care of me?" And Joe answered.

When I awake in the middle of the night to use the bathroom, I sense Joe waking in the next room, too. I expected him to be vigilant. He calls out to me.

"You OK? Need any help?"

"No I can do this." I truly do feel safe. I manage to make it down the hall to the bathroom with my walker, and back again. I get myself back into bed, and return to sleep.

We both survive the first night. It's a first step.

The next day I relish the idea of putting all my occupational therapy to the test. I am up early, as usual. I've always been an early riser. With my walker in front of me, I gather my clothes for the day and head toward the bathroom. I look forward to taking my first shower at home and dressing myself. How do I think I can do this without waking Joe? Will the walker make too much noise on our beautiful hardwood floors? It must be those plastic wheels. It couldn't be the tennis balls that have been split to fit over the aluminum ends on the walker. Oh, well. Joe wakes. He's up and bounds out of the guest room to greet me with a kiss. Our first morning kiss in our new life: over, above, through the walker. Eventually we'll work it out with this third party intruding!

"Need any help?"

"No thanks, I'm going to be fine. I need to try things on my own." Sounds like a piece of the independent woman in me. Before he can reply, I add, "But, I'll yell if I need you."

All goes well. Things are slow, but I expect that. No water on the floor like my first shower in rehab. I am lucky we already had a handheld shower in our downstairs bathroom. Joe has purchased a shower chair identical to the one I used in rehab, and Mr. Grab Bar has installed his grab bars. I am grateful for those because I use them often. I am successful in taking a shower and washing and rinsing my hair—yes, I soaped all areas of my hair—drying it with a towel and dressing myself. It takes an hour. My hair is naturally wavy, no need for a hair dryer today. I notice my hair is getting long, too long. It needs to be cut.

I am pleased with myself. I see the purpose of rehab and understand why the folks there felt confident in discharging me. I remember back to last week and my anxiety about leaving too soon. This morning I am overjoyed with my accomplishment. I meet up with Joe in the kitchen where he has taken out the cereal bowls and a banana. I pour my cereal, peel the banana, cut slices onto my cereal, and pour the milk. I can put the milk away. These small actions may sound trivial, but today they are milestones for me. Joe carries my breakfast to the table and we eat another meal together. Thirty-two days after that errant seizure smashed into our lives, we're ready to begin anew. We read the newspaper and wait for the VNA nurse to arrive for my assessment.

The next step: we begin the restoration.

———

As a family we've always enjoyed watching the Olympics on TV. In winter it's ski racing, ski jumping, the luge, skaters racing, ice skating, and ice dancing. In the summer games it's swimming, diving, the track races, the high jump, the pole vault, and the marathon. My favorite segments are always about how these athletes train to be their very best; those were phenomenal. I marvel at the young women and men who train for the gold.

When Tim and his new wife, Joanna, moved to Vermont, he told me he discovered the right sport for him—running. Tim had played many sports as a youth, and in his young adult life he competed in late afternoon street hockey games or evening softball leagues. Now that he works for a newspaper, it means most of his nights are taken up with the paper. "Running is perfect for my body, my lanky frame," he said. "And I run whenever I can fit it into my schedule."

He's right about his body and his frame. He takes after my father. Of the four of us in the family, Tim is the tallest at 5 foot, 9 inches. And to the dismay of the three of us, he can eat all day long, anything he wants, and not gain a pound—just like my father.

Once he began, Tim discovered the love of running and took it a step further. In 2003, he trained to run the Boston Marathon: 26 miles and 385 yards. I was impressed at his goal. He worked at it every day. He ran different strides, took long runs one day, a break another day, a short run the next. He concentrated on his breathing, his water intake. He pushed himself to run faster, in a burst for a minute or three, then slow down. He probably didn't know I was paying attention, but I was. I listened to everything he told me on our phone calls.

In order to qualify—and he wanted to qualify so he could obtain a bib number—he had to run a marathon within a specific time for his age group. At age 36, he had to run it in under 3 hours and 11 minutes. He ran his first marathon in Philadelphia, missing his mark by 2 seconds. Two seconds. What a heart-breaker! His second marathon, a few months later in Keane, New Hampshire, was a success. Tim ran the race in just under 3 hours, at 2 hours and 59 minutes. We lived a two-hour drive away at the time and drove up to cheer for him. Joe and I made a sign, "GO TIM-DAWG."

I admire the way Tim trained for the marathon. In rehab, I used Mick Jagger as an inspiration *to start me up*, now I turn to my own son as an inspiration to *keep me going*.

———

My discharge papers say an assessment nurse from the VNA will call within 24 hours. She arrives as scheduled and introduces herself as Janice. She is a pleasant, slightly-built woman in her early forties with short blonde hair and blue eyes. First she needs to obtain a sense of us and our overall living situation. I am considered housebound—unable to get out on my own—all services for which I am eligible will come to me in my home. To continue my rehab, Janice determines I will require physical therapy twice a week and occupational therapy once a week. In addition, there will be nursing check-ups each week.

My training at home begins with an assessment, and then goals. Janice says I need to have a clear understanding of what has happened to me. That is, the nature and complexity of my medical problem: the diagnosis and surgery, etc. Boy, I sure would like to know what the hell happened.

She sits comfortably on the couch with me while I wrestle with what has occurred during the past four weeks. She readies her laptop, and for the first time after rehearsing it in my head so many times, I tell my story out loud.

"I experienced a seizure in the middle of the night approximately one month ago. After a ride in an ambulance, another seizure alerted hospital personnel to perform a CAT scan, followed by an MRI. Both scans showed a tumor in my brain, the size of a plum, resting near my motor cortex, and pushing through my scalp—the bony part of my skull. The tumor, a benign one (thankfully), was confirmed to be a meningioma. It was removed surgically, and the deteriorated bony skull replaced with a piece of titanium mesh. After spending two weeks in rehab trying to jump start my left side, I know I need more rehabilitation to work on my left side, and to continue on with my life." When I am finished speaking a sense of relief comes over me.

"It sounds like you've got all the facts. I'd say you've a good understanding of your medical problems. Any further questions?"

"Not right now." I'm not so sure, I think to myself. I am still trying to wrap my arms around the whole big thing.

The second part of my plan is about safety. She walks around the first floor of our home. Joe and I both know what she's doing. Joe chimes in before she can say anything further. "I removed the scatter rugs in the living room and the runner in the hallway, and any clutter before Martie came home from rehab."

"I'm noticing. You've done a good job at that."

I say to myself, I need a clear path for my rolling Broadway walker. The nurse returns to the couch and her laptop to make more notes.

Another part of the safety plan is identifying and understanding all the medications and the frequency with which I take them. That's easy. Before my brain tumor, I took two prescription meds: one for high blood pressure and one to stall osteoporosis. Now I will add an antiseizure medication, Dilantin, which must be monitored closely to ensure an accurate amount remains in my blood. Both Joe and I review the list. We discuss the next Dilantin blood draw, which is tomorrow.

The third goal is health maintenance. That means monitoring my blood pressure levels with the goal of keeping it within normal limits. Janice will be assisted by another nurse, who goes by the name of Tellie.

It doesn't take long for me to get acquainted with Tellie, a grey boxy-shaped nurse. Every morning at 10 a.m., like clockwork, she speaks to me with a "Good morning. Please step up on the scale." I do. Next she instructs me, "Place the blood pressure cuff around your upper arm and the clip on your finger." Tellie is insistent I become self-sufficient in these tasks. I comply, and wait as the cuff pumps itself tight around my arm. Once the pressure on the cuff deflates and the oxygen level in my finger registers with a beep, I hear the dial tone on my phone. This is followed by the boops and beeping sounds of my medical data, which is carried over fiber optic lines of the telephone. My grey boxy-shaped nurse is just that—a large grey box, a computer!

118

Her full name—Tel E-Med. I like her, even though every morning she startles me with her "Good Morning!"

———

It's my first week home from rehab, and I am aware of the importance of my blood count. One of my discharge orders is for blood testing to ensure my blood count does not slip below the desired level. (I don't want to add another blood transfusion to my worry list.) Also, I need to keep an eye on the Dilantin levels in my blood. Once we discovered that the antiseizure med, Keppra, brought on an awful itchy rash, I started on Dilantin. It puzzles me why it took the nursing staff so long—from my hospital stay through my stay at Spaulding—to discover my allergic reaction to Keppra. A rash is one of the primary side effects.

My first outing is to C-Lab, one of the local blood testing laboratories on the Cape. I discover new obstacles along the way. I struggle out of the car just like I do when moving my body out of bed. By the time I stand up, Joe has brought the walker around. I push the walker ahead, but it struggles. I'm used to its easy flow on a hardwood floor. The surface in the parking lot is rough, and the wheels don't traverse well over the uneven and bumpy patches. I'm grateful to see a ramp, but it has bumps and small potholes. I have trouble maneuvering myself and the walker as we move up the ramp. Joe helps me through the doorway. I think about others who are disabled and have been for years. I think about the disabled population and their families and all they have done to help reduce barriers and restraints so that ramps like these have been built for folks like me.

Joe needs to help me off with my coat. I take a breath and prepare myself for the dance routine, the same in all medical offices: state your name...date-of-birth...what's your insurance...change partners (only kidding)...take a number...take a seat...then wait...wait...wait. We leave the blood lab with the results and the directive to "see your primary care doctor to review them."

I call my doctor's office the next day to make an appointment and get a surprise. He has undergone open-heart surgery and will be out of the office for an undetermined amount of time. I'm stunned. My primary care doctor is a young man, in his late forties.

"What should I do?" I ask the receptionist. "I need someone to interpret these blood results as soon as possible."

"The doctor has three physicians covering for him on different days." The receptionist lists which doctors cover each day of the week, and on weekends. I am madly writing names and phone numbers on yellow stickies, and growing anxious. This is overwhelming, I feel dizzy and confused. I need to sit down. Then she adds, "And these doctors have requested that they be called on their specific day only."

That's when I toss the pencil up into the air and say into the phone, as politely as I can, "OK. Thanks for your help. Bye now." Then, "Grrrr." I could drop an f-bomb now! And I do, as loudly as I can.

I never call any of those doctors. Can't do it. I don't feel good or safe about calling someone who has to be called on a certain day. That's just where my head is right now, thinking about myself and my needs. My vulnerable state is still in bloom. Brain-injured or not, I am an intelligent woman, and I can figure out the blood count. I look at the results. In the middle of the report is a column for ranges that show the normal value. I view the categories and the ranges. It looks like my blood count and the Dilantin level are normal. I run the numbers by the nurse on her next visit for verification. She concurs: "all within normal limits."

———

Physical therapy with Pam happens twice a week. Pam is a tall, slender woman in her mid-thirties. She has short dark hair, brown eyes, and enjoys the outdoors. On our first visit she performs an assessment and goals are established. My mobility and strength are limited; my gait is unsteady; my activity tolerance is fair; and I need rest after 10 minutes. Nothing new there. In my words: I'm weak, I tire easily, and my balance is rickety. As for strength, I'm going to have to dig deep for it.

Pam's goals are fashioned under the umbrella of my Home Exercise Plan or HEP. And that's what it means—exercise, exercise, and more exercise. These movements will boost my strength and balance, right my unsteady gait, and strengthen my limbs. Over time I will need to decrease my dependence on the walker. And that will mean additional leg exercises. "Oh no, not more!" But I am determined to walk on my own, that's *my* goal. In rehab the walker was not "clunky." Here at home where there are more walls and furniture, I feel it is always in my way. There are more walls and furniture.

———

Occupational therapy starts later in the week. Following the protocol of Janice and Pam, Susan, my occupational therapist, begins with an assessment and the creation of goals. Susan is in her fifties with a salt-and-pepper crown of curly hair, sparkling hazel eyes, and a British accent. Her chief concern is my ADLs, my Activities of Daily Living. She wants to know how well I function as I move about in my life. Can I shower, bathe, and dress myself without any support? "Yes, I can." She's also concerned about safety; are there items, like rugs or clutter in my way that might cause me to slip or fall? "No, there aren't, we've removed them." She watches me use the walker, checking that the split tennis balls fit tightly. I'm impressed with the importance of safety.

Next she assesses the motion in my left hand and fingers—the area where the work will be done. I will be manipulating different grades of clay, or putty, similar to the type used at rehab. I try them out. My Play-Doh. She hands me two sheets of exercises, which describe what I must do with the putty. I need to roll it, squeeze it, pull it, punch it, pinch it, pound it, rub it, make it into a ball, make a snake, make a small bracelet, and spread my fingers wide to open it. My fingers hurt doing those exercises. No pain, no gain.

———

The night of Martie's surgery coincided with the first class of the graduate course I am scheduled to teach spring semester. It's scheduled for 15 consecutive Mondays. In addition, I am obligated to be on campus at Bentley University for two days a week, usually Tuesday and Wednesday. That means being away for two nights each week. Once the surgery is scheduled, I call to cancel my first class. I can make up the time over the course of the semester.

I will not be able to leave Martie alone at home for a few weeks. There is no telling how long that would last. While she was recovering from the surgery and in rehab, I had a chance to think about my options. I can't cancel the class; the course is required. I can't ask someone to teach it for me because it's a specialized course that, I believe, only I can teach. It's

not easy to teach a graduate course you have not prepared for. I can't ask a colleague to face that.

It doesn't seem feasible to drive Martie up to the Boston area and have her stay at the Red Roof Inn where we stayed overnight before the surgery. It's not clear she could handle the two-hour drive each way, and then I would have to worry about her during the day. The only viable option is to ask people to come to us and stay with her on those nights. It's a lot to ask of a friend or relative. Most of our friends have jobs. I can ask our son Ken. That might work for the first week, but I can't expect him to repeat that every week. Then there's the issue of compatibility. There are some people who mean well but who can't deal with the anxiety of being away from home and taking care of someone else. They are high maintenance; you have to take care of them. They spread their anxiety to everyone around them.

I need people who are nurturing and care enough to be willing to take a couple of days off work. I also need to deal with Martie's reaction to having someone stay to care for her. I am sure she hasn't thought of that issue yet. Her first reaction may be to resist and feel that she can take care of herself. She may be right, but I can't take that chance. It's the unexpected that worries me. What if she has a seizure? What if we have a snow or ice storm? What if we lose power? On and on, I list the potential disasters in my head.

The way to deal with her reaction is to present the solution as already decided with the people scheduled. She is not likely to want to call people and convince them that I was wrong about her needing help.

I need to line up several people to share the load so that each one only has to stay once. I need nurturing friends. As I go over the list of candidates, two names jump out almost automatically: Beverly Beverly and Anna. Both are close friends and caring people. On the other hand, both have full-time jobs. Both had come down to visit Martie in the hospital the first week after the surgery. I decide to call them a couple of weeks before I need them. I am not sure how to approach the topic. I have no practice at asking for help. How do you start? What if they can't, or won't? How do I make them feel that it is OK to say no?

The conversations are easier than I expected. Asking for help is not that hard once I overcame my fear of rejection and my shame at having to ask. I just ask if they would consider coming down to stay and that I would understand if they can't. It turns out that Anna can't make the first week but can do the second and Beverly can do the first. They both are excited about the prospect. Taking time off work is not an issue. They both see helping us as more important. Instead of feeling shamed about asking for help, I am elated that they are so willing.

Later, the other friends and relatives I ask are happy to help. They like being on the list of people I would ask to perform such an intimate task. I learned I am not alone, or I don't have to be. People seem to want to help if you give them a chance. I never knew.

———

Love comes in all sizes, shapes, and means of delivery. And in surprising places. When I was in the hospital, I was overwhelmed by the feelings I experienced as love flowed around me. That love emanated from family, friends, and the hospital folks who cared for me. The physical and occupational therapists demonstrate the same kindness during their home visits. Now I discover, from Joe, there is more love coming—over the bridge—to me.

It's time for Joe to return to work. He took a short leave of absence while I was in the hospital and in rehab. Joe works at Bentley University, where he teaches and consults on a part-time basis. Bentley is a two-hour drive from here and, because of the commute, he stays overnight. Even with the VNA schedules in place during the daytime, he feels uncomfortable leaving me alone at night.

"I'll be OK. You don't have to worry about me." My old, familiar reply.

"To begin with I've arranged with your friends Beverly, and then Anna, to take the first two weeks. The plan is for them to arrive on Monday, stay over a couple of nights, and then go home on Wednesday. I'll feel better that you won't be alone."

Secretly I am glad. It will be fun to see my friends and spend time with them. I start to plan what we'll do together. But "Whoa, Nellie." There I go again. Slow it down. The two selves are vying for my attention: the old self, who claims I will be OK and starts to plan, and the new self, who catches me and reminds me my friends are coming down to *help* me, not to have a pajama party.

This helping me stuff is a difficult concept to accept. My old self did things on her own, without any help. Anxious feelings crowd around the new concept. The newness of self reminds me of a landscaper creating a new walkway with large slabs of stone. These slabs are enormous, heavy, with misshapen edges, suggesting the edges may not fit together. The slabs of stone are dumped on the ground. Eventually they will be arranged into a walkway. The landscaper's challenge is to push the stone slabs together to fit, pound them around if necessary, and chisel some of the edges to create that walkway. It's a lot of strenuous and backbreaking work. It's the identical challenge to my recovery and reconstruction.

I use pieces from my old life to fashion a new one. I look for objects that belong to me, even my rough edges, to fit. I'm trying to fashion a new world—Martie's world. I take a deep breath and begin to settle a piece into place—*accepting help from others*. But I'm having trouble making it fit. Perhaps there's some shame attached. That will need to be chiseled off in order to fit. Then I see a larger piece that won't fit at all, it has remnants of guilt on it. I'll just discard it completely and look for another piece. Joe's course resumes tomorrow, February 19, and runs through the first week in April. Maybe I can fit that new piece—accepting help from others—into place during that time.

———

Beverly and I have been friends since 1985. We met while working at the corporate offices for T.J. Maxx in Framingham, Massachusetts. She worked in the computer division as a software developer; I was in the finance division working on budgets and financial reporting. Meditation was the first connecting strand of our friendship. Bev was just beginning to meditate. She was looking to de-stress, to ground herself, and to become centered. I had been meditating for nine years. We were good for each other. She was going through a divorce; I was able to support her. She, in turn, could listen to me and support me through difficulties in my work. And even though she didn't have children, she had an uncanny knack of understanding and providing solutions to my kid problems. Although there is a six-year difference in our ages (Bev is younger), our friendship has endured.

I feel the cloak of her friendship as she walks in the door. She reaches to hug me and whispers in my ear.

"I thought I was going to lose you." That's when my body crumbles and starts to shake.

"I thought I was going to die." We cry together for a moment. "I'm glad you're here," I finally say.

"Me, too." She wipes at her tears. "I was happy Joe asked me for help. I wanted so much to do something. I remembered the time you came to stay with me when I had my hysterectomy. I never forgot that."

I feel many feeling about her being here: happiness, warmth, and love. Bev is a great friend to do this for me. I feel her love, but I also feel a twinge of unworthiness. Why is that? Not sure. Maybe an understanding will surface later.

A previously arranged dental appointment is scheduled for the following day, and I am grateful Bev is here to drive me. As cumbersome as the walker is, Bev and I manage.

I am a new patient to Dr. Robert Lynch, and I will be difficult due to my fear of the dentist. I chose Dr. Lynch because I heard he is a kind and patient man. On my first appointment in December he agreed to administer Novocain without the epinephrine (my body has an allergic reaction to the adrenalin rush). Today I'm here for a filling.

It's my second time in his office and three days since my discharge from rehab. My vulnerability spills out and I am weeping as I explain my recent trauma. Dr. Lynch's staff are also kind. His office manager, Allison, provides a drink of water, and a tissue for my tears. The filling is grossly deep and needs much work. Bernadette, the dental assistant, rubs my arm and speaks in a soothing manner.

Because of the extensive work more time is needed, and after the first hour, Dr. Lynch goes to the waiting room to inform Beverly. I'm exhausted at the end of the two hours, but before I leave Judy, the dental hygienist, introduces herself.

Back home, Bev prepares hot soup and tuna sandwiches. I take a nap. Afterwards we catch up on our lives. Bev and I always talk what I call *"soul"* talk. We discuss in detail what has happened to me, how it may affect my life, and how I'll manage going forward. I have no answers, neither does she, but our conversation, guessing about the future, and our laughter leave me with our usual sense of comfort. The nights are thankfully uneventful as I retire to bed early. I am filled with much love when she leaves, and grateful to her for leaving her space of reality, her job, to come to mine and care for me for a few days.

———

By the second week of physical therapy, Pam, my physical therapist, instructs me in the use of the straight cane. There are two types of canes: the four-pronged cane with four tiny legs on the bottom and the straight cane. I will use the straight one. The four-pronged, or the quad, is used for folks who have trouble with their balance, like those recovering from a stroke. I count myself lucky. Using this straight cane feels different from pushing the walker. There's no object in front of me on which to lean. But I continue to feel the need to work on my balance.

"Place the cane in your right hand, the hand opposite your weak leg. Now, move the cane forward, and at the same time, take a small step forward with your weaker leg while supporting your weight on the strong, right leg. As you move forward, transfer your weight off of the stronger leg and at the same time use both the weaker leg and the cane to support your weight."

"I think I can do it." I've got my balance. I place the cane in my right hand to guide my right side and use my left leg to walk forward with the cane. This is cool. I like it. I am doing it. Those leg exercises are paying off.

Pam notices I tire after cane walking for five minutes. "For now, use the straight cane along with the rolling walker during the day." And then she adds, "Gradually build yourself up to cane use all day."

This ping-pong action between the walker and the cane and the cane and the walker continues another 10 days.

Exercises accompany the cane walking. I pore over the pages of home exercises. They're daunting. I hold onto the counter for balance and begin. Legs up, out to the side, then to the back, a crouch here, a bend there. Rise up on my toes, back on my heels. Keep my legs straight, bend while holding them together. Do a kick. Twenty times for each. Repeat on the other side. My kitchen counter is getting a good work out.

I continue day after day, but these exercises are boring and monotonous. To counteract the monotony, I think of myself in training, like an athlete preparing for a competition, like Tim training for a marathon. I need to do this—for me. A layer of weariness flows over me after working my leg muscles. But I feel like I am waking them up and sending signals to my brain and creating new pathways. Those are the thoughts I have while exercising. And I repeat to myself: "I am in training, not to run a marathon, like Tim, but to walk again."

———

Susan, my OT, has a to-do list for me. She would like me to accomplish tasks in the kitchen like boiling water for tea or an egg, making toast and English muffins, and heating soup. And always, always pay attention to my need for rest. I must learn to pace myself. She says I don't do that very well. I could've predicted that.

Part of my resting is taking a nap every day between 1 and 2 p.m. Joe fields the phone calls for me. He knows when I am feeling low during the day or not up to talking. He also knows which callers take a lot of energy from me, and which are nurturing. He excels at tuning in to my needs.

When I wake from my nap, it's time for the other set of exercises. These I do while on my bed; they help me wake up. I begin sitting in an upright position with a pillow behind me. Bend ankles up and down, bend knees, tighten thighs, squeeze buttocks. Straighten legs, lift hips to ceiling. Chair exercises: bend leg, straighten leg, 20 times. Repeat on other side.

They may be boring but part of the entry fee for my new self.

———

Anna lived across the street from me in Natick. We became best friends. We are the same age. Anna is petite, looking like a little doll with dark brown curly hair. We called ourselves the "snoop sisters" because we liked to go to real estate open houses and check out other places around town as we took walks together. Anna discovered an interesting gym called Easy Motion. Up to that time I never thought I'd be caught dead in a gym...but if my snoop sister said it was great, I believed her. For the first time in my life, I became enamored with strength-training equipment. I joined. We drove there together on Sunday mornings.

We become close, like real sisters. It was difficult telling Anna I was moving away to the Cape. She took the news hard, and I thought she would turn her friendship away from me. She didn't. She's coming down today to help me.

After I greet Anna with a hug the tears start. "I'm glad you're here. It means a lot to me."

"You mean a lot to me, too, even if you're not just across the street anymore." She's holding on to me and not letting go. I laugh at her bittersweet comment and notice she's holding back tears. I'm holding on to her, too.

Anna draws back to get a good look at me. "You look so good, much better than when I last saw you in the hospital."

"Everyone is saying that, I guess I looked pretty bad."

"Well, we weren't sure you were going to make it."

"I wasn't either," I whisper, "especially in the ER." Now we are both crying.

"We both could use a cup of tea," she says. "Do you have our favorite, apricot?"

"Uh-huh."

We sit for a while and chat, reliving some of what I have been through, and I listen to her thoughts about my ordeal. When she is through, it's lunchtime.

"How do you feel about lunch at the beach?" I ask.

"What! Don't you think it's a bit cold?"

"Not the way I have in mind. Here's what we do. We go off to the sandwich shop, buy sandwiches and chips. I have the iced tea here, then we drive to my favorite beach—Corporation Beach. We eat lunch there, in the car, of course. And come back home. You game?"

"Let me grab my coat, snoop sister."

I have been longing to see the beach since I got home. After being out with Beverly last week, I felt a sense of freedom and energy, a yearning to do more. An outing to the beach will be great. I feel like a little kid.

We are ensconced in a warm car, watching the roaring waves as the tide rolls in. The seagulls are floating on the updraft, and my favorite little shorebirds are skittering along the tide line searching for food. The whole time is soothing. Anna enjoys it, too.

"That was breathtaking," Anna says as we drive back home. "I've never seen the ocean or the beach like that. It has its own beauty in the winter. And it's so soothing; I may take a nap when you do after we get back to the house."

"Fine with me. I am glad to show you my world on the Cape, and to have you enjoy it so much, but more importantly, to have you with me."

———

By now it's March; February is behind me, as are two weeks of physical therapy. Pam, the physical therapist, stuns me with her greeting.

"Let's go outside!"

"Can we?"

"What's to stop us? You look ready."

Although it's March and cold, there's no snow or ice. I feel shaky. Pam takes my left arm; I have the cane for my right side. I feel in balance. Off we go down my street. I feel timorous at first, but after not falling in the first few steps, my confidence increases. It feels good. Another taste of freedom. We walk past one house and then I tire. We turn around for home.

A milestone.

We move into March, and with Pam's encouragement, Joe and I venture out into the neighborhood. I circle my left arm into his right arm and, with the cane in my right hand, we walk. First we go as far as one neighbor's mailbox and turn around. The next day we try two mailboxes. That's how I measure my distances. Counting mail boxes to measure how far I can go. It's fun. A few more days and it's five mail boxes. I get stronger. We stroll now to the first crest of our street (which is probably three tenths of a mile), and then back. My legs are becoming conditioned, along with my heart and lungs. One day, probably two weeks into this new sport of ours, I/we make it to the top of the hill—four tenths of a mile! Instead of turning around to walk back, Joe convinces me to walk a bit farther and meet the street behind to make it a walk around the block. I'm game. After three-quarters of a mile, I am tired but victorious.

Another milestone.

———

My brother Billy and his wife, Barbara, are here for the first evening of the third week because Joe was unable to get anyone to stay with me.

Billy gives me a long hard hug and doesn't say a word, he doesn't have to. I just hug him back.

They won't stay overnight but are here for the late afternoon and supper. Barbara brings her tuna casserole. Billy raves about it and says he "licks the bowl every time."

Billy is recovering from his BKR—bilateral knee replacement. He continues his rehab on an outpatient basis. Unlike me, he is able to drive. We talk a bit about our father.

"I still can't believe he's gone," says Billy.

"I know. It's not even a month since he's been buried. And we weren't there!"

"I don't think I'll ever get over that part."

"That's gonna be a tough one for you." Billy spent 30 years as a funeral director, owning his own funeral home. It was hard for him when our father died while we were both in rehab. Billy wasn't able to call on his old-time resources to assist with any of the burial arrangements.

"I'm ready to put this casserole in the oven," says Barbara, changing the subject.

Barbara is a few years younger than Billy. She has a great laugh and is full of energy and delight. It's hard to believe she's a cop. She's a member of the police force in a suburb west of Boston. She's tough, and good at her job, too.

After supper we sit around and watch one of my favorite TV programs, *Without a Trace*. I watch the female agent, who was shot, be lifted into an ambulance. As soon as the ambulance doors are shut tight, from out of the blue, I burst into tears. Billy and Barbara come closer to me on the couch.

"What's the matter, Martie, you all right?"

"Honey, you OK?"

I hide my face in my hands. I can't stop crying, can barely breathe. I can't believe this is happening.

It is difficult for me to stop crying. All I can think of is that night. That night I left my home in an ambulance and the ambulance doors, just like the ones on that TV program, shutting tight with their loud impact. I hear that loud slam over and over and over. I can only guess that sound is poking around the feelings of trauma which are beginning to break loose in me. What are those feelings?

Terror? The terror of what was happening at the moment, what was going to happen, and would things work out all right. Would I be all right? Lots of anxiety and fear...all of it unspeakable. Unspeakable at the time, and now being stoked by a TV program. That scene in the show hit me hard.

"Uh, I can't believe that just happened!" I wipe my tears with the backs of my hands. "The shutting of those ambulance doors...that sound in my head. I guess my brain remembers the sound, and it set off triggers of the ambulance ride in January."

Billy puts his arm around me. "You've been through a lot. More than you realize, kiddo. Time to take it slow."

I nod my head in agreement. "But, what a surprise...the ambulance doors... the *sound* of those doors shutting..."

Later, when they leave for the evening, I reassure them many times that I am all right. I have recovered from my crying outburst.

———

Kindergarten was a long time ago, almost 60 years for Margo and me. That's where we met. Over the years we ran into each other again and again. Our most recent encounter occurred in 2005, two days after I moved to the Cape. She was coming out of the supermarket. I was going in. I yelled out hopefully, "Margo?" Sure enough, it was her. Because it was cold, we sat in her car for a while and took up from where we had left off 20 years earlier. Now we live in the same town.

Margo looks forward to being with me for the second evening of this week, she won't be staying over. She is a sweet person, and I am lucky to be among her collection of friends. And this meeting is especially meaningful; it's the first time I've seen her since my hospitalizations.

My tears greet her and I reach for a big hug. Our hug saying so much.

"I'm happy to be laying eyes on you, Margo. I didn't think I'd see you again."

"I was so scared for you, all you've been through, and Joe, too."

"A lot of unexpected things have happened, but I'm glad you're here with me tonight. What's this?" She hands me three white silk flowers in a glass vase. "Margo, this is beautiful. You find the nicest things." Another hug passes between us. "I just love it. Thank you so much."

"It's just a little thing I found. But you, look at you. You look wonderful. Tell me how you are feeling. Tell me everything."

From there we talk about my journey and my emerging new self. We enjoy talking about her grandchildren and her many retirement activities. She and her husband, Phil, live close to a small beach and walk there two to three times a day. I admire them for that effort. Margo is a retired English teacher. She reads everything; she's in two, sometimes three, book clubs. She's always recommending great books for me to read.

She stays into the evening, and I introduce her to one of my favorite TV shows. No surprise reactions, no sobbing, no outbursts on my part this evening, just enjoyment for well-written drama. Afterwards she says she is now hooked on my crime show.

"Remember, if you feel scared, or anything, or if you need us, call immediately. Phil and I are a stone's throw away. We can be here in no time."

I give her a hug. "I promise." But I feel like a little kid. She is a loving friend to soothe me as she does. I know she's not pretending when she says I "look great." She is genuine, a kind person who means what she says. I am filled with love by her concern for me. And I will call if I need her.

Susan, my OT, returns the next week with another to-do list, activities that are simple for most folks but not me. They involve using the fine motor skills of my fingers by putting on my pierced earrings and paging through a magazine one page at a time with my left hand—to bolster dexterity in my left hand. And lastly, I must make an *O* by touching the tip of my left thumb to my left index finger, then middle finger, ring finger, and little finger. And repeat as fast as possible.

But I have an agenda of my own. It's been over a month, and my clients have yet to hear from me, personally. I have 16 clients in my Natick practice and two in Yarmouth Port. I would love to talk with them, but that would be too overwhelming (for them and for me). At the same time, I feel a sense of urgency to get letters written to them. Most of my clients have been coming to me for help for a long time.

Many people know a lot about psychotherapy. Today a plethora of self-help books is available to guide the uninitiated through the maze of therapy with many practical ideas and useful theories. Typically a set of games or multistep guidelines from self-help books are useful and educational. But those types of books cannot fix the situations I deal with: violent domestic struggles, stalemated divorce disputes, alcohol and drug dependency failures, suicidality, and chronic relationship conflicts.

When an individual takes the plunge, makes that first phone call to me, it's usually after a difficult situation and with a high level of anxiety. That's what I hear in their voices when I invite them to make an appointment. The self-help books also imply that our adult problems stem from childhood conflicts, mirroring the theories I learned in graduate school. One of the most notorious problems stemming from childhood hits us all—abandonment. Because of the unexpected visit of seizures, brain tumor, and paralysis that has incapacitated me, I feel I have abandoned all my clients. I need to reach out to them. I have been composing letters in my head to each of my 18 clients for a while. It's time to put my words on paper. I discuss this idea with Susan.

"You have a lot of patients."

"For a part-time practice, I guess I do. I refer to them as 'clients.'"

"Well, I think that's a great idea. Will you be using the PC to type your letters?"

"Why do you ask?"

"It will be a wonderful exercise for those last two fingers on your left hand, you know, the pinky and the ring finger. Those two fingers need more work. Typing will be great finger exercise. I have one thing to caution you about."

"Yes?"

"When you type your letters, do a little at a time. From what I know about you already, I have a sense you'll do too much. Am I right?"

"Yes." I probably will do more than she advises. "What do you suggest?"

"Let me think about this." She closes her eyes and tilts her head to one side and then the other, and finally says, "No more than 10 to 15 minutes a day."

"Uh-huh, sounds about right." There's no way I'm going to keep to that schedule! It takes 10 to 15 minutes to set up at the PC, gather my papers around, and check to see to whom I am writing. But I politely nod my head in agreement, playing the good girl role for all it's worth.

"I'm glad we're in agreement. If you don't keep to this type of schedule, you'll tire yourself out, and we don't want that."

"Oh, no." I have a feeling we're playing a game here. She knows I will overdo it, and I know I have to try to push myself to get all of the letters done. At 15 minutes a day, it will take forever. And it's just typing.

I begin drafting my first letter as soon as she leaves. Of course, I spend 30 minutes and longer. And just as Susan promised, I get very tired. Some days I stop when I feel tired, and on others I push through the tiredness. I pay for it. My walking suffers; I don't walk as smoothly or as easily. My balance suffers; I walk crookedly and weave around. My thinking suffers; I can't think at all. My decision-making suffers; just forget about it. My brain shuts down. Sleep is the only way to get back my functioning.

I change my approach to the client letters by parsing out the time in smaller and smaller portions depending on what my body is telling me. I return to listening to my body. Could this be another piece to restoring my new self?

In the end, I feel pride when I finally finish the letters. Each client receives info telling him or her some details of my misfortune, and that it will be awhile before I can return to the office. I urge each one to keep in touch with the clinician I chose to cover for me. And in the final paragraph, I write something special and personal that relates to them alone. I end by saying that I will be in contact with them again.

While I am happy the letters are done, they were hard to write, harder than I imagined. There is a piece of unreality floating somewhere in my brain that leads me to believe I can continue my practice in Natick, but I suspect that in reality, I cannot. On some level the letters are the beginning of saying good-bye to my clients. But what about Yarmouth Port? I was just beginning to network, place ads in newspapers, and talk up my practice to business professionals and other clinicians in the area. Is the Yarmouth Port practice a possibility? I can hope it is for now. I need something to look forward to in my profession. I am a psychotherapist, a clinical social worker who loves her work.

The letter-writing exercise is long, slow, and tedious, and raises new questions. Will my brain connections improve? Did I create new pathways? Wake up old ones? I am frustrated with myself and cry a lot. I realize I am trying to reach the "old self"—the person I was before the brain tumor. Why wouldn't I? I have no other life. I was successful at the old model I aspired to—do it yourself, do it right (a.k.a. perfectly), be in charge, get it done. Now. What do I do now? Time spent crying and working through my frustration is not for self-pity. It's to clear my thoughts and feelings. That's when I come to a conclusion, reach an idea. I am reminded again, I must reinvent myself.

I have done that several times in my life: from wife to mother to career woman, to the juggling act of keeping a household and Joe and motherhood and career simultaneously in synch, to graduate student, drastic career change, and to plummeting income. But this time it seems different. Why? The physical aspect. I have little control, right now, over limbs that don't move the way they used to or the way I want them to. The times I reinvented myself in the past, I took the movement of my body for granted. Now I require more time to present myself to the world. Getting bathed and dressed are major activities in my day, not swift movements like they were in the past. Moving from one object to another—bed to chair to bathroom to toilet to tub to hallway, etc. takes time and effort. Another set of activities. And decisions. Will I use the walker or the cane?

I notice improvement in my walking and helping around the house and in the kitchen, trying to help Joe with meals, to capture normal again. *Normal.* I am forever chasing normal. What is that? If I am walking on my own, will that be it? I don't know. If not that, then...what? There's so much I have lost. I can't get a pulse on it. I still feel vulnerable and weak. There's got to be some emotional fallout from all this. Right now that seems too huge to even peek at, even after six weeks. And there's the physical healing from the surgery. When my hands drift upward to my head I can tell my incision is healing, but what about the inside? My brain? That sagittal sinus vein? The neurons and their pathways? What about them? There has to be a lot of mix-ups and circuit interruptions occurring. I feel it. I say the wrong word sometimes, actually a lot of times. The word I use often begins with the same letter as the one I intend to say, as in "pass the stone" instead of "pass the salad." And I always surprise myself! Like where did *that* word come from? It's as if I have a drawer full of words that begin with "s," and my brain reaches in to retrieve a word and comes out with any old word, and it's the wrong one. But I tell myself, at least it is going into the correct drawer, the "s" drawer. I bet a neuropsychologist would raise an eyebrow over that theory.

———

March 5th finds us at another medical visit. This time it is the six-week post-op check-up with my surgeon, Dr. Anderson. Going out for those blood tests earlier has been good training for me, and my walker. Still this is new territory, another road to traverse with the walker, another set of doors to get through to where I need to be. I feel like Alice in Wonderland. But instead of falling down an eternally long and winding rabbit hole, I am stumbling through doors and uneven and potholed parking lots while pushing a walker before me. And, like Alice, I feel disoriented and tired as I stand in a new line. I am number five to check-in and begin the familiar information dance. It feels strange standing in this waiting room. The people around me look old, bent over; they have walkers or canes—like me. Do I look that old? Do I look bent over? Yes, to that question. I don't want to think about looking old. My eyes begin to tear up. Don't cry now! I have to start the information dance in a few minutes. Oh, the line is moving up. "Can I help you?" I state my name, date of birth, etc., etc.

Finally we get to what Joe calls the "little waiting room." He borrows this phrase from a *Jerry Seinfeld* episode. After some time, a nurse practitioner enters and asks her questions. I find them hard to answer (I'm trying not to cry); they bring back memories of the hospital and the surgery. After more time waiting, Dr. Anderson finally enters the little waiting room. I look forward to seeing him. Like any patient, I feel enamored of him; he saved my life. He took that awful tumor out of my head. He replaced my damaged skull and fixed me, and I am whole again. By that I mean: I can see, I can speak, I am learning to walk, I can swallow, I can think, I can compute. He didn't mess up my brain. I am thankful and grateful to him for that. I intend to tell him.

So much happens when he enters the room that I forget everything. He says a warm hello to both of us, as he shakes our hands. Right away he checks my incision and says it is healing nicely. Next he checks my eyes with a light. He asks me to follow his finger, he asks me to close my eyes and touch my nose. Then I am told to watch his fingers as he waves them on either side of his head, asking me if I see them? I do. He asks me to hold my arms out in front of me with my palms up and outstretched, then to close my eyes. Dr. Anderson watches this motion of mine for quite a few seconds; I'm not sure what he's observing. Strength measurement is next. He presses and pulls and pushes against my arms, my hands, my feet, my legs on each side. On each limb he tests he makes a note, probably a rating on a scale.

"You look great. The scar on the top of your head is healing well. I notice the weakness on your left side has improved somewhat since your hospital stay. Are you continuing rehab at home?"

"I have physical and occupational therapy twice a week, and it's going all right. They both will continue for another few weeks." It's nice to have someone notice my improvement.

"Everything's looking good. Pretty soon, you'll be using just the cane."

"I'm using it a bit already."

"Good work. About the remainder of the tumor left in your brain. Has anyone contacted you about it?"

Joe and I give each other surprised looks. "No."

"There's not much of the tumor left. It's just I couldn't get at it surgically without the risk of putting you into a stroke."

"Thank you for that," I laugh.

"There's something called a CyberKnife, which from what I know, with one to two treatments could handle the leftover tumor."

Joe and I don't know what to say, we don't understand what he's talking about. It feels too overwhelming. But Dr. Anderson stands up, signaling the office visit is over.

"I'll walk you out and have you see Jill. She'll set up your appointment for a month from now." He shakes our hands and says good-bye.

———

Joe, I notice, has taken on a new role. It shows in the way he is treating me, which is new in our marriage. He's taking care of me. It's a nice feeling, a loving feeling. But a different approach in our relationship from the time I had my first seizure. Now I feel *"less than"* in our relationship; I feel dependent. It's a change-up of roles. As a woman and a caretaker, it was always me on the lookout for ways to take care of him.

At this time, I simply cannot. My first priority is me, especially in the physical sense. It's all I can do to take care of me. I am self-absorbed. Will I stay this way? Will I become narcissistic? Will I lose my nurturing sense? Are these pieces to be placed alongside the new ones I am attaining to be part of the new self? I hope not. Self-care is different from being self-absorbed.

———

Self-care is a familiar theme, and one that I've taught my female clients for years. My goal in therapy is to help them discover a new and deeper sense of themselves, a spiritual sense. And while planting seeds and coaching these clients, (I assist the men in my practice with self-care, as well.), I take stock of myself in order to discover what I need. It's important for me to truly make "taking care of me" a regular routine. If I can do that stock-taking for me, then I can turn around and teach it to my clients.

Back around the time I began my psychotherapy practice, I introduced several new things into my life: a meditation practice, yoga, piano lessons, and social time with friends via lunch and dinner. I also remember setting aside time each morning for spiritual (not religious) readings to keep me grounded and for reminders throughout the day. And it worked for the most part. Presently, most, if not all, of those practices are impossible.

I experience dizziness and fall over in bed when I try to meditate. My poor brain, what is going on up there? Yoga, with its stretching postures and movements to get up and down on a mat, is out of the question. My fingers are not strong enough for piano playing, and after the brain disconnect with the piano in the family room at rehab, I am hesitant to try for the present time. Lunch with friends I am trying slowly, but I must limit the time. I always enjoyed the lunches. They were not only fun but supportive. I never realized how much energy I put into them. Two- to three-hour lunches were common. Now I have trouble with an hour. My brain rebels and starts to shut down. I can't think; I stop listening. Forget figuring out the check and the tip. I need to get home and sleep. Going out for dinner in the evening is out of the question for now. Did I mention I go to bed around 6:30 p.m.? Spiritual readings don't work either. Can't understand why just yet.

What I am enduring diverges dramatically from the past. I guess I am working the rebuilding of myself from the outside in. I begin with the primitive pieces, the fundamental pieces of self-care—bathing and dressing. The next building block is the muscle building/brain retraining exercises. I have plenty more to do, more building blocks to fit together to find out who I am. And how do I become the woman I am meant to be? Is she a new woman, my old self, or pieces of each?

In searching for the spiritual piece, I use a moment one morning to jot down familiar phrases on a piece of paper. For some reason they seem to flow automatically.

I am a woman regaining my power.

I know I do not have to do this all by myself.

I can ask for help.

I accept help when it is offered.

I am learning to let go...especially of the small stuff.

I observe and see the love everywhere.

Joe is the "healthy one." I am not.

I am ready to gag. In rereading these words, I feel angry. I slash a line across the page and write in all caps: THIS IS CRAP! I AM TRYING TO BE SOMEBODY ELSE'S SPIRITUAL DUMMY.

That's not me. Not now. It seems my spiritual thread has unraveled. Currently, I haven't got a clue as to what's going on. I'll leave things alone for the moment, and take things a step at a time, literally. For now I'll concentrate on the physical stuff.

———

Joe and I are sitting talking one evening. I am playing with my hair, which is getting long, and frequenting a nervous habit of fingering my skull, drumming my fingers on my scalp in a rhythm. Good exercise for my fingers—if I were using my left hand. My skull now has a fuzz of hair growing where my incision is, and I am playing with the fuzz. Suddenly as my fingers run over the scalp, I notice the different crevices through the skin. My scalp around the incision feels different from the rest of my skull. I notice there are tiny holes in a pattern, and there's a hard irregular substance that follows the horseshoe-shaped incision. Earlier that morning I stood in the shower for the first time, holding on dearly to the grab bars. The timbre of the sound of the water when I let it pour over me while I moved my head around was different from what I remember hearing when I did this before the surgery.

"Joe, something's weird on the top of my skull around the incision. What is it?"

"Don't you remember? It's where the tumor ate through you skull."

"Ate through my skull! Gross. Did I know that?"

Joe laughs. "Yes, I told you a few times. Dr. Anderson told you in the hospital. *You* have been telling everyone about it."

"I have no recollection. I never saw the connection between my reinforced skull and the tumor eating into it. My skull feels so weird. Come over here and feel it." Joe comes off the couch. I direct his hand over the top of my head to feel the hard irregular substance. "What is that?"

"That's the cement. You wouldn't want the top of your head to cave in, would you?"

"Very funny. Sure feels weird, though." I continue to play with my new skull. "I can't believe I don't remember any of this."

"Me either. You sure told enough people. That's where the titanium mesh is located."

Joe and I go back to watching the TV program, but I can't concentrate on the show. I feel a bit weepy. Something foreign in my body. Something necessary in my body, a new skull. Something new to process—more new information. Why don't I remember being told about it?

———

I've known Donna since she was 14 years old and dating Eddie, Joe's nephew. Donna and I have an unusual relationship. We jokingly consider ourselves the *"outlaws"*; she is a daughter-in-law, as am I, in Joe's family. We have fun with it. She is 10 years younger than I am, and we share common interests. Over the years, and we've known each almost 40 years, we've consulted with each other over home design—pillows, couches, wall colors, etc. We have a mutual love of home decorating and colors and textures. We've had a lot of fun conspiring with color. When Donna discovered Joe needed coverage for me, she didn't hesitate to rearrange her schedule (she is a nurse manager at her local hospital) to come down to the Cape.

My tears greet Donna. She wipes them away and says, "I'm happy you are OK, Martie, we were all worried."

I hug her hard. "I'm touched you came down to be with me. It's easy to be myself with you."

"I brought the ingredients to make lasagna. We can have it the night Joe comes home."

Donna gets herself settled in the kitchen, the place where she loves to be.

"You interested in lunch at the beach?" I ask. This is getting to be a good habit now that I have people driving me.

"Oh, you know I am. What time? Shall I make some sandwiches?"

"No, I've got it all planned. How's 11:45 sound?"

Donna enjoys the beach as much as I do, and Corporation is her favorite beach, too. She and her husband, Ed, often drive down to the Cape on a Saturday in the spring or early summer and visit Corporation. Today she's looking forward to viewing it on a cold and calm March day.

We enjoy our lunch watching the gulls sitting. They are not flying up in the wind today. There wind is quiet. The tide is going out. I am glancing at the sand, the hard sand near the water's edge.

"In rehab they told me not to walk on the sand, but I'd sure like to try it. Do you think we could manage it somehow?"

"Let's give it a try."

Donna helps me out of the car. I show her how I walk on the street with Joe while I use my cane. We stroll along the parking lot.

The soft mushy sand is particularly challenging. "Uh-oh. I guess this is what they meant."

"Just hold on to me. We can make it down to the harder sand. Then it will be easier."

I feel the loving gesture from Donna. We make our way down closer to the water. The sand is more acceptable to my footing, and to the cane's. We are doing it. I am walking on the beach!

"Donna, this is a glorious feeling." I hold on tight to her and breathe in my new freedom, another milestone conquered.

When we arrive home, I am quite tired and I nap.

The next day Donna busies herself in my kitchen with the lasagna. I awake to a delicious aroma. Donna won't accept any help, and I allow myself to be nurtured. When Joe arrives home we enjoy Donna's gourmet Italian meal, prepared with skill and heaps of love.

———

An additional set of exercises is added to my leg repertoire. Stand at the bottom of the stairs. Step up to the first step with my right foot, bring my left foot up to meet it, then down with my right foot, and down with the left foot. Repeat 10 times on the same step. Then repeat with my left foot. That's much harder. Oh, and repeat with the left foot 10 times. In the beginning it's like those stairs in rehab, but after two to three weeks of performing this exercise twice a day, I feel a difference. There's strength returning in my legs. All the leg exercises are coming together to make these muscles wake up, jump to alert, and work again.

The following week I discover the reason behind those exercises. Pam, the physical therapist, takes me up, and then back down, the stairs with my cane. Another leap, another milestone. Later that same week I am able to perform the standing exercises—all seven of them—without her support. More progress.

Now I am using the cane all the time—even outside the house. It's the last week in March, right around the time I took a stroll on the beach with Donna. When Pam takes me upstairs with the cane, and then downstairs, Joe comes nearby. He joins us at the bottom of the stairs. He's impressed and joins in the celebratory feelings. Pam proclaims me "stair ready." Ready enough so that Joe and I can move upstairs to the master bedroom. Another milestone.

———

I became acquainted with Anne's two sons before I met her. Joe and I had just bought our first home in Natick and heard about the two brothers from the neighbors. Indeed, they were great. In the mid-1970s they made great sitters for our boys. David, who loved the Beatles, often brought his guitar and played songs for Ken and Tim. When David outgrew sitting, Andy stepped in. Andy and Tim shared a love for sports. This love has them connected in a friendship they share today.

During one of my "can-one-of-your-sons-come-and-sit-for-me?" phone calls, Anne and I began talking. We discovered some interesting things about each other: We are close in age; Anne is three years older. She married young, also, and we grew up in the same town, not far from each other. Our paths hadn't converged because she attended the public schools in Newton while I went to a parochial school in Waltham.

142

Anne is of Scottish origin and enamored with the British. She loves the queen, and growing up adored Princess Anne, hence her insistence of the spelling of her name with an *e*. She once had a small business selling novelty pins. The name of that business: "Anne with an *e.*"

To know Anne is to know someone born with a sunny disposition. She always has a smile on her face, a song in her heart, and mirth in her eyes. If you find yourself down in the dumps, you won't feel that way for long around Anne. She will cheer you up quickly. That's the way she is. It's the way her heart is.

Anne followed her dream and retired to Maine—Kennebunk. She and her husband, Bill, who died at the young age of 52 about 16 years ago, always talked of moving to Maine like Joe and I talked of moving to the Cape.

Today she's driven three and one-half hours to be with me. She enters my kitchen with her overnight bag and a thermal casserole dish.

We exchange tears with our long silent hugs. She whispers, "I was so worried about you." We stare at each other for a moment. No words. No need. Just happy to be looking at her and she at me.

"You look wonderful. So much better from when I saw you at the hospital." She gives me another big hug, and we wipe our tears.

"I am thrilled you could come. What's that you have that smells so good?"

"My own mac 'n cheese. It has ham and asparagus in it."

"What do we do with it?"

"I'll take it out of the thermal skin and put it right into the fridge. And then I'm going to make us some tea. You go and sit down."

We have our tea—our favorite is apricot—we always have it, right back to our Natick days, which seem so long ago.

We catch up on everything and everybody: her family, my family, and then Anne, and then me. We talk about what we will do the next day.

That night we have a stew prepared by one of my neighbors; we save Anne's mac 'n cheese for tomorrow evening, when Joe returns home. I talk to Anne about lunch.

"Do you want to go out to lunch tomorrow at a restaurant?" I know she will agree. Anne loves to go out to lunch as much as I do.

"Yes, but do you think you can manage it?"

"I'm sure I can. I'd like to try it anyway. It will be like old times. You and me going out to lunch together." I do feel a bit stronger, and I really want to do this, to prove...what?...to myself. I don't know? Probably to get some sense of normal back.

"Where will we go?"

"There's a lovely restaurant just down the road in Dennis called Scargo Café."

It's amazing the things I hadn't noticed when I wasn't disabled. I manage with my cane to use Scargo's ramp to get to the restaurant door. I need Anne's help to open the heavy door and then step over the threshold. I never took notice of thresholds before. Now they take an important place for me upon entering any establishment. Walking with a cane over floors that are not smooth or straight or suddenly become carpeted can be unnerving. I have a cane to ensure my balance and assist in my walking, but my eyes need to be on the floor as well as looking up to see where I am headed for a table.

Moving my body into a booth and keeping track of my cane at the same time is another issue that I didn't plan. I notice my left side is weak. I have difficulty pushing it along the cushion. Perhaps I should have entered from the right side. Thankfully it is leather and not fabric. Anne helps with the cane. But where to put it? The booth is large enough to accommodate resting it on the cushion. For some reason I feel possessive about it, don't want it on the floor. I'm fearful I might forget it. I'm feeling anxious. Going out to lunch was my idea. I need to stop a minute, take a breath. I want to enjoy this with Anne.

Lunch is divine. Another feeling of normal.

On the way home we pass Smuggler's Ice Cream Shop.

"Oh, look, the ice cream place will open in a few weeks. A sure sign of spring."

"I love ice cream," says Anne.

"Ah, so do I."

———

What am I doing behind a tree on a cold November night?

It started about a week ago when Martie told me that her mother and father were going away for the weekend, leaving Friday night. Could I come over after her sisters and brother were in bed? With us both being almost 18, it would to be our private time.

Now I knew that we were not supposed to be in her house alone. Her mother had made it clear that we had to be under parental supervision. It

felt a little like spying to me. But when her parents were in the house, they didn't seem to pay us any attention. So what's the difference if they weren't there? Still I knew it didn't matter what I thought. I would be breaking a rule. On the other hand, Martie and I didn't have much chance to be alone. Maybe the cuddling would get more serious. Maybe without the fear of her parents walking into the room, she would be more relaxed, be under my thumb so to speak. Also, she would be the one in trouble, not me. I'm the guy. I'm supposed to be in pursuit.

On Friday, I head over to her house. On the way, I stop at Brigham's for some of her favorite ice cream, Mocha Chip. A sure way to gain some points with her. As I drive up to the house, Martie comes running out to the car.

"They haven't left yet. Go."

I get out of there. It's after eight o'clock. Why are they still here? I take a drive to nowhere. Amazing how time moves so slowly when you want it to fly. I drive and drive and then head back. Almost 8:30. I cautiously coast down the street. I can see that the car is still in the driveway. Martie appears from beside the house.

"They are almost ready to leave. Just a few minutes."

I drive around the block and park my car in a place they are not likely to see it. I grab the ice cream and walk back to the house. Car is still there. God, they are taking forever. It's pretty dark out so I walk around the back of the house. I can see into the living room. They seem to be getting their coats. I step behind a tree. I position myself so I can't be seen from the window or the front porch when they come out. If they ever decide to really leave. Do they suspect something? Expecting their daughter's boy-friend to ring the bell? What if they open the door and yell, "What are you doing here young man?"

My hand is getting tired from holding the ice cream. I put it on the ground.

"Woof."

Oh God, the dog next store.

"Woof, Woof."

"Get out of here," I whisper.

He comes closer. "Woof, Woof, Woof."

I am afraid to run. The dog might chase me. I can't just stay here.

I look over at the porch. Mr. Hayes is standing there.

Maybe he will ignore the dog. Maybe he is scared and will wimp out.

He walks down the stairs toward me. I'm dead. I don't want to scare him. I don't want him to think I'm a prowler or a Peeping Tom. But I am a Peeping Tom. I pick up the ice cream and move from behind the tree.

"Hi Mr. Hayes."

I make him a peace offering, "I brought you some ice cream."

"What are you doing here?" He smiles with relief. It's only me.

The four of us gather on the porch.

"So you couldn't stay away," says Mrs. Hayes. Her tone is scolding. Her look is piercing. Her stance is aggressive.

"Sorry Mom," says Martie, contrite.

"You can stay until nine, then you have to leave," Mrs. Hayes' concession to the fact that we are adults, sort of.

They get in the car and leave us without another word.

"Why are they leaving for the weekend so late?" I ask Martie.

"That's actually next week. I got my dates mixed up."

This could be a very short relationship.

———

Love. It's a short word, but holds an enormous amount of power. I am filled with love as each person—friends and family members—enters through my kitchen door. I'm honored and humbled as they arrive to take care of me. I don't feel I need to be taken care of, but Joe does. He says he will feel comfortable having someone here.

The love that walks through my door each week is powerful. I cannot muster the range of feelings within me, or fully express in words how profoundly I am touched by this love. I wish I could. That's another piece to the new me I would like to make mine. Instead, the wall of bewilderment that shielded me from my feelings the past four weeks so I could heal is rising again.

Learning how to construct that wall began early in my life, in the 1950s. I grew up in a family, and a generation, where feelings were nearly taboo. I wasn't supposed to have any. Therefore, I didn't learn to express them: anger, grief, sadness...even love. Nobody's at fault, really. It was the practice of our lives in those days. Over the past several decades I've made an effort to learn how to experience, and express, feelings. I'd been working on just that for years before the brain tumor. But it seems as though, along with the impulses that retrain my muscles and brain patterns, I have to jump-start the reactivation of my feelings, too.

Each week when a friend or family member walks through the kitchen door I choke up inside. I feel their love strongly. But I don't know what to say, or how to express what I feel for them. They have kind words, whispers of love, hugs, tears,. The food they bring to prepare is another expression of their love. I return with my own big hugs, tears, words of love. I am happy to see them, but at the same time, feel unworthy of their love. Perhaps that's what is keeping me from sharing my deepest feelings and thoughts with them. My unworthiness. But I do know this. My heart is like a deep well—going all the way to China—and it is filled with love for all who come to help me. Slowly, I am reaching into that well, and searching for how I can respond with the full measure of my love for them. Do they know it? Can they feel it?

———

Then there's Joe. He's the love of my life. I'd be lost without him. Those two statements sound clichéd and simple, but they are not. They hold all my feelings of love for Joe. We've been together a long time—43 years—and weathered the many storms that roared through our relationship. Typically we were both able to be at the head of these storms guiding things along together. Sometimes one of us was less strong than the other but not incapacitated, like I am now.

How is it that he manages to think of such an idea—having friends and family here to care for me? He's relieved to have someone here, a thoughtful and caring act. Joe's been thoughtful and caring and loving throughout this part of my recovery. That can't be easy for him, watching me endure surgery, paralysis, walker, cane. He has to do everything around the house. And he is becoming my caretaker. A new role for him. Our roles are reversed.

I have not heard an angry remark, a door slam, or even a long sigh to indicate anger or resentment. There are times he has to be mad, feel angry. How could he not? I feel angry. Our whole life, our relationship, has been turned upside down. One thing I learned years ago when I discovered my feelings was this: I can feel anger at the situation and hold love at the same time. And that's what I feel from

Joe during my rehabilitation and recovery at home—love. I am at my weakest physically and emotionally, and all the while Joe remains kind and gentle, and ready to do more. I am grateful to him for that, and I appreciate all that he does. That is love. The depth of my love for him goes through the depths of all the oceans of the world.

———

Two weeks later I receive an unexpected phone call from the office of Dr. Lincoln. We met the radiation oncologist when she swept into my hospital room about a month ago. The secretary in her office wishes to set up an appointment. I tell Joe about the phone call and my surprise. What I'm really feeling is fear.

"I'm not having radiation."

"Well, what makes you say that?" Joe replies in a comforting tone.

"All those scary stories I've heard about it. I just don't want my brain FRIED. And besides, one of the options she talked about in the hospital was that we could just wait and see."

"I think you're getting ahead of yourself. Let's just go and see what she has to say."

"I'm not sure about this at all."

"Let's at least give it a shot. It can't hurt."

The following week we arrive at Dr. Lincoln's office in Hyannis. By now it is the middle of March, and while I use the cane full time in the house, I'm still using the walker when I travel outside. At Cape Cod Hospital, where her office is located, there are new bumps and little potholes to maneuver.

It is our first time at the Cancer Center at Cape Cod Hospital, and we sit in yet another large waiting room. I am struck by the number of sick people: the sunken faces, the bald heads, the scarves, the hats, the decorative wraps that hide bald heads, and the eyes that lead right into the soul. I don't have cancer. I am one of the lucky ones.

My name is called and we are escorted to Dr. Lincoln's office where she meets with us immediately—bypassing Joe's "little waiting room." And no more waiting. I don't remember her at first; we spent little time with her in the hospital. Dr. Lincoln has a pleasant, heart-shaped face, and light brown straight hair that hugs her chin. She welcomes us as she shakes our hands, and her pleasant smile puts me at ease.

She asks about my progress from the surgery, my recovery from the paralysis, expressing surprise at how well I look. I tell her I am working hard on my exercises.

She wastes no time with details. "Radiation is not an option, it is a necessity." Her words strike me in the chest like a fast ball. How could that be? She goes on to discuss my case as she presented it to the *Tumor Conference Bureau* in Boston. I am impressed that she did all this work for my tumor. With all the work and research, she came back quite strongly with the decision that the remains of my tumor should be removed—by radiation. She continues by stating that I should not wait around for something more to happen, that is, for another tumor, or tumors, to spawn.

"Today there is a new form of radiation called radiosurgery," Dr. Lincoln says. "It's a high-intensity radiation that destroys tumors in one, possibly two, visits."

This sounds familiar, like something Dr. Anderson mentioned at my post-surgical visit.

She explains further, "These machines are huge. They are special x-ray machines that hone in on a tiny area, a specific area of the brain, with an accuracy of one millimeter. In your particular case, this type of x-ray machine would be a good fit."

I'm feeling anxious and overwhelmed.

"Unfortunately, this machine is not available at Cape Cod Hospital. What we have here cannot pinpoint radiation in smaller areas, and a wide area of radiation could create collateral damage."

"*Collateral damage.*" I don't like the sound of what that might mean. What I do understand is that areas in my brain around the tumor material could be damaged.

I'm dizzy. Radiation was not supposed to be on my radar, and now it is. And I am hearing new words like "radiosurgery" and "collateral damage," and they scare me. I don't need any more damage than I already have, and some damage I don't even know about yet. I am still healing, for crying out loud. Stop. Hold it. We are going too fast. Whoa, Nellie. Let's slow this down!

It is our decision in the end; it has to be. But Dr. Lincoln makes a compelling argument for finding out more about radiosurgery. And Joe and I both feel the urgency, the urgency of making the decision while in Dr. Lincoln's office about having her make the call to her Boston colleague. After discussing both options with her, Joe and I both agree to look into the radiosurgery option.

"All right, then. I will pass your name on to my colleague at Brigham and Women's Hospital in Boston."

We will wait for word from them.

———

Before the brain tumor, I never accompanied Martie when she went to see a doctor. And she never accompanied me. She always went with a list of questions and usually had them answered. Like most guys, I never bring a list.

Visiting doctors together became the norm after the tumor. The nature of the visits changed in several ways. The issues discussed were, of course, more serious and the procedures more complex. In addition, Martie had a difficult time focusing on her needs and the questions she wanted answered. She still made lists. They just didn't get used. When the doctor arrived in the waiting room, she forgot why she had come. She seemed hesitant answering the doctor's questions and appeared to me to be saying what she thought the doctor wanted to hear because her thinking was lagging behind. Most often, when asked she just said, "I'm fine," even when she wasn't.

I had a hard time understanding her behavior; she had always been so self-sufficient. We would talk before the doctor arrived and agree what we needed to report and get answers to. I had the advantage of being the observer in the room. So I could focus on what the doctor said without the pressure of having to answer his questions or respond to his requests to squeeze his hand or walk in a straight line while he talked. But in the presence of the doctor, Martie acted as if we had not planned at all. At first I thought she was covering up the real issues. "Is she purposely lying?" I thought. After the visit, we would talk about what happened. Martie couldn't explain it except to say, "My mind when blank when the doctor walked in."

This is another example of how my role as caretaker grew because of Martie's cognitive deficits at the time.

The few minutes you have with a doctor are very valuable. There is a limited opportunity to comprehend what the doctor is saying and to ask about what you want to know. Unless you ask, doctors generally don't provide much information beyond the narrow issue at hand. You really have to think quickly to get additional information. I am not being critical of doctors. They do what they have to do to treat a lot of people in a limited time. The doctors we saw would answer our questions but without adding new information.

We devised a strategy to overcome Martie's difficulty keeping focused. First of all, after discussing this issue, Martie agreed that I should speak up if I felt she was not reporting something accurately or if she forgot something. I handled this by talking to Martie, not the doctor. I would say, "But remember that last week, you couldn't get out of bed one day?" These comments allowed all three of us to take a step back and reassess. Second, whenever there was a major decision to be made, we would say we needed time to talk together and asked the doctor to come back in a few minutes. Then we would go over what the doctor actually said. We often had different versions. Martie often had the substance right or close to it, but she missed the subtleties, the exceptions, and the unexpected—those key words or phrases like "this will get worse over time" or "swelling is normal."

The appointments could have been a source of conflict for us. I know that I do not want Martie present or making comments when I talk with my doctor. Martie seemed just the opposite. She wanted to learn as much as she could from the visits. I made a conscious attempt to downplay my role. I never wanted Martie to feel like she was helpless, like a child that needed a parent present. And, in truth, she was not like a child, she just could not think fast enough under stress to take in everything that was happening. She didn't need a parent; she needed a translator to pick up the words that were spoken too fast for her to comprehend.

THE MYSTERY OF THE LOWER LEVEL

Trot, trot to Boston,
Trot, trot to Lynn,
Look out, little girl,
'Cause you might fall in!

This short nursery rhyme originated in the New England and is often sung to little ones as they are gently bounced on an adult's knees. Once "in" is reached, the adult parts his or her legs and pretends to let the child fall between them. That action almost always stimulates a laugh. The thrilled child insists, "Do again!"

Trot, trot to Boston. Joe and I are off to Boston today. We are not trotting but rolling along in my Toyota Camry. I notice changes in myself as we ride along the Mid-Cape Highway. I am sitting straighter, and I don't have to lift myself up to see out the passenger-side window, as I did about five weeks ago on my return trip from the rehab hospital. I've improved. I notice a change in the season, as well. The cold winter is reluctant to vanish, and spring is yawning its way in like a slowpoke. No buds on the trees yet, but the scenery along the highway looks different, as if something important is about to happen. Spring is on its way. Spring on the Cape is always a slow process. The vernal equinox came two days ago, but the road shows remnants of winter, with dirty snow piles and oak leaves clinging to their limbs, afraid to let go. Once we ride over the bridge, I see that the off Cape towns have more snow than us.

Trot, trot to Lynn. The city of Lynn is north of Boston by about 15 miles. Right now I wish we were driving to Lynn—and beyond. I'm scared of what we are going to discover at our appointment with the Radiation Oncology Department at Brigham and Women's Hospital. I don't want to go. I know, I know. If I find out for sure, then I will have the facts, and I can deal with them. But I am feeling much like a little girl right now, and my scary feelings threaten me.

Look out, little girl. Last week, Craig from Radiation Oncology called on behalf of Dr. Kahn to inform me that the doctor could see me at 11 a.m. on March 23. There was no question as to whether that was a possibility, or convenient, for me. It's convenient for him. I am to be there. So here we are on the road to Boston— Joe, me, and my fears. After my office visit with Dr. Lincoln at the Cancer Center at Cape Cod Hospital we investigated different radiosurgery and radio oncology treatments for brain tumors. Many of the machines used in treatment involve screws that hold masks or appliances in place. Viewing pictures, I could see that these screws went directly into a person's skull. I was horrified. At the visit with Dr. Lincoln, I asked her about this notion of "screws in my head." Was this true? "Oh, yes," she said, without further explanation. I was stunned. Nothing more. No elaboration.

Tears well up. My chest knits itself into its familiar pattern of anxiousness. It feels tight. I can't do this. Even if it is only one or two sessions like Dr. Anderson said. Screws into my head. Going through my skin and all. What about infection? What if they hit a bone? My fears are convulsing inside me. Softly I cry. I can't even talk about them with Joe. Perhaps if I did...

I notice he is quiet, too. There's only the hum of the tires as we roll along the highway at 75 miles an hour. He looks tense. Both hands grip the steering wheel, eyes straight ahead on the road in front of him. I leave things alone. That's what I usually do in situations like this. I leave it alone, and watch and see how things evolve. A little voice inside screams, "Do something! Say something!" But no, I hang out with my anxiety as my only companion.

I learned to do that as a child. In my household there was much shouting and yelling. I learned to be silent and wait until my mother's anger subsided. She was overwhelmed at times with four children and little help from my father. He was working all the time. He had to. That's the way it was in the 1950s. I learned that if I talked too soon, the shouting started up again. So I sat with my anxiety.

Joe does not yell, but I've learned that interrupting his thought process too soon doesn't work for him or me. We both end up arguing and sometimes misunderstanding one another. He needs to figure things out for himself, just like I do. I'm aware that Joe is thinking and that he is scared, too, afraid for me. We both don't know what to expect. We have talked and talked and talked about it. It is time for silence.

'Cause you might fall in! We've lived near the renowned Boston-area hospitals for over 30 years. This is our first time seeking treatment at one of them. The directions provided by the hospital say there are 10 traffic lights to go through once we exit the expressway. And we hit a red light at all 10. It's arduous finding our way through the downtown streets. We finally roll into the valet parking at Brigham and Women's Hospital. Young men wearing red pinafores with the valet company's insignia wave us in. Joe takes a breath, and I hear his sigh of relief.

"We made it, and how nice I don't have to worry about finding a place to park."

I love the city, but in my vulnerable state and using a cane to steady myself, which also alerts others to *please be aware*, the hospital seems forbidding. We enter through a huge revolving door, as big as I've ever seen. Instead of being divided into quarters, it's divided in half with plants in the middle. I suppose that from the designer's perspective it appears not only aesthetically pleasing but also easier to negotiate. To me it looks intimidating. I walk through slowly.

Once we get into the hospital, it's like we have landed in a different world. "Toto, we're not in Kansas, anymore." That's just how it feels. It's as if we stepped off a plane into a foreign country. What appears to be an army of people is milling about, going to and fro, some with a purpose, some not. The languages are diverse. Not much English. I hear German, Spanish, Chinese. They are not munchkins. These people seem to have different roles: visitors, doctors, nurses, pharmaceutical reps, business folks, and others. My anxiety has subsided for the moment. The crowd, moving in what seems like six different directions simultaneously, is like a living thing. We have to get ourselves into that crowd. We have a purpose.

We follow Craig's directions: "Look for a bank of elevators to the right of the revolving door and go to the second lower level." How can there be two lower levels? We enter the elevator and see buttons marked L and LL, which must mean Lower and Lower Lower. Or is it double L for light n' lovely, long lasting, lite lager, or Double L Dude Ranch? Commercial jingles pour through my brain. They keep my anxiety at a low volume. The double L is for the second lower level. Folks in scrubs, business suits, and casual clothes, like us, crowd into the elevator. At L, everybody, with the exception of a woman in a business suit, walks out. The elevator continues down into the underbelly of the building. At LL, the woman in the business suit steps out and takes a left turn, clearly knowing where she is going. Joe and I step out and stare at the walls, looking for signs.

A petite Asian nurse wearing surgical scrubs and a smile approaches. "Can I help you?"

"We're looking for Radiation," Joe says.

"I have an appointment with Dr. Lamb, er, Kahn," I say hesitantly. His unfamiliar name is not rolling correctly off my tongue.

"Follow this corridor," she says, pointing to our right. "Radiology is directly at the end. You can't miss it."

We extend our thanks. The ceiling on this level feels low. At 5 feet 2 inches I am not a tall person, but I feel the closeness of the ceiling as we walk. It is a long way down. I wonder if this is really a cave that was dug for the radiation machines. The radiation equipment has to be in the basement of the building, in the ground. All that radiation. Fears are rising.

I lift my slipping purse back onto my right shoulder. The cane in my right hand is supporting my gait. I am a three-legged woman. I grab Joe's hand. He turns to me and smiles.

———

I fish into my pocket and find his business card. Kahn. That's it.

We find our way to the reception desk and are greeted brusquely, without a smile. Forms come our way. The receptionist gives me an ID card, and we sit in the waiting room. Cancer patients are waiting, just like at the Cancer Center at Cape Cod Hospital, but here they appear sicker. I spot a couple of visitors in the corner. It looks like they are piecing a puzzle together—one of those thousand-piece ones.

There is a short hallway off this small waiting room. Along the hallway is a built-in fridge that holds water, juice, and milk for coffee. A coffee maker is perched on the counter, and there is hot water for tea. A basket cradles sugar packets, along with saltines, graham crackers, and Lorna Doones (my favorites). Restrooms are here. But I spy a closed door at the end. The door opens and a nurse emerges with haste in her step. I glimpse a number of women in hospital gowns sitting in hospital beds with IVs attached to their arms. Looks like they are receiving a type of infusion. Possibly chemotherapy? I have a lump in my throat, feeling scared for them and for me. When I look back in the waiting room to the other patients, most of the faces are down, no eyes with which to make contact, a number of shining, hairless heads. I shiver and send thanks to an unknown presence in the universe that I have no cancer, but I wonder again about the radiation treatment.

We are called to the second waiting room—a much smaller room—with a PC, a whiteboard, examining table, and two chairs. I wonder where the doctor will sit. The door opens and a short man dressed a white coat steps inside. He has jet black straight hair, wire-rimmed glasses, and light brown skin. He introduces himself.

"I'm Dr. Kahn. I'm happy to meet you." He shakes our hands and instructs one of the two people accompanying him, also dressed in white, to grab a few chairs from outside the room. He takes one of the chairs and sits down opposite me. He introduces his intern. When she greets us, she sounds like she may be from Eastern Europe or Russia. She looks young, in her twenties. The second introduction is for his nurse. She is Caucasian and fortyish. "They're part of my team."

"I've read all the surgical notes and diagnostic materials about you. Is it true that you never had a headache before the surgery?"

"Yes, that's correct, no headache."

"I see you've been through a lot." He flips through pages in a folder. "Your surgery, a new piece in your skull, and left-sided paralysis. I'm surprised you are not in a wheelchair. You must have worked hard."

"I have." I feel more at ease.

"Let's talk about what we here at Brigham and Women's can do for you in the next phase of your treatment." He has a soft but compelling voice. He is promoting his wares. He continues by giving us a further education about meningiomas, in particular atypical ones, like mine.

"They are *nasty*," he says. "Every area in your brain, every part of your skull that the tumor touched is fertile, a potential spot for that tumor to grow back, to return into your life. That's why we have to not only get rid of the tumor pieces remaining around your sagittal sinus but also irradiate *all* the areas that might have been touched by the tumor."

"Wow, this is new information for us. We never knew that." I think he knew he had us then, and went on to explain: "We have a Novalis radiation machine that performs stereotactic radiotherapy—SRT. It's a method of delivering accurately focused radiation treatment over a predetermined time span." He makes use of his hands as he talks, brings them both together with the fingers arcing and almost touching to emphasize his point of the accuracy of the stereotactic process.

"Is that the machine that takes one to two visits?" Joe asks.

"And will there be screws put into my skull?" My burning question.

"No. The amount of time will be computed by me. I will design a specific treatment just for you, just for your specific case. And each time you come for a treatment, you will receive a fraction of the total, which decreases the chance of killing nearby healthy tissue."

"So, how many visits?" Joe asks.

"From 27 to 35."

Wow! The numbers startle me, especially after being told one or two visits by our other two specialists. The stunned look on my face registers on his.

"Remember I will be designing your treatment on two levels. First, to rid the remaining fragments that could not be removed surgically by Dr. Anderson, and two, to irradiate all areas—brain and skull—touched by the tumor." Dr. Kahn looks over at the top of my head. "I notice your hair is beginning to grow over the incision. I suggest you buy a wig. You *will* lose your hair. There's a lot to consider here."

If his marketing speech was meant to dazzle, it did. I am floored with the information, especially the number of treatments. We know from the list of degrees on his business card that he is a distinguished scientist.

"My radiation therapists are the best in the world. They can fit you with a mask today, and we can start next week."

"A mask? For what?"

"The mask is made to fit the features of your face. Its purpose is to stabilize your head during the treatment. Each patient has his or her own mask made up ahead of time."

"So, no screws into my skull."

"No, my dear, no screws into your skull. We have moved quite a way from that early technique."

"That's a relief."

Dr. Kahn is right about one thing: we have a lot to consider. He looks across at us as though waiting for something. It appears he has completed his marketing spiel and is waiting for us. Do we get a bonus—like an extra radiation dose if we sign up in the next 10 minutes! I half expect one of the team to say, "But wait, there's more!" But this is not about a vegetable slicer on a late-night TV commercial—this is treatment for my brain we are talking about here—and every move, every thought, every word, every decision, is crucial.

I don't know what to do or say. My healing brain is vibrating from all Dr. Kahn's information. At the same time I'm trying on the idea of radiation *not being optional*. From Drs. Anderson and Lincoln I heard maybe one or two visits. Now I am hearing 27 to 35, the same number that folks with cancer receive. No screws, thankfully, but a mask. What will that be like? They can fit me for a mask today. How can they do that? Did they know I was coming? Don't they have anything else to do? Not enough patients to zap? Did they know I would say yes, that I would sign up for this great deal he is offering?

"This is too much," I say. I feel overcome with so many feelings that I am light-headed and dizzy, signs of overwhelm for me. I want to cry. I look over at Joe. It looks like he is trying to process and make sense of it all. I don't want to get zapped. What if my personality changes, what will happen to my brain functions...in the long term...what about so many things? Before I start crying, I turn toward Dr. Kahn.

"I think we need some time alone to talk about this."

"Of course, use this office. Take all the time you need. When you are finished, just open the door."

That said, Dr. Kahn and his team leave.

———

I'm a bit weepy. Joe starts talking right away, which helps me get myself together. I need to process all the info I have heard, and I need a sounding board.

I've always been a sounding board for Joe. That began when we were both 17 years old, Joe walking me to the bus stop in Central Square in Waltham, Massachusetts. We were in our senior year at St. Mary's High in Waltham. I lived in Auburndale—a village of neighboring Newton—and took a city bus to get to school. Joe lived in Waltham. Every day when we were dating, Joe walked me to the bus stop at 2 p.m. We talked and talked about our future. We planned to get married after Joe completed his education, which would include eight years after high school. Joe planned to be a research psychologist and teach at a university.

Many buses went by before I finally climbed onto the 4 p.m. local. I easily slid into the sounding board role, asking questions, becoming an active listener, putting myself in his shoes, donning the devil's advocate role, wondering why we were waiting so long to get married. As it turns out, we didn't. We married while he was in college.

"What do you think?" he asks.

"I don't know."

"I thought we had all the big events behind us, the surgery, rehab. Now this."

"Me too. This is so unexpected. He scared me with 'they are nasty.'"

"Yeah, I didn't know about the areas the tumor touched...seems bizarre... we've never heard that before."

"I'm going to lose my hair again. Did you catch that?"

"It was the way he said, 'you will lose your hair.'"

"I guess it's good we've been recommended here—to Boston—where the best are."

"He seems like a bright guy."

We review every aspect of Dr. Kahn's talk. Joe's calm demeanor helps me, and my fears lessen. Slowly, I realize that this is the next step in my journey, albeit an unexpected one. We can't determine how I will get to the Brigham from the Cape—a 90-minute drive *without* traffic—on a daily basis.

"One thing at a time," I say to Joe. "For now, let's open the door and tell them our decision is to go ahead. I will have the mask fitted today. We can go from there."

"OK." Joe opens the door, and we wait.

After about 10 minutes, the doctor returns and we inform him of my decision to undergo the treatments and have the mask fitted today.

"I think you're making the best choice," he says, looking straight into our eyes. "Oh, doctor," he calls out to his intern as she walks past the door, "will you catch Barbara and send her in, please?"

I notice he is courteous with his staff. He produces forms from the folder he is carrying. They are the consent forms that give him permission to perform the specialized stereotactic radiation on me, along with any necessary tests. HIPPA forms are included, stating who and what facilities have access to my medical information.

Once I sign the forms he hands me another with details about the treatment. In particular, it lists the potential benefits, how the treatment will be administered, and the possible side effects. He has penciled a star beside one of the side effects—radiation damage to the brain or other parts of the body. I stop. We discuss it further. He tells me there are no guarantees, and that there's a 5 percent chance of damage from the radiation. I feel scared by his words and begin to question my decision. I weigh the possibility of the tumor returning, surgery again, paralysis and rehab again, versus this radiation treatment and a small chance of radiation damage, the likes of which I don't know. How and when would it show up, and what would it look like? I think of all these possibilities in a flash. I initial the form where he drew his star.

On cue, it seems, Barbara returns. He tells her to arrange the mask-fitting. Dr. Kahn asks if I am claustrophobic. I relate my story of needing a Valium in the hospital before I could undergo an MRI.

"We can take care of that here, too," he says. "You might find the mask-fitting process a bit claustrophobic, but there's no need for concern, my radiation therapists are kind and they will take good care of you."

He leaves and we are alone again. "Well, I did it. I made the decision. Now I feel shaky." Joe leans over from his chair and takes my hand. I feel tears start to bubble along my eyelids but I blink them away.

Barbara brings the Valium. "Take it now, and we'll wait about 20 minutes before I walk you down to the fitting room." The *fitting room*? Too bad I'm not getting fitted for a lovely ball gown. It's not a ball I'll be attending.

I feel myself getting drowsy. I'm glad the Valium works so quickly. No wonder the Rolling Stones had a great hit with "Mother's Little Helper," that little yellow pill. I notice my brain is keeping me distracted so I won't cry—the Rolling Stones...a ball gown. I don't need to be crying now, but I sure would like to. This is hard stuff. Making a decision like that. Getting zapped, getting fried, my brain. What's really going to happen to it? Yes, I want the tumor remains gone, but what will happen to the rest of my brain, later on down the road? My thinking...my cognitive abilities...my focusing...my memory...and those are the abilities I know about. What about the ones I don't know. Go home, think about it more, and then come back? I don't know. I guess I'm doing the right thing. Using Joe as a sounding board helps. Dr. Kahn made a big deal out of radiation damage. What's that about? Joe's answer would be "lawyers." I wonder if there are people who don't sign by his penciled star. Then what? Does he stop...say bye-bye...leave the room?

Barbara escorts me to the mask-fitting room. Dr. Kahn is right. His radiation therapists, or RTs, are extremely cordial and kind as they greet me. I meet two young men, Ron and Charles. They will be with me during my treatments. On their days off, Clare and Christy will assist me. They ask if they can get me some water before we start. I tell them no, thank you. They are very careful as they help me onto a table and place my head in a cradle-type basket. Before each step the RT explains precisely what he is doing.

First, he wets a piece of white gauze-like fabric in warm water and places it alongside my head, to meet the back of the mask. Now the front. Again gauze-like fabric is wetted, but this time it is placed in strips across my forehead. Another strip is placed across my lower face, beginning on one lower cheek and extending under my nose to my cheek on the other side. The next piece of the fabric looks like the wishbone from a cooked chicken. It begins at the midpoint of the strip placed across my forehead, travels down to the bridge of my nose, splits to go around my nose, and meets up on the strip previously placed under my nose. The last piece is a whole piece of the fabric cut to go over my entire face, beginning at the top of my forehead, coming down along the sides of my head, covering my eyes, nose, and cheeks, but curving up by the lower sides of my cheeks to the upper lip. There is a small, flat tab fitted into the mouth of the mask. The mask will not cover my mouth, and there will be an opening for my nose. I will be able to breathe.

The pieces of fabric feel warm. When the last piece, which covers my face, is put into place along with the mouth tab, I feel claustrophobic. I am grateful for the Valium. But I wonder what will be happening with the actual radiation treatment? When the mold is complete, the whole large piece is lifted from my face. It's still soft. I am told that this is the mold for a hard and durable mask that will keep my head from moving during the radiation treatment.

The fitting is over. The RTs suggest I get a prescription for Valium for my treatments. When I leave the room we meet Dr. Kahn. "My RTs tell me you did very well."

A thank-you is about all I can muster.

"Now it's time for my work to begin. I will be designing a treatment especially for you, and I will call you when we are ready to begin. It should take a couple of weeks. For now I will say good-bye."

———

Our 20 minutes or so with Dr. Kahn and his staff help clear up our misinformation. I learn a lot about why atypical meningiomas are so dangerous and how stereotactic radiation really works. Nice that the head frame with screws is no longer used. Thank goodness for the mask. I had no idea that the whole area where the tumor had been needs to be irradiated. Once Dr. Kahn explains it, it makes sense. I'm surprised by the idea of more than 25 treatments. We came for the consultation to hear about how the one-treatment method works. It doesn't for Martie's situation. How will we deal with six to seven weeks of radiation?

Martie seems impressed with his knowledge, but I'm a bit uneasy with his aggressiveness. If he were a used car salesman, I'd consider his pitch on the border of being unethical. But as a national expert on meningiomas and on radiation, I believe he wants to win in two ways: he wants to win Martie as a patient, and he wants to destroy the "nasty" atypical cells in her brain. I admire his determination. And I feel lucky that we live close enough to Boston to take advantage of this wonderful technology and talented man.

One choice is between six weeks of standard radiation on Cape Cod and six weeks of stereotactic radiotherapy in Boston—about two hours from our home. The choice seems clear to me from a medical perspective. The stereotactic radiation seems safer because it is more precise and more likely to kill the tumor cells because of its power. But, having the treatments in Boston five days a week presents a logistical nightmare. It is clearly going to take over our lives for a month and a half during a period when we are both working two to three days a week. Can we drive up every day and then continue on to work some days? We were told that fatigue will become more of a problem as the treatments continue. Can we both take a leave from our jobs? That seems impossible. Can we stay in a nearby hotel for six weeks? In addition to the many thousands of dollars it would cost, we would have to eat out at restaurants and live out of suitcases. Can we stay with our son, Ken, who lives nearby, for six weeks? A lot to ask. Could we stay with several people, moving from place to place like gypsies? Just the thought is exhausting.

We drive home. Martie sleeps. I worry. Another unexpected turn of events. Every time I think this phase of our lives is in a steady state, it rocks and rolls again.

———

A short diversion about radiation, again from my layman's perspective. Radiation works because it damages a cell's DNA. Because abnormal cells reproduce faster than normal ones, they are less able to recover from the damage and lose their ability to reproduce and retain fluids. In a typical schedule of treatments, the total amount of radiation to be given is calculated and divided—the term is "fractionated"— usually into a number of equal doses given five days a week until the total is reached. The relatively small once-a-day dose and the weekends in between give the normal cells time to recover. The total amount at the end is determined by how much the patient's body can handle. It's a calculated risk; kill the bad cells but not the patient.

Over the past few decades, new technology and procedures have made the delivery of radiation more precise, thereby reducing the collateral damage to healthy cells. But adjacent tissue still can become damaged, which is a real, if low-probability, risk when irradiating the brain. That is Dr. Kahn's 5 percent. The availability of the MRI has made it possible to see a tumor in detail. Stereotactic radiation uses the imagery to target tumors more precisely. The term "stereotactic" means aiming a beam in three dimensions. These beams can be aimed with a precision of one millimeter—about 1/25th of an inch. That technology can be used to irradiate tumors that cannot be removed surgically, as was the case with the remains of Martie's tumor.

The linear accelerator–based radiotherapy machines, like the ones at the Brigham, are more prevalent. One benefit of this technology is its ability to easily treat large tumors by treating them over several sessions, called

"stereotactic radiotherapy." Linear accelerator machines are not restricted to treatments only within the brain. They can be used throughout the body, as well as on the head and neck.

That exhausts my knowledge of radiation except for the common side effects of loss of hair and fatigue and the uncommon ones, like collateral damage.

———

My mind is getting restless; it needs to be exercised along with the other muscles. On April 2, I resume my psychotherapy practice in Yarmouth Port and begin seeing clients again. I feel ready, I am walking with a cane, and my hair—albeit fuzzy—is growing in. At home we are under the pause button waiting to hear when the radiation will start, which is beginning to affect not only my state of mind but our relationship. It's good to have the office to go to, even if Joe has to drive me there.

I was fortunate in finding the office space and Bill, my landlord. He is also a social worker. He owns the building and has furnished it beautifully. I began renting from him in August 2006 with my first referral. My rental arrangements include one day a week—Mondays. Bill has been sympathetic to my current situation and provides encouragement in getting my practice off the ground. My networking has stopped for now, but after these radiation treatments are finished, I will start again. I have plenty of ideas.

For the present I have a couple of clients and one I see regularly. She has been patient while I have been recuperating and rehabbing. We are currently back to our Monday 2 p.m. weekly sessions. Lori is pleased to see me and to be talking about her situation. (All client names and situations are fictional to protect their identity and ensure confidentiality.) I inform her about the next unexpected step in my treatment and casually state I will be able to arrange things at the Brigham so I can return to Yarmouth Port for our 2 p.m. sessions.

———

"How am I going get to Boston, Joe?"

"We haven't even heard from them yet, and it's been over a week, now. Didn't he say 'within a week'?"

Here we go. I am on one wavelength, Joe is on another. It's all about getting our needs met. We're each experiencing anxiety over something we can't control: Joe wants the radiation schedule in place, and he wants knowledge and information about it *now*. I want a different kind of plan in place. How will I get to Brigham and Women's Hospital five days a week for seven weeks? I want someone to figure it out for me. And I want it done *now*. I want Joe to do it. Which one of us will change our wavelength and come across to the other's? Maybe it depends on who is needier. When you get right down to it, it's a dance with familiar steps. Who makes the next step, the next twirl, the next back bend? Which step is that? Or, who's going to give in first? That'd be me. And because it will be me, it also shows progress in my recovery. Why progress? I am remembering my steps and automatically following them. That is not to say these steps cannot change—in the future.

"He said, 'a couple of weeks,' which sounds vague to me. And besides, I don't see how we can count on what he said. I got the sense there was a lot he had to do. It's a pretty big task, you know." That's my next move in the dance.

"What's there to do? You've already had your mask made."

"I know, I know." I hear the frustration rising in Joe's voice. You'd think it was his head to be irradiated. For me, I'm glad we haven't heard yet. We still haven't come up with a strategy for transporting me to the Brigham. I don't have a scheduled radiation time yet, but my priority is who will get me there and how.

Initially, I had the idea of staying at a hotel in Brookline, like a lot of out-of-towners from around the country who have no other place to stay. The hospital sent me 10 pages of hotels, motels, B&Bs, and inns, all prohibitive in cost. How do these out-of-towners handle the costs? We are a semi-retired couple from an average middle-income background. That option is out of the question.

A Plan B is kicking around in my head. It involves serious consideration of the many generous offers from our friends to drive me up to Boston. That would give Joe a break, especially on the days he's needed at Bentley. Les, our good neighbor next door, has offered; my friend Nan's husband (he was one of the first); maybe Margo (don't know if she will drive to Boston); then there's Jon and Jan (they're back from Florida). Not sure if there's enough friends on the Cape. There will be seven weeks of driving. I'll need five people a week. I don't want to erode their kindness. It's a long, arduous, and tedious drive from the Cape to Boston day after day. Even as a passenger, I don't look forward it.

Plan C is traveling every day on a bus. A medical bus runs to the Boston hospitals that leaves the Cape daily at 8 a.m. from the Sagamore Bridge (I will need to get to the bridge) and picks up people from the Boston hospitals at 4 p.m. I am a fan of public transportation but not now, not for this reason. I am too vulnerable to depend on the unpredictability of a bus. With the fatigue that may overcome me as the weeks go by, I don't want to be on a bus.

Another week goes by and we still have not heard from Dr. Kahn. Joe wishes I would call, but I don't. If Dr. Kahn is not ready, what can he say? I am still working on my travel. Another idea is starting to germinate. Our son Ken and his wife live in Brookline. They have suggested we stay at their home one of the nights toward the end of the week. Two of my friends off Cape have offered to have us stay with them.

I try to engage Joe's help to consider the options. He's not cooperating. I feel his resistance. I can't figure out what's going on. Slowly, my anger fuse is beginning to burn. He's sitting on the couch across from me.

"I just don't see how…," he begins.

"But it *can* work." I interrupt. "There are many people around us who've offered their help, who want to help us."

Joe looks at me. "Nobody's going to want to drive you to Boston day after day."

"We won't call on the same people. Let's see who we have. Our neighbor, Les, said he could…"

Joe cuts me off. "He doesn't realize what it's like driving into Boston. He doesn't do it that much."

"I plan to ask Margo and Phil."

Another sigh. "How do you know they will…"

Impatiently, I don't let Joe finish his thought. "I don't, but I'll ask them." My voice is going up a notch. "And Nan's husband, Jon. He specifically stated he wanted to give you a break."

"Yeah, and then who?" Joe's frustrated. I can hear it in his voice. "You're going to need a whole lot of people if you don't want to, as you say, 'use them up.' We shouldn't be asking people to do this. We should do this ourselves. I don't see how…"

My brain is starting to fold, I'm getting tired. "It *can* work. Of course we can ask people. There are friends off Cape who said they're willing to help. Maybe we can work some of them into it, too." My mind is feeling muddled. I can't talk anymore. I'm feeling frustration. I want to stop.

"How? I just don't see how that can possibly work."

"I don't know. That's why I'm asking for your help."

Joe gets up and walks away, indicating the conversation is over. That pisses me off, because the conversation is not over. Now my fuse is in full burn. I'm angry. My head feels cloudy. My brain shuts down. I can't reason or think anymore. I storm out of the room and go upstairs. I slam the bedroom door shut.

I'm crying. I'm hurt and upset. Why won't he help me? I can't do this by myself. We have plenty of people willing to help. The biggest barrier I see is Joe.

I do a lot of crying. That's something I have noticed lately—the crying. It happens frequently when my brain gets on overload. Am I waking up new brain cells? Creating new pathways? Don't know for sure, but whatever's happening is emotionally painful to me.

It seems I can't think too much, reason too much, use my brain too much. That can't be it. Must be something else. I am thinking and reasoning now. I have discovered, since the brain surgery, that I cannot journal my thoughts. Don't know why, I'd always written in my journal in situations like these. Instead I spend time thinking and reasoning things out. I think about what my brain has endured so far. The surgery and the physical interference—gloved hands, surgical instruments, specialized saw to the bone, and cement. All that medical meddling in my brain has to have had an impact. My brain was manipulated and moved around. It's still recovering. There's more intrusion expected with the radiation.

I think back to the argument Joe and I had. In the past we hardly argued like that. We were always able to talk it out. Talk it going back and forth. Now I am often at a loss for words. Get confused easily, become impatient and interrupt him, then stir the angry pot because I can't get my point across in an intelligent way. That's it! I can't compete with Joe, anymore. I feel that after what's happened with my brain, I'll never be smart again, or his intellectual equal. Again I cry. I quickly get a sense of myself and stop. I am smart. The surgeon did not take my smarts out with the tumor. My brain and I are still in recovery mode. It's only been three and one-half months.

"Joe," I yell as I come down the stairs. "I need to tell you something."

"Yeah." He looks up from what he is reading.

I sit on the other end of the couch. "First, I'm sorry for storming out on you like that; I don't usually do that."

"No, you don't."

"But I've figured out what's going on with me. I'm trying to compete with you."

"I didn't know we were competing, but...I'll have to think about that. I've been doing some thinking, too." He puts his book down. "We were both brought up by parents who believed in doing it themselves."

I add, "We're in a situation now where we find ourselves needing other people."

"It's hard for me to ask for help—makes me feel weak."

"I know how you feel, Joe, but try looking at our situation another way. We are lucky to have so many friends who want to help. What do you say we let them?"

"Well...maybe...but I don't know where to begin. You have something drawn on that paper there. What is it?"

"Some notes. I have some ideas. Let me go and play with them, and see where we stand."

"Fine, go ahead."

Back in Buffalo when we were in our twenties and I was getting my PhD, Martie started taking courses at the university. It was not clear what they would lead to, but she needed the stimulation and to let me know that she had a brain, too. When we moved to Michigan and I was teaching, she took more courses. A few years later, after we had moved back to Boston, she "announced" one night at dinner that she was quitting her part-time job and going to Framingham State University to get a degree in economics and computer science. I put announced in quotes because that is what is sounded like. She later admitted that she thought I would either resist or make fun of her decision. But I didn't. I think I wanted her to have a professional job because it would make her and our relationship more interesting to me, a selfish motive, but it kept me from resisting.

Years later, after having a successful job in the IT Department at T.J. Maxx, she left again to pursue a Master's degree in clinical social work. That was a big step. She was in her forties and had a job that paid well. By moving toward social work, she was following her dream. It was clear that she would never be able to make the same salary, and that getting the degree would require more than $20,000. I was not sure where this was going, but she had supported me through years of college and graduate school. I believed that it was her dream and that she would make a great social worker. This time my motive was her career.

There is a reason I bring up those earlier decisions here.

During the time we are trying to figure out the logistics of the radiation treatments, I am sitting on the couch reading. Martie comes through the living room yelling, "I have to do everything myself! I figure it out! Nobody helps me! I should know better than to depend on anyone!" She stomps upstairs and slams the bedroom door.

Well...While I was not specifically named, I am clearly the intended target. Give me a break. I am learning to be the caretaker. I don't deserve this. It's not fair.

After a few minutes of feeling the anger boil within me, I take a breath. Why should I be angry? This is not about me. It's about something else.

After about an hour, Martie comes down to "talk." She had spent the time trying to figure out what is going on. She says something profound.

"I can't compete with you."

Wow! I didn't think we were competing. But watch us try to solve a problem together, like trying to figure out why the TV sound won't come on. Competing is part of the relationship. That is why Martie kept going back to school. She wanted to compete in educational achievement and in the income she could provide and, I think, wanted to present herself as an interesting person. I had a PhD and a series of jobs with increasing responsibility. She went after similar goals and achieved them. Now the balance we had worked out without ever saying it out loud is lost. Martie has not just lost her physical balance; she's lost her sense of being my equal. All of a sudden I'm the nurturing caretaker and she's dependent. Does that mean she is also less interesting? I don't see it that way now, but I don't have any idea what will happen over time.

Figuring out the logistics of where we will stay during the six weeks of radiation brought this conflict to a head. The planning is not easy. We know we cannot drive to Boston every day. We are still working. She needs to close her practice in Natick. Figuring out this puzzle is a challenge that Martie wants to solve.

The surgery has changed the equilibrium we had established over 43 years. That change has the potential to cause a major rift in our relationship. If I were to belittle her abilities or make fun of her deficits, it would be a blow to her self-esteem. But I can't just ignore her deficits. So I continue to be cautious about what I say. I don't know yet how to handle the sensitive subject of her limitations. What I really want is the old Martie back. I was comfortable with her. I liked her independence and that she stood up for herself. She's tough and loving, a great combination. And I love her. The new Martie is unsettling. Will meltdowns become part of our relationship? This sucks.

—————

Once feelings from our argument have cleared, my notes transform into plans. If we travel off Cape on Monday and stay over with a friend that night and Tuesday, two nights are covered. Ken and Danielle have offered one night. I 'll ask, how about we stay two, as in Wednesday and Thursday nights? After Friday's treatment we can return home for the weekend. Three phone calls later, to my friends Anna in Natick and Beverly in Dedham, and our son, Ken, and the plan begins to take a shape.

The nights are covered, how about the days—who will drive me into the Brigham? Joe can drive on Mondays, Thursdays, and Fridays. What about Tuesdays and Wednesdays when he works at Bentley? The empty spaces keep staring back at me, like we're in a let's-see-who-will-blink-first contest. I finally put my notebook down. As soon as I do a name flashes in my mind—Linda! Linda lives two doors down from my friend Anna. She is a neighbor/friend I helped several years ago when she successfully endured cancer treatments. A young woman now in her late forties, I know she would love to help me. When I lived across the street from her she did not work, choosing to be around for her kids. Perhaps she is still free during the day.

Linda answers the phone, and I explain the latest stage of treatment and what I need for transportation.

"I'd do anything for you. I'll drive you in every day."

"No, no, Linda," I laugh. "Not every day, just Tuesdays and Wednesdays. That's what I need. You'd be a godsend."

"When do I start?"

"Not sure yet. Waiting on the doc. I'll call you when I get word. I am just so happy you can drive me."

The transportation plan is in place. Joe, however, is not convinced it will work. He has questions. They are all about "what ifs." And the what ifs are typically about things that are out of his control. I understand. Our life has been tilted off its center recently; even the illusion of control is impossible to own these days. And it's the middle of week three and we have yet to hear a word from the Brigham.

"Will you please call him?" I couldn't answer Joe. We had been over this many times. I believe in letting things be, letting it alone. "Leave everything alone in its fundamental simplicity, and clarity will arise by itself." That's paraphrasing a quote I found a long time ago, and I strive to live by it when things in life are out of my reach. I'm sitting on the couch thinking about things and the whole process. Suddenly I realize that if I'm letting go, I am retrieving threads of my lost spirituality. The recognition of a piece of my spirituality causes me to smile. That's another lost piece integrating itself into the new me.

When I first returned home after rehab I wrote what seemed like foreign-sounding phrases on a yellow sticky: regaining my power, not doing it myself, ask for help, accept help, learn to let go, see love everywhere, and Joe is healthy, I am not. Then I remember how I put a slash through the words and wrote, "THIS IS CRAP!" It was not me then. Looking back, I recognize how right I was to understand that I needed to heal on the physical level first.

It was crucial that I felt a strong sense of safety and security before I could focus on the spiritual. First, my body needed to heal from the physical assault of the seizures and surgery. The incision on the top of my head is healing, and my hair is growing back. Walking, left-side functioning, and strength have returned through the arduous physical work. I can now attend to concepts like personal power, or letting go, or looking for the new me. Those views on my spiritual side are slowly coming to life as I feel stronger about my physical self.

My spirituality is how I relate to myself and the world. It's my soul—how I connect with the people in the world around me, how I relate to the "big picture." I believe there is something big, something whole, something divine. My spirituality is how I explain this phenomenon. I call it the "Divine Universe." I call upon and refer to the universe often in my language, as in, "The universe is trying to tell me…," or "I look to the universe to…," or "I ask the universe for help in…" I had possessed a formidable spiritual sense for many years before those seizures pierced my brain. And, a few years before my surgery, my friend Karen, convinced me to take the "Course on Angels" that she teaches. I became enchanted by what I heard. Now I often ask my angels for help when I need it. I notice that I did not reach out to the universe or my angels during my early time of recuperation or rehabilitation. Upon reflection, I see I needed to heal the physical part of my body before I could invoke the spiritual part.

My spirituality is not religion based but love based. Since the brain tumor and all its ramifications for me, and for Joe, I am convinced of the significance of love—especially its outpouring from the Divine Universe. I remember my time recovering in the hospital when I was on the receiving end of an outpouring of love from my family and friends. It was palpable then, and transcendent. I remember telling everyone, "There is nothing else but love!" As I heal, love drives everything, and I strive to hold on to that thought and have it lead me.

———

Two events unblock the impasse. First, one of Joe's colleagues does some investigating and finds Dr. Kahn's email address and gives it to Joe. Second, while I am still in my *"let everything be"* mode, my friend Martha calls. She talks to me about my personal power and questions me about losing it to Dr. Kahn by not calling him. She makes me consider that perhaps I am just a number, and what if I fall through the cracks? I wonder. Am I giving my power over to him? What if I *do* fall through the cracks? I know for sure I have a number—but am I *just* a number? There are so many people who are treated at the Brigham, people who have cancer. I do not. Will they come before me? Oh dear, what should I do? I am in full anxiety mode. Almost over the top. My chest feels tight. It's tough to breathe. It is Thursday of the fourth week of waiting.

What is the universe trying to tell me? I think it's time to act.

I need help with the wording of the email and discuss it with Joe. I send an email to Dr. Kahn—a better mode than a phone call.

"We have a chance of getting to him directly," Joe says.

"You're right. If we call, we'll get Craig or voice mail."

"I'm going to write something about feeling I've been lost in the system, what do you think? I want to make myself heard."

"Sounds good. Go do it."

I press Send. The message is on its way.

The next day a call comes from the Radiology Department. I have an appointment for the following week to begin the radiation treatments. That's four days from today. Was the timing of the call a coincidence? Or did my email move things along? We'll never know.

"Joe," I shout. He's in the house somewhere. "That was the Brigham." Joe comes up from the cellar. "You probably didn't hear the phone, but that's the call we've been waiting for."

"Yay! What did they say?"

"It was Craig. He says I start next Tuesday, the 24th at 2." I wait for Joe to say something; he doesn't. I know he's processing this info. I can tell by the rapid blinking of his eyes. I can't wait. "Joe, I'm starting to get nervous, now."

"Wait a minute, let's talk about this."

And talk we do. There's so much to discuss. Tuesday is not a good day to start. Joe will be working at Bentley that day. Two is not a good time. I won't be able to see my client. I must remember to take Valium. And on and on.

"I feel so narcissistic about all this," I tell Joe.

"What do you mean?"

"Well, thinking that the schedule should revolve around me. I guess with all the healing and recovering so far, everything *has* been *all about me*, and I expect the next phase of my recovery to be that way, too. Now I have to rearrange times with my client, and I haven't figured that out yet."

"I know what you mean. This whole thing—the radiation—is a mess. That schedule you devised is already off course. As for your client, don't worry. Something will work its way out for her and you. It usually does."

Because of his support, and also because I feel heard, there is no anger clouding my thinking, and I come up with a solution for a driver on the first day. Joe works at Bentley on Tuesdays and will not be able to drive me to my first treatment. With whom will I feel comfortable driving me up to Boston from the Cape? My brother, Billy, who lives nearby. Joe nods his agreement. Billy says, "I'm there, what time?" I'm lucky to have him as a brother; he would do anything for me.

Billy and I use the driving time as a way to catch up with our respective families and each other. The second time driving to Boston seems smoother, the directions clearer, the valet parking easier. Billy reminds me as we exit the expressway to take my Valium.

Before check-in I glance in the waiting room and see a familiar face. I check in first and then approach him with a big smile.

"Hello there, imagine meeting you here!" I am standing in front of one of the senior executive officers of T.J.Maxx. He was there when I worked as a financial analyst, and I spent many budget conferences and financial reporting meetings in his office. My role consisted of explaining budget numbers and assisting him in the revision of those numbers. He is peering at me as if he knows me, or should know me. His face lights up in recognition as he thrusts out his hand.

"Martie Dumas, how the hell are you?" He's pumping my hand.

"I might ask you the same. What the hell are we doing in this joint?"

"Ah," he says, as he waves his hand. "It's the best place to be if you've got that C-word." He leans forward and says, almost under his breath, "prostate."

"Oh, I'm sorry."

"Well, I'm in the best place there is. Right? I wanted to be up here, in Boston, where the best doctors are."

"You are living on the Cape, too?"

"Harwich. What's with you?"

"I'm living in Yarmouth Port, moved there full time two years ago and love it. Had a brain tumor in January. Not cancer, luckily."

"I see you've got a cane, you must've gone through a lot—with the brain and all."

"Yeah, paralysis, a two-week stint in rehab, learning to dress myself and walk again, but I'm getting there."

"You know, Martie—how long ago was it that you left?"

"Oh, a long time—'92."

"Hasn't been the same. You did a great job when you were there, working for me, a very good job. I want you to know that."

"Thank you, that's kind of you."

"No, I mean it."

As I walk away and find a seat in the waiting room I ponder our conversation. I'm not sure what that praise is all about. Whether it's his cancer or his retirement mode, I'll take his compliment. I never received any acknowledgements like that during my seven-year tenure at T.J. Maxx. It was not a place generous with its compliments.

I sit and wait to be called. The Valium has cast its soothing net of calmness. I look around. The waiting room is crowded with patients and their families. I'm happy to have Billy with me. If Joe can't be here, Billy is the next best person.

To my surprise, I wait no more than 10 minutes. The executive is called just before me and wishes me good luck. I do the same. Today is his first treatment, also. Carey, my assigned radiation therapist, guides me to the treatment room. I meet the other radiation therapist, Ron, whom I met when I had the mask fitted.

I also meet the Novalis machine for the first time. It's mammoth, taking up space from the floor to the ceiling. It has a large black circle in the middle and strongly resembles a monster. One that comes to mind is a Cyclops—a one-eyed giant from Greek mythology. The Novalis Cyclops has its eye in the vicinity of its navel. The irony does not escape me that the mythological Cyclops forged weapons for Zeus—lightning bolts.

The room is about the size of the small waiting room I just left (20 feet by 20 feet) and to which I want desperately to return. It's cold, surely made that way for Cyclops, no comfort for me. Cyclops is a behemoth hanging from the ceiling, pure white. I imagine it carries a beam from where the radiation will blast my brain, like Zeus' lightning bolts. Even with the Valium, I shudder.

"Are you OK?" asks Carey.

"Yes," I lie. How could I be OK? This is fucking scary. If I don't get eaten alive, surely I will get burned alive. Oh, oh, there go my irrational fears. Did I say irrational? This *room* is irrational. My feelings fit the occasion. I remind myself to breathe.

Ron and Carey both notice my anxiety and immediately go into protective mode.

"We know this is your first time, and everything is new to you, even downright scary, I'll bet," offers Ron.

"Yeah, it is." I am swallowing tears now. I'm not sure I want to do this. All the papers have been signed. Can I change my mind? Run out of the room? Unsign them? Rip them up? I heave a big sigh.

Carey takes my hand and puts her arm around me. "All patients feel like this their first time—especially in this room."

"Everything is going to work out for you, we promise," Ron chimes in. "Dr. Kahn is the best in the world; people come from all over to consult with him. He won't let anything go wrong for you. He has designed a program especially for you. That Novalis machine will not hurt you. It's state-of-the-art and has been tested thousands of times over. Everything here, all of us on the team, are ready to help you through your treatments, and there will be no pain."

"That helps, a little." I wipe away my tears. I appreciate their words. I try to let the Valium work. Usually I don't let strangers see my tears. Look what I received in return—wonderful support. I like this part of the new me.

"Are you ready? There's no rush. The first time usually takes longer."

"Let's go."

Ron escorts me to the table located in front of the machine. Carey helps me onto it. I have difficulty due to lack of strength on my left side. Once my body is settled on the table, I feel cold and ask for a blanket. A strap is then tightened around the table and me, so I won't fall off, I presume. At this point, Carey mentions that the table will move during the treatment, as will the Novalis machine. Swell, I think to myself. Carey also suggests music, and I choose new-age music for its calming effects.

My head is placed into a cradle similar to one used when my mask was fitted. I discover it is the back part of my mask. Screws tighten the mask to the cradle, not me to the mask. The front part is placed over my face. Talk about claustrophobic! This piece of the mask is far from the loose white gauze-like fabric I felt at the mask-fitting appointment. It is hard as a rock, inflexible. My face cannot move. It feels frozen in place. My eyes are closed. There is a gauze opening near my nose. A plastic tab is placed in my mouth to keep it open. And, thank you Valium. Otherwise I might be hyperventilating.

A large plastic depth helmet is placed on the back of my head. The depth helmet encircles the top of my head. I can't feel it, but it resembles a beauty salon hair dryer, only shorter and with small openings for the measuring instruments. These instruments are crucial. They are long, thin tubes that are inserted into the depth helmet. The therapists take several measurements. These measurements are to ensure that the mask is in the correct position for the radiation beams. Carey calls out a set of numbers to Ron and he, in turn, verifies them. If any number does not agree with what he sees on his computer, I must shift my body on the table—making the mask tighter. Ugh. But I know the importance of getting it right. The mask takes the place of the screws of earlier times in keeping the patient's head immobilized. When Carey's numbers on the depth helmet match Ron's on the computer—finally—the first treatment begins.

It feels strange lying here, my eyes are closed. I give in to the Valium and try to drift off to sleep but can't. Carey starts the dreamy music and tells me, "We are ready to begin, good luck."

"Good luck?" Cripes! But she is being kind. I drift off, and the table does its dance. Did they discuss this—the table moving? They must have. I'm not remembering. It sure has jerky movements. I didn't know I'd be in for a ride. Then it stops. I realize I don't know how long the treatment will last. Someone may have told me that, too, but with the information overload I don't remember. I'll just have to wait. The table moves again.

It's an odd sensation to be traveling around a room, all alone, strapped to an examination table, eyes closed, hearing whirring noises, whining noises, loud, strange sounds. Could be somebody's worst nightmare or someone's plot for a science-fiction movie.

Just when I think the mother ship may be landing to take me up to somewhere, the door opens and Carey announces, "Your first treatment is done. How are you doing?"

I don't answer. I'm relieved it's over. She removes the mask. Thank goodness! One down, how many more to go? Carey undoes the strap and blanket and helps me sit up. It takes a few seconds to orient myself. Ron comes over and checks in with me.

"Are you all right? How are you feeling?"

"I'm OK. I'm sure glad I took the Valium. The bed moving around is a bit weird, but I guess I'll get used to it."

"Well, you're an excellent patient. We were able to get through the first treatment without stopping. Congratulations!"

Ron hands me a sheet of paper with my schedule. I notice that tomorrow's time is 8:30 in the morning.

"That's awfully early. Is there any way I can change that to around 10?"

"If you take a look you'll see that by next week, on Tuesday, May 8, where I've placed a star, the schedule shifts to 10:30 in the morning. You're lucky to start now. The 8:30 slot opened because someone finished her treatments earlier than expected."

"Oh, and there'll be no treatment Friday, April 27. The machine is being serviced. We'll see you for two more treatments this week."

Carey guides me back to the waiting area. I need her arm because I am feeling a bit shaky.

As part of my scheduling plan, Billy drives me to Ken's home in Brookline—a 15-minute drive. I discuss my schedule with him. He is, of course, willing to drive me to my 8:30 a.m. appointments. I count and there will be eight—six after this week—before the 10:30 a.m. ones begin. I thank him, but tell him no, I am working on something else off Cape. I guess that will be Plan D.

We expected wrinkles in the schedule but not on the first day. Phone calls to Anna and Robert, our first sleepover, and Linda, my driver on Tuesdays and Wednesdays, smooth this wrinkle away. Anna and Robert are early risers due to their respective jobs, and Linda is up early with her children.

It is Friday of the first week and, as the schedule dictates, we are in Brookline with Ken and Danielle. The first week of treatments is complete and all has progressed smoothly. The 8:30 a.m. treatments occur on time. We have our first weekly meeting with Dr. Kahn. It is short. It's obvious he's observing me. I inform him everything is going well, no headaches. He is excited about his design for my treatment, reminding me of a budding inventor after a discovery in his garage.

"Instead of beginning with a low dose of radiation in the first few weeks," he begins, "and building up to the highest dose by the end of the treatments, I invented a different approach." Here he uses pencil and paper to display it graphically. "My design constitutes generating a low dose, a medium-strength dose, and a high dose for each of the 27 treatments."

"That *is* different from what you described earlier," says Joe.

Joe's answer excites him and he proceeds further. "In this way I can be sure to irradiate all places in the brain and skull touched by the meningioma."

I don't understand the physics of all that is involved, but I do know it means I will get zapped with more radiation and heavier doses than previously planned.

At the same time, I am impressed with the work he is doing and pleased Dr. Kahn is working to help me.

———

Dr. Kahn describes his treatment plan to me and explains why we had to wait four weeks to start. The MRI data he had from Cape Cod Hospital was not compatible with the software in Cyclops. Consequently, he couldn't just give the disk to his physicists to do the computations. He ended up doing them himself—that's why he is so proud of his solution. Every day Martie has three different levels of radiation, each aimed at a different location. The lowest dose is aimed at the widest area, the area where the original, plum-sized tumor sat. The next-highest dose is aimed at the area where the meninges, the membranes that cover the brain, had been cut during the surgery. The third and highest dose is aimed at the remaining piece of the tumor, which had been too risky to remove surgically. That kind of precision and power could not be done without Cyclops and Dr. Kahn. We have, indeed, made the right choice in coming here for the radiation treatments.

———

It's Friday, so we head home. Along the way we discuss how we can manage the next two early Monday treatments, and we agree to take advantage of the special medical rate provided by the Brigham at a hotel in Brookline for Sunday night. That way I will be there at 8:30 a.m. with no worries of driving through Boston traffic. We plan to do this for the following Sunday as well.

Arriving home we're exhausted. I've just begun, and the fatigue that Dr. Kahn mentioned as the treatments occur feels like it's arriving early, like a premature infant. A message on our telephone dismisses that fatigue. My friend Margo is promising a meal. Could we please call?

"I got your message."

"Oh, glad you're home. You must be exhausted." She draws out the word "exhausted."

"Beyond tired."

"How did the week go?"

"Pretty well. Lots of things to tell you, though. Will save it for another time. What is this about a meal?"

"I'm cooking a roast, with potatoes, a salad, and a vegetable. I just need to know how you and Joe like it done and what time I can deliver it."

I'm overwhelmed. She's filled with surprises. Most people would do a casserole, like mac 'n cheese or tuna, not a four-course meal. Too much. Tears flow. "Margo, I don't know what to say. You are too kind."

"Oh, stop. How do you and Joe like your beef done...medium, rare, well?" she persists.

She is serious. She has made a meal for us. I feel as if I don't deserve it. Why? Because I am walking around. I feel fine. I do not feel ill in any way. I am not on my death bed. I finally get a grip on the situation and give her an answer.

"Medium rare. And six o'clock is good, if it is for you."

"It's perfect. I'll see you in a couple of hours."

Joe is staring at me. He has a sense about the phone call. I fill in the details and he expresses not only surprise but gratitude. And he's also hungry. I laugh. That's my man.

Shortly before six o'clock Margo and her husband arrive. The roast is hot from her oven. Everything looks elegant. Sides of mashed potatoes and squash along with a salad of field greens are included. We are introduced to Gorgonzola cheese and Emeril's raspberry vinaigrette dressing. Dessert includes her wonderful brownies. I know the secret in the recipe (she once told me, but I'll never tell!). If the brownies aren't enough, Margo includes two pints of ice cream.

"I didn't know which flavor you like." Finally, she pulls out a bottle of Italian red wine. If I felt overwhelmed talking to her over the phone, I don't know how to describe my feelings now.

"Margo, this is incredible, a gorgeous feast. Thank you, thank you."

"Yes, thank you," adds Joe.

"Oh, but it's my pleasure."

"This is too much."

"And I'm bringing dinner every Friday until your treatments are done."

"But, Margo..." I begin, trying to tell her she can't. I'm not...what? sick enough? worth it? I am speechless. That is love.

After the first week of treatments I realize I cannot continue taking Valium daily. I will be a zombie the rest of the day, and I wonder what I'll feel like by the end of seven weeks. Will I need to increase the dosage as the weeks go along? I need to manage my anxiety another way. For 27 years I practiced meditation. When I returned home from rehab I tried to meditate but couldn't. First some dizziness, then I could not get into the meditation zone, so I stopped. I am ready to try again.

On the Monday morning treatment at 8:30 a.m., I am greeted by Charles and Christy. The routine is becoming familiar. I am strapped to the bed, the mask on my face feels tight, but already I discern from the numbers Charles is reading that I will have to move my body to make the mask fit tighter. I move down a bit. Numbers match computer. Small thin tubes taken out. Depth helmet removed. Lights off. Charles and Christy leave. Music starts. Cyclops begins its whir. Table stirs and shakes. Treatment commences. I try meditation.

I start by taking long slow breaths—in and out, in and out, exhaling long and inhaling long. Next I try my mantra over and over. I am aware of the music in the background. It is soothing. I feel the table jerk as it moves. I hear the machine whir. Back to my mantra. I seem to go deeper and deeper in consciousness and feel less anxious, breathing in and out, in and out. The table jerks again. A whoop from the machine. Back to my mantra. Exhale long, inhale long and slow, back to my mantra, over and over. The table jerks again. Another whoop from the machine, plus a whirring sound. Inhale long and slow, exhale long and slow, back to my mantra, over and over.

The door opens, lights flicker on, and Charles shouts, "All over." Christy helps me sit up and move off the table. Charles is quick to change the sheet for the next patient, a familiar routine now.

"I didn't take Valium today," I announce.

"Really," says Charles. "How did you do during the treatment?"

"Pretty good. I used meditation. I have practiced it for many years and thought I'd give it a try. And it worked. Didn't want to keep taking Valium."

"Hey, that's great."

As Christy escorts me to the waiting room she says, "We often have patients who take Valium the whole 27 treatments, so it's great you found something that can help you."

181

During my walk back to meet Joe, my eyes glance in at the control room where a twenty or thirty computers are arranged in a row. It's astonishing to see that many. Several radiation therapists hover around them laughing and joking. I wonder about their frivolity and if mistakes can be made.

Spending five days a week in the Radiation Oncology waiting room provides me the opportunity to people-watch. On the surface, it all looks calm and orderly. Martie's appointment time is the same each weekday morning, so I see many of the same people, those with times close to hers and the people who come early hoping to get out early.

The first day I notice the heads and hats. Most of the patients are receiving radiation to the head. Some are also receiving chemotherapy elsewhere. Many of the guys wear Red Sox caps. The women's headgear is more varied: hats, wigs, or nothing—proud to show their baldness.

Almost every new patient is accompanied by a friend or family member. I try to figure out who is the patient and who is the companion. The difference is in the eyes. The patients look straight ahead, hoping not to be seen. Their companions tear up seeing a full waiting room. All "eyes" are on the goal: making it to the last day.

Our mates are incredibly resilient. As they tell their stories, it seems to me that, for most, there is little hope for their recovery. But every day they show up for their treatment—we all do.

We are all hoping that the invisible "Force" will defeat or maim the power of disease. You can't see or hear or smell or feel radiation. Somehow it enters the brain and, we hope, kills the enemy cells. The Obi Wan Kenobi doctors also hope the Force is with them. While the treatments are ongoing, they can't tell if what they hope for is happening; they can't see whether the Force is killing the dark cells without doing collateral damage to the healthy ones. The resolution of this battle won't be known for months. The doctors depend on the clinical symptoms reported by the patients to make their guess about the status of the battle. When Martie's only complaint is that she is "as tired as I have ever been" or that the skin on her head where hair once grew feels like a constant sunburn, the doctor

seems relieved that the treatment is proceeding with no signs of serious collateral damage. No headaches or dizziness.

The waiting room has a table with a jigsaw puzzle in progress on it. Once Martie is called for her treatment, I sit and try to fit a few pieces in. It passes the time and gives me a feeling of community; I am passing my limited success on to the next person who sits at the table. When Martie comes out of her treatment, she sits for a few minutes with me at the table to give herself a chance to recover and eat some graham crackers with apple juice. I'm relieved she made it through another treatment. The day can begin now.

Periodically, there's a celebration as one of our mates hits graduation day. The display of feelings is genuine, if muted. Sometimes, the companion will bring a helium-filled balloon. Lots of good wishes all around. I know I will never see them again. You don't voluntarily go back to a Radiation Oncology waiting room to see how your mates are doing. You hope you never will be there again.

It feels good to be working again—at a job I love. And it's a little piece of "*normal*" returning to my life. At the same time my mind is filled with my Natick practice and my clients there. I know what to do. Much of my thinking lately, and some grieving, has been about my practice. Sadly, I must close that office—the one I developed and maintained for almost eight years.

Closing a psychotherapy practice is as difficult as opening one, maybe harder. When do I decide to close? There are all those *good-byes* to clients. In my case, Mother Nature is responsible for the when; it has to happen now. As for the good-byes...

Saying good-bye to a therapist is not the same as saying good-bye to a primary care physician, or a hair stylist, rabbi, or acupuncturist. In my field we have a name for it—termination. While the name may be off-putting, I learned in graduate school, and in my internships, terminating with a client is to be taken seriously. Why? Because of all the deaths and losses we each endure in life. In most of those circumstances we do not get a proper chance to feel the feelings of loss and say a proper good-bye. As we approach termination, psychotherapy work gives both my client and me an opportunity to search for feelings of loss, be they old or current. I encourage the client to feel those feelings. That way the client can safely move on. That's the theory.

Clients are afraid to say good-bye. Who can blame them? We all are. It's painful. The losses in their past hurt again and are painful. Clients present behavior called "acting out." Appointments are made with sincerity and then cancelled at the last minute, or clients don't show up for their appointments. And there are no phone calls to explain. Clients can't be reached by phone. Or, a client will make an important life decision impulsively—with the intent of alarming me. It usually works; I am alarmed. But what can I do? We are discontinuing treatment. Those folks usually show up for the last session—with the sole intent of informing me of their news. Then there are the clients with serious conditions, those who act out by hurting themselves physically. The idea of terminating with me is horribly painful to them. They would rather cut themselves...make a suicidal gesture...or put a hot cigarette to their flesh.

As a therapist, I have been on the receiving end of these type of situations. But now, I feel I am facing the hardest type of termination. I am proud of my practice in Natick. Beginning in 1999, I grew it from nothing. Today it is—was—thriving. But I must end it. I have to say good-bye to all I've built, and then a good-bye to my clients, the people I have treated, served, and helped over the years.

While waiting for the radiation to start, I spent some time grieving over the closing of the practice. Now I am concentrating on my clients. They are in limbo, but probably, correctly presume I will not be returning to Natick to continue working with them. It is critical that I provide clarity as to where things stand.

I confer with my colleagues who are covering for me and inform them of my plans to close the practice. I ask that they wait for my letter to be received by my clients first. After that, my colleagues can begin discussing any feelings my clients may have about closing the practice.

It's a difficult letter, much harder than the first one. It's vital I incorporate several key thoughts. How can I tell them I am closing the practice? All 16 of my clients are troubled in their different ways. I loved working with each of them week after week, or in some cases every other week or once a month. I felt privileged to become a part of their lives, to go deeper with them into their souls and spirits...to provide guidance, empathy, and/or emotional assistance. And sometimes to watch them grow. That was an honor I received in return.

As a therapist, my role encompassed many things, but the main component was listening, in order to create a relationship with them. If I had to give one theory I followed or believed in it is this: building of relationships. If I did not listen earnestly and concentrate deeply on the content of their words, I would lose a sense of them. I needed a true sense of who they were inside—not the surface self they presented to others—in order to help them become unstuck in their dilemmas. I needed to communicate trust so they could feel safe with me. Once the relationship was built, I offer them with tools to cope.

Most of my clients presented symptoms of depression and anxiety. Those symptoms—while real—typically masked something deeper. Over our weeks of meeting together, I would encourage further talking. I am very focused and good at keeping my clients on track. For instance, I am adept at catching clients when they begin a thought but do not finish it. My task is to gently coax them to finish. As in, "No, please continue, you're on a roll." Or, "I think you need to complete that thought, don't you?" Or, "Why don't you finish. I have a feeling it may be important." In addition, I have a good memory. I remember just about everything clients tell me. Often my clients have said to me, "How do you remember all this stuff?" I do not take notes while in the session; I write them after the client leaves.

Once we—the client and I—reach a deeper level, the therapy becomes harder. The real stuff, the hard stuff, the secrets, come out in the open. Once that occurs, it is difficult. After a time, sometimes a long time, of suffering, the problem reveals itself. After some more time—maybe weeks, maybe months, and sometimes not at all—comes painful extricating of information and feelings. Then tears, lots of them. In some cases old behaviors occur: acting out, or clamming up.

I treated people who carried the scars of childhood sexual abuse—men, as well as, women. It's surprising how many triggers occur in their lives, especially when they begin to have children. That's when the most feelings came to the surface. Often those folks begin to act out. They may show regressive, old behaviors, like resuming drinking or tardiness at work, or display new behaviors such as shoplifting, lying, or classic symptoms of depression or moodiness. When that happens, they may not realize what's really occurring. What they need to do is stop, slow down, recognize the feelings that are emerging, and ask why. Once we get to that place, their lives and their children's lives can begin to settle down. But that discovery—of the early abuse—can be a long process. Clients with those wounds are fragile and scared, and I treat every one of them with great care, empathy, and support. One client struggled to retain her oldest child—she lost her three youngest to state custody—because she felt overwhelmed, and she feared she would act out with reckless behavior. Another client had difficulty with her teenage daughters. Both noticed the connection to their childhood abuse and bravely chose to deal with it.

Substance abuse—alcohol and drug abuse—was a tough burden for my clients to carry. Any addiction reminds me of Pigpen, one of the Charlie Brown characters. He's the one with the cloud of dirt that continually surrounds him. No matter what he does, he can't lose it. That's what having an addiction is like—a cloud constantly around you. I've treated clients with 1 day, 30 days, 7 years, and—in one woman's case—7 years of sobriety. Maybe the urge to drink is not there, but the thought is. With an addiction—be it drugs or gambling or hoarding—it's always there. To date, AA is the best recovery aid proven to work. The 12-step program works for many addictions and many people. Sometimes AA was difficult for my women clients because the meetings seem geared toward men. I have attended the meetings to see for myself, and they are right. But I urged them to go anyway and find suitable sponsors and keep an ear open for the AA messages. They need to be there because of the sobriety message, the feelings that are expressed, and the support that can be found.

Early in addiction treatment, denial plays a huge role. That's the hardest wall to break through, especially with a family that refuses to believe their daughter, my client, has a drinking problem. In a case like that, I referred the parents to a colleague and we worked together. That was our plan. Often it doesn't work the way I learned in graduate school.

Loss and grief are devastating issues. Many people come to my practice grieving over a spouse, a parent, a sister, a child—sometimes it was a job. Loss of a child, physically or symbolically, is the hardest to bear. I provided lots of education about grief. Our society is geared for living—not for dying. And when dying occurs, the feelings are "supposed" to go away after the funeral. But they don't; that's when they begin. Most of my clients are surprised at what I teach them about grief. Our work together involved help with coping skills. I gave them permission to feel their feelings when their grief makes an appearance. Anniversaries of special days, such as birthdays, provide occasions for grief. I remind them there are many triggers in their lives, and sometimes grief just makes an unannounced appearance.

Couples counseling presents a different challenge. Often I feel like a ping-pong ball as I listen and watch two sides of the argument/problem. As a therapist, I was taught not to take sides, to be neutral. I find that to be not always helpful. I get better results siding with one partner, then the other. In other words, giving the couple the ping-pong action. I also take sides to teach the other spouse, to force an issue, to empathize with the other spouse, to create a situation, to recreate a situation, allow them to fight, sometimes assist a spouse in recognizing the suffering in the other...all in an effort to effect a change.

Sitting with couples and helping them is often like a dance. My role was to observe and learn their steps before I could participate and work to help them. Specifically I watched how they expressed their feelings, held back their feelings, or sabotaged their feelings. Sometimes the dance worked for them, and they didn't want to stop. What most couples needed was time to be with each other to talk things out. Over time their pain and suffering might dissolve. Hurt feelings and neglect are discovered and atoned for. In one instance alcoholism was unearthed. It had been well hidden, and it took some time to dig it out. But many couples refuse to change. The dance followed a cyclic pattern that, in spite of the pain, they found it easier to deal with than facing what change might bring.

———

My letter begins with the progress in my recovery and the unanticipated complication of radiation treatments. I then announce my deep regrets about closing the practice. The letter goes on to say I will be meeting with them during May and June while I am undergoing my radiation treatments. I stress the importance of meeting to say good-bye, and that I will be calling each one to arrange an appointment. I express my sadness again over closing the office and stopping our therapy together. My letter closes with personal words for each individual client. Each letter begins the termination process for me; I am heavy with grief. Each is a chore to write.

Another wrinkle has creased the schedule. Because there was a month-long wait for the beginning of the treatments, Anna and Robert's guests will be arriving next week, and will be at their home for the month of May. Next week, when we are at Beverly's, I will talk with her about staying more than we had planned. I hope she can fit us in. I hate to ask for more.

My friend Beverly has a warm and generous heart. She gives up her bedroom with its queen-sized bed for Joe and me. When we discuss with Bev the current snag in our accommodations plan, there's no problem.

"You know," she says, "that gives me an idea. I've always wanted to try out those blow-up mattresses. Know which ones I mean?"

"We sleep on one at Ken's house. His is quite comfortable."

"I often have company over, like my nephew, and this would be good for him, too. I could put it in the cellar. Would you and Joe mind?"

Mind? We are thrilled. "Bev, I appreciate this so much. It means a lot to me."

"I'm happy to do it. Besides you and Joe will be my guinea pigs for the blow-up bed."

Friday is the designated day for my weekly visits with Dr. Kahn. I look forward to them, and today I am eager to talk to him. Besides presenting himself as an intelligent and learned young man, he is gentle and welcoming. Today, after my second week of treatments, he asks about my post-op healing and my left-sided weakness. He asks about headaches and other problems I might be experiencing. The familiar neurological diagnostics are next: following his finger with my eyes, pushing my strength against his with my arms and legs, and holding my arms up and out with my eyes closed. He is checking to see if there is collateral damage or a recurrence of the tumor.

"Any questions?"

"I saw the computer room the other day with the radiation therapists." I surprise myself as I start to cry. "What if they make a mistake?" I can hardly talk as my head falls into my hands. I look up at him with tears in my eyes and ask, "What if they push a wrong button?"

Dr. Kahn leans his body forward in the chair. "My dear, you do not have to worry. The program I have designed for you is *foolproof*. No mistakes can be made. First off, the Novalis machine is highly precise and accurate. And, we are the

188

best in the world. People come from all over to study the way we do things here. Because of my design, nothing can go wrong. The people who work for me, my radiation therapists, are skilled technicians. I assure you, no wrong button can or will be pushed."

Relief.

Fridays are also the days Joe and I let out a big sigh. The week is over, we are going home. My treatment time is now 10:30 a.m. That time has more flexibility for all involved in the administration of my treatments: friends who offer sleeping arrangements and my friend Linda, who drives when Joe works at Bentley. This new time allows us to leave the city early on Fridays—before noon—avoiding heavy traffic. We are home at the Cape a little before 1 p.m.

We arrive home to another meal from Margo—mountainous lasagna—such comfort food. She prepared many layers of noodles and loads of hamburger and sausage. The sauce is thick and plentiful. There is so much lasagna that we will freeze it for leftover meals. Fresh blueberries and raspberries accompany the salad of romaine lettuce, with an introduction to a new salad dressing—Margo's own vinaigrette. It tastes nice and sweet. I'll need to get that recipe. This plan of hers—cooking a meal for us every Friday—is a godsend.

———

The following week—week three—I decide to bring my healing shawl into the treatment room. The room is cold. I am surprised that both radiation therapists, Ron and Charles, notice it.

"I've never seen anything like this," says Charles. He caresses the soft weave and carefully places the shawl on me.

"Me either," echoes Ron. He is preoccupied with placing my head in the mask cradle and preparing the face mask.

I'm still able to speak, so I add, "I'm surprised you haven't, especially in a cancer facility and with this machine giving cancer treatments."

"Where'd you get it?" asks Charles.

"My friend from high school, Martha, made it for me when I was first in the hospital."

"It's beautiful, the colors are radiant. You're lucky to have a friend like that."

Before I can agree with him, Ron places the mask over my face. The depth helmet is positioned over my head, measuring instruments inserted, numbers called out. We're back to business.

A few treatment days later as I walk back to the waiting room, I meet Barbara, the team nurse. She notices the healing shawl.

"What's that you are carrying? It's beautiful."

Before I can get a word out of my mouth, I hear a voice from inside the crowded computer room. It's Ron's. He yells out, "It's a healing shawl!" We look at each other and smile. I think to myself, Ron is so business-like and matter-of-fact. I never would have guessed he paid attention to my conversation.

We meet with Dr. Kahn again. He asks about my paralysis, and I mention the continuing debilitation of the fingers on my left hand and the work I am doing to strengthen them.

"What are you doing?"

"Well, besides using the putty, I am playing the piano."

"Oh. Tell me, what are you playing?"

I hesitate because I can't remember. "Right now the name escapes me, but it's the second movement of a Chopin piece. It's for the left-hand only, and the theme sounds like 'I'm always chasing rainbows.'"

Dr. Kahn sports a gleam in his eye and his face lights up. "*Fantasie Impromptu,*" he says.

"Yes! That's it." I am excited about his interest in music. He talks further about his own piano playing.

"Chopin is my favorite. I love to play his pieces."

Dr. Kahn and I have made a connection, different and deeper than just doctor-patient. That warms my heart.

"I hope you will continue playing."

"That's my plan."

———

During May and June, while the radiation treatments are proceeding, I'm ending my job at Bentley University. I have a contract there as a part-time faculty member and consultant that will end on June 30, and I have already chosen not to renew it. The consulting work I do is for a unit called

the Design and Usability Center. They offer services to help companies make high-tech products easier to use. A lot of the work is on the design and assessment of websites for companies who want to make them easier for customers. Over a 30-plus-year career, I have specialized in methods for assessing the ease of learning and use of products, mainly computer software. I have written three books on topics related to those methods, so I have a solid national reputation, which helps Bentley obtain contracts for me to apply those methods and makes me qualified to teach graduate-level courses.

During April I was asked to lead a project with a client that I will call Ajax Company. The design center had previously conducted projects for this company that did not go smoothly. Ajax has a reputation for asking for much more than normal service. For example, the previous contract provided for a final briefing on the project to be given to Ajax senior managers. The PowerPoint presentation for that briefing went through more than 10 iterations and ended up with more than 80 slides. There were additional tasks that we had not agreed to beforehand. The design center lost money on that contract. Consequently, when the opportunity for this new contract came, I was asked to manage it. The hope is that my experience and reputation will allow me to manage the work within our budget. Also the project manager on Ajax's side had been a graduate student in two of my courses, and we had given a professional conference paper together.

I am confident that the project will go well, and I take pride in being asked to manage a tough client. But I will have to stay on top of it and maintain control over keeping the work within a reasonable scope. My Bentley colleagues know what Martie will be going through and offer to shift the project to another senior manager or have it co-managed. I reject their offer. I am an experienced consultant. I don't run away from challenges.

Martie and I talk about the project and the timing. It's a discussion we've repeated over the years.

"Why are you taking on Ajax now? Let other people do it. You've earned the right to coast for your last two months. You can help out without running the project."

"I'm not convinced that anyone else can manage it. Ajax likes to eat contractors. I know I can work with their project leader. He's a reasonable guy. Everyone else is busy, and no one else wants this project because of past history. It's what they hired me for. I slay the fiercest dragons."

"That was before I needed you to take care of me. I need all of your attention, not half of it."

"I just can't coast. I will have two smart student interns working with me."

"There's a reason they're students and you're not."

"You're doing two jobs too: closing your practice in Natick and having the radiation at the same time. We both have professional reputations that we've built over years. We can't just drop our responsibilities. I know you won't, and I won't either. We'll figure it out."

"This feels different."

See, we do compete.

I meet with the Ajax project manager, and we have a frank discussion. He is in a new position and wants to do a good job for his company. He needs to listen to his managers and please them. Part of my job is to help him look competent by following his lead and giving him and Ajax a little extra. During that discussion, we set expectations for each other. I am willing to forget what happened between the organizations in the past, and he agrees to work with his managers if they try to expand the scope of the project without adjusting the cost or schedule.

Years ago I read a book titled *Managing the Professional Service Firm*. In it, the authors make a persuasive argument that a good consultant asks him or herself each day or each week, "What more can I do for my client today?" It's amazing how many useful activities that question stimulates. The successful consultant does more than what the contract specifies or what is normally expected, but without breaking the budget. That strategy is what I will use with Ajax.

Having graduate student interns on the project is a mixed blessing. They are bright, motivated, and fun to work with—as well as inexperienced. I will need to use them wisely. I meet with them and make it clear what each person's role will be and that I must see all emails and slides before our client does. I will lead all phone calls, and I need to know immediately if there are any problems. And, I explain, there will be problems.

"Don't be afraid to bring them to me. The key is finding a solution that works for both companies."

I know I am taking a risk leading this project. If it turns out that I have to work many extra hours, Martie has a right to be upset. I need to support her emotionally, now more than ever. My reputation should be a lower priority. The brain tumor has shifted the balance we had in our careers. In the past I could be confident that she would handle her practice and work out any problems between us. Now I can't be sure what the problems will be and how she will handle them. If she is challenged making dinner, how will she deal with the complex feelings that she and her clients experience during termination? I need to keep the pyramid from falling: at the base is taking care of her emotional and medical needs, then I need to do my contract work professionally, and, just one more block on top, watch over what is happening with her practice.

———

By the third week things seem to be moving smoothly, like today's newer automobiles with their computer chips. All chips are in place and functioning as planned. With the recent calamities—seizures, brain surgery, paralysis, rehab, and now radiation, life feels like it is spiraling out of control. I need to control something. That's why I have a plan. Sleeping accommodations: intact. Drivers to Brigham and Women's Hospital: in place, and on time, and substitutes easy to obtain. Like understudies for a play, they are ready to step in at any time. Radiation treatments: on time. I feel more relaxed using meditation and not Valium. Weekly meetings with Dr. Kahn: exciting piano music discussions. Letters to clients: written and mailed. Phone sessions with Yarmouth Port client: occurring on a weekly basis, and going well.

Joe and I adapt to this new routine. It's our new life. We've gained some balance, if somewhat fragile. Having a structure and a routine that works helps lessen the anxiety of our current situation. It gives me a sense of control over the small day-to-day things, because if I look over the big picture, I have no control.

I know where I lay my exhausted head at night, who will drive me to the Brigham, and that the treatments start on time. The treatments and the day of the week drive my life. If I know which day it is, we both know how to proceed. For me it's easy. For Joe, there's another layer of complication. Bentley College is another aspect to his life, and an important one—it's part of his impressive career. His working group has been awarded a large contract with Ajax. It's also an important one for Bentley. That's providing him with some anxiety, but at the same time I suspect that it's taking his mind off me and all the other commotion in his life.

I begin the termination process and start the phone calls. Everyone is happy to hear from me. I spend phone time recapping my long medical journey, catching up with issues in their lives, talking about closing the office, and finally arranging our last appointment. Initially I set up six appointments a week—two each day on the three days I have office time. The two each day have a space of four hours between them. That will allow me to sleep between client appointments. The fatigue Dr. Kahn promised is beginning to envelope my body. That fatigue is not like any tiredness I have known. The fatigue I am getting acquainted with now, and it is only beginning, is like someone is draping a heavy metal blanket over my body, and closing my eyes—against my will. I feel I have to fight against it. An added annoyance, my hair is coming out in clumps. Soon I will sport another horseshoe-shaped bald spot.

During my first week back to the office I can't see the six clients I scheduled. I see two. Not because any of them cancelled. I cancelled. Physically I could not meet with more than one client a day. I was overcome with fatigue and had to sleep. But the sleep doesn't take away the fatigue. My body is pushing me down, and I am in no condition to talk or listen to anyone. It's typical of me to do more than I can manage. I rearrange my client calendar and reschedule half of them. Those clients experience first-hand my treatment ramifications, and they are angry. Then *they* cancel, causing more rescheduling. I understand. They've been through a lot. I wonder if some will ever show for their last appointment.

——————

Martie and I go through the radiation experience together, sort of. I do everything she does except have the actual treatments. And, of course, I

didn't have the tumor. It's like a research experiment: she's the treatment group and I'm the control group.

These seven weeks of treatments are one of the hardest challenges I've ever faced. I now know what it's like for all of those people who have had a series of radiation treatments. Ironically, my father had a series after his operation for colon cancer. That was back in the mid-1970s. I didn't pay much attention at the time. I can't believe he drove himself to Mass General for six weeks of treatments. I wish I had offered to help, a lost opportunity.

We live out of suitcases during the week and sleep during the weekends. We were told that fatigue was a side effect of radiation. I had no idea how exhausting radiotherapy to the brain really would be for Martie, and me as well. Martie mentions it at our weekly meeting with Dr. Kahn, but he doesn't react. He is listening for other side effects, those that might mean the tumor is growing or that there is collateral damage. It sure feels like he doesn't get how debilitating the fatigue is.

I do some reading about fatigue and discover that there is quite a bit of discussion about it in the medical literature. Most of the articles say it is a common side effect of radiation, but its cause is not well understood. It may be due to the tumor or the radiation. It may also result from lowered blood counts, lack of sleep, pain, stress, daily trips for treatment, and the effects of radiation on normal cells.

Fatigue is not the same as tiredness. Everyone gets tired. In fact, it is an expected feeling after certain activities or at the end of the day. Usually we know why we're tired, and a good night's sleep will solve the problem. Fatigue is less precise, less cause-and-effect. Fatigue is a daily lack of energy, an unusual or excessive whole-body tiredness not relieved by sleep.

There is even a term for this kind of fatigue, "cancer-related fatigue" or CRF. Even though Martie does not have cancer, her tumor had abnormal cells, very active ones. The articles I read say the fatigue starts about three weeks into radiation treatments and usually stops somewhere from three weeks to three months after the treatments are over. It seems that the older the patient, the longer the recovery. And there's this unsettling caveat: some people never get over the loss of stamina that results from radiation.

I am the control condition. I have the same schedule and, I believe, as much stress as Martie. But I am tired and I recover some of my stamina with my 10 hours of sleep every night. Martie does not. She has a couple of long naps a day but is still fatigued. Even though I sleep, I am about as tired as I have ever been in my life. I don't wake up during the night. I am gone for 10 hours. I can't imagine what she's feeling.

Here is a typical week's schedule for me during the treatments.

Monday—up at 6 a.m., finish packing, leave Cape Cod by 8 a.m., drive two hours to Brigham and Women's (B&W's), park, wait with Martie for the 10:30 treatment, retrieve car, drive 30 minutes to Beverly's house—thank you Beverly! Unpack and make lunch. Check my emails using Beverly's computer. While Martie naps, go out to get ingredients for supper. Make supper with Martie, have dinner with her and Beverly, clean up kitchen with Beverly. Make up bed and get in it by 9 p.m.

Tuesday—Up at 7 a.m., dress and work around one bathroom for three people. Drive Martie to Wellesley to meet her friend, Linda, who will drive her to her treatment. Thank you Linda! Drive 30 minutes to Bentley, work 9 to 5 on the Ajax project. Drive to Beverly's, picking up ingredients for dinner on the way. Make dinner together, eat with Beverly. Pack up suitcases. Make up bed and get in it by 9 pm. Too tired to read.

Wednesday—Up at 7a.m., dress and work around one bathroom for three people. Load up the car. Drive Martie to Wellesley to meet Linda, who again will drive her to her treatment and to Ken's afterward. Thank you Ken! I drive to Bentley, work 9 to 5 on project. Drive 45 minutes to Ken's in Brookline, unpack. Decide what to eat, go with Ken to get take-out meal. Eat with Martie, Ken, and Danielle. Get in bed by 9 p.m. Too tired to read.

Thursday—Sleep till 8 a.m.! Dress and drive Martie to her treatment at B&W's. Wait with her. After treatment, go to patient services to get reduced fee parking tickets for the next week. Retrieve car and drive back to Ken's. Work on project from my laptop computer and make calls about project. Check emails on Ken's wireless network. Too tired to take a walk, even though I should. Decide what is for supper and go out to get ingredients. Help with supper and clean up. Spend time with Martie, Ken, and Danielle talking over the week's events. In bed by 9 p.m. Too tired to read.

Friday—Up at 7 a.m. Dress and remove sheets from bed. Pack and get suitcases, etc. into the car. Drive to B&W's. Wait with Martie for treatment. After treatment, wait to see Dr. Kahn, always good to see him each Friday. He checks Martie out and asks if all is OK. Retrieve car and drive two hours to Cape Cod. On the way, talk about week's events, fill car with gas. Arrive home about 1 or 1:30 p.m. Open house, get a wash started, and take a long nap. More wash. Margo comes with dinner—thank you Margo! In bed by 9 p.m.

Saturday—Get the week's mail from neighbors. Sort it. Pay bills and go to bank and post office. Take trash to dump. Do minimal house cleaning. Do a food shopping run. Make calls to update my sisters and Martie's siblings. Screen calls for Martie, making sure she has the energy to talk, or I fill in the caller on progress. Make a meal, which tastes good after eating other people's food all week.

Sunday—Read the paper and take a short walk with Martie. Cut the grass and do minimal weeding. Nap. Finish my work on my laptop computer. Catch up on emails. Call Tim in Montana to keep in touch and fill him in. Pack for the next week and in bed by 9 p.m., exhausted. Too tired to read.

———

The first two weeks fly by, and while they are tiring, the novelty makes them easy to deal with. By the third week, the tiredness begins to overwhelm me. The 10 hours of sleep every night are not enough. I feel like I am always going uphill. I can't imagine how Martie feels. Watching her I can see her slowing down and sleeping more, morning and afternoon naps. The uphill climb each day starts when the alarm goes off.

Some days it's hard to keep my concentration at work. The client for the project is demanding, though not unreasonable. It is nothing I haven't dealt with many times in my career. But these days, I just want to curl up under my desk and sleep. My Bentley colleagues are great, offering help. But they have their own projects, and I want to show them that I can deal with a demanding client. I don't think they ever doubt that, but I am not one to ask for help—ever my mother's son.

I begin to dread Monday mornings. Getting up and out of the house is a challenge. As the weeks go on, Martie slows down and has trouble making decisions. It seems to take her forever to get ready. She has not learned yet that she needs to plan for extra time. It's hard to be calm and not show when I am annoyed. She doesn't need more pressure. But for me, there's no way to let off steam. Getting mad at her doesn't make sense. She isn't the problem. But what do I do with the anger? Stuff it for now.

While Martie is more tired than I am, she is calm and emotionally grounded. I don't know how she does it. My guess is that she is blocking out everything except what she has to do next—a valuable protection for now. Keep putting one foot in front of the other and don't think or feel. No time for anything that gets in the way of moving forward.

———

"Now's your chance to be a blonde."

"Get one with straight hair."

"You can get a fall and have a pony tail."

Fun and positive comments come from friends and family when I announce that I'm shopping for a wig. Dr. Kahn said I will lose my hair and suggested I buy one. Here I am, with Joe, at Robert's Hair Salon. I do not feel enthusiastic. It's not fun. My spirits are low. Some women may find this part of the treatment enjoyable. I do not. In my younger days my scalp sported beautiful dark chestnut brown hair with a natural wave and some curl. Over the past 20 years, it has transformed itself into a nice salt-and pepper look for which some women pay dearly at the hair salon. Right now it has a ragged, tired look—probably reflective of what my body is enduring.

Mr. Robert has a gentle way about him, and he is patient. He's sees that I don't know what to do or how to proceed. He brings one, then another. Finally I announce, "How about a white one, about the length of my hair." I try it on. It looks great, but it reminds me of my mother-in-law. I can't wear that. I try a blonde wig, and I look ridiculous. It clashes with my skin tone. The end of blonde for me. Many sighs and wigs later I decide on a model called "The Nancy." What a stupid name, but it looks exactly like my hair style.

"I will probably never wear it, but I'll have it just in case," I tell Joe as we leave the salon.

"Just in case of what? Rain?" he teases.

"Who knows?"

———

"How's the *Fantasie Impromptu* coming along?" Dr. Kahn begins our Friday meeting.

"Quite well. The fingers on the left hand are becoming stronger, particularly my little finger. I think I'm ready for something else. Any suggestions?"

"If you have any Bach, he has some pieces stressing the left hand."

"I have his *Two-Part Inventions*. I will look in there."

Dr. Kahn nods in agreement and then proceeds with the medical and neurological probing. He tests the strength and agility in my limbs and uses his light to command movement of my eyes. He inspects my horseshoe-shaped bald spot and notices the redness. He sends Barbara to the apothecary for cream. I report no headaches.

We head home to the Cape and look forward to another meal provided by Margo. Joe and I find that we look forward to her meals and realize the magnitude of her generous offer—week after week. She prepares fried chicken for our third week home. Talk about finger lickin' good! And it's hot. It's complemented by an iceberg lettuce salad with Paul Newman's raspberry vinaigrette dressing. Margo wasn't sure which dessert we would like. She brings two: her homemade butterscotch-oatmeal-raisin cookies and ice cream.

The following Friday Joe and I are unbearably fatigued. The effects of the radiation are hammering me harder, and the routine, plus the Ajax contract work, is showering a tiredness toll on Joe. We are fortunate we can nap instead of worrying about a meal. It's a whole roast chicken with a brown crust, accompanied by mashed potatoes, au jus gravy, and Margo's own broccoli-raisin salad. She never forgets dessert; today it's her own recipe for key lime bars.

———

It's Tuesday of week five, my client calendar has been rearranged, and it is working better with one client a day. My plan is fixed—again.

Joe and I are taking our usual morning walk at Beverly's before he takes me to meet Linda.

My cell phone rings. "The machine is broken," says Ron, my radiation therapist. My mind goes to the Cyclops, and I picture it crumbled to the ground dropping a tear from its one eye. "You don't need to come in today."

I don't know how to react. I feel like throwing the cell phone on the ground. Instead, I burst into tears. I cry hard as I mumble my words. "Joe, I can't do this anymore. I've tried, really. This is too much. All these things in place, and now the machine is *broken*. This is going to extend the treatments well into June. Can't do this...Can't do this...Not gonna do this...How can they expect me to? I'm so fuckin' tired. Trying to close my practice...All my plans to make this work...I give up." I cry so hard I hiccup. It's as if all the emotions I have held in since January are bursting through the dam, and I am willing to let them roar out of my body in this purge. Everything is falling apart.

Joe is befuddled. He's not sure what's happening. But he's trying to console me. At the same time he is trying to pull information from me so he can understand what just happened.

"What was that call all about?"

"The radiation therapist..." My words mingle with sobs. "No treatment today...machine broken...getting part from Europe...call tomorrow." Now I am freaking out. "I can't do this." I sob into his chest and he just holds me.

Finally after more minutes of sobbing, I take a breath and wipe away the tears.

"Start over," he says "Ron says the machine is *broken*, how many times do I need to say it?" I blow my nose. "They're waiting for a part. It's being FedExed from Europe. Maybe tomorrow. I have to call to see if the part arrived and if the machine is fixed and operational for a treatment."

Now Joe feels the impact of this new and is stunned. "We're almost at the end...two weeks to go. Our plans depend on it ending in two weeks. What does this mean?"

"I don't know. But right now I need to catch Linda before she leaves the house, and tell her what's going on."

After reaching Linda, Joe and I talk more about our latest bombshell.

"If the part's coming all the way from Europe," I say, "It's hard to believe Cyclops will be up and running by tomorrow. I'm thinking of going home."

"You could be right. It's a chance, though."

"It's a chance I'd like to take. The client I had today rescheduled, and it's a beautiful day in May. Let's go home to the Cape and have lunch on the beach."

"I'm not sure. Hmmm. I do have writing to do for Ajax. I could do that at home. Lunch on the beach sounds great. I think we've earned it. Let's go."

I'm sitting on my favorite beach, Corporation, with my toes playing in the sand, and it feels heavenly. It's just warm enough to not need a coat. I'm reading a book, but at the same time, I savor the scene. I breathe in the sea air and watch the sea gulls hover. The tide is going out, and the waves travel gently across the sand. Blue sky surrounds me with a dozen dancing puffed out clouds that drift in the breeze. It's the week before Memorial Day, the time before the official start of summer, and I feel like I'm playing hooky.

With all my planning, my fretting, working so hard to get all the pieces into place, the one thing I never counted on happens—the machine breaks. I am reminded of a kindergartener using blocks to make a tall building. She builds each block up to a new level, and someone comes by and pulls a block out, crumbling her structure. She persists as another pupil takes a block from her foundation. She continues to build up, replacing the lost blocks each time, until finally she achieves her desired height. Her building is finished! Along come two bullies, running around the corner, and they smash into it. Her building falls to pieces, and she cries hard in frustration. Just like the machine, my bully smashed into my plan. And just like my kindergartner, I cry—a lot. I give up—and I give in—to the situation.

Joe is in the chair beside me soaking up the beauty. I thrust my arms up toward the sky in a stretch, relinquishing all to the universe. I bask in its beauty and enjoy this free day. Tomorrow...who knows?

———

Two days later Joe and I sit in the waiting room. It's Thursday. I did not have a treatment on Tuesday or Wednesday, and today all the staff is hoping the machine will be fixed. My rescheduled appointment is for 6 p.m. I don't know how the earlier part of the day went for the other patients, but I notice the overflow in the waiting room. I can't imagine their long wait. Now I'm part of the mix. And no one knows what's happening.

Reminds me of being in an MBTA subway car. Unexpectedly, the car jolts to a stop and the lights go out. Passengers are sitting or standing, holding onto straps. They are packed tightly together, all wanting to get home, be somewhere else. Nothing is happening, and no one is telling them what's going on. All they want is information.

Right now there's nothing to do but unite with the others here...and wait. The body language of the other patients speaks loud and clear. Heads bowed, arms folded, eyes closed: do not talk to me. Joe joins a couple of family members at the table, and together they pass the time fitting together the 1,000-piece puzzle. I note the irony to myself. I have many fragments in my life that I am struggling to piece back together. It seems as though Joe and I were just beginning to shape a life together—albeit a new one—when we learned: *radiation is not an option, it's a necessity.*

That news put us into another tailspin, knocking down the few new pieces we had fashioned together. Ever since that train wreck of a tumor came roaring into our life, we have been changed forever. That first seizure, heralding the fast-growing tumor, smashed into our orderly life. No, I'll say it like it was—a perfectly ordered life. I admit: I was a perfectionist. Had to have everything just so, and in place, and in order. I like order and knowing where everything goes. That way when I want something I'll know where it is. I like things clean. I like to be on time. Call me compulsive. I admit it. My perfectionism and need for order helps reduce my anxiety. Recovering from brain surgery and paralysis, learning how to dress myself in a different way and discovering how to walk again change my perspective. As I recover and heal, my perfectionist attributes—some of those pieces—will probably be put back into my life. Perhaps in a different manner. It's part of who I am.

Today our life together feels new and at the same time strange, like untested terrain. Joe is in a caregiver role, always vigilant and helpful. I am in a vulnerable role and need his care and protection. That's the reverse of the independent two-career-couple life we lived and thrived on. We have a table full of pieces to put together in our life puzzle—our new normal. We're discovering that some of the pieces we find from the wreckage don't interlock the way they used to. Our reconstruction continues.

As it happens I do *not* have a treatment. Around 8 p.m. we are informed. "Definitely tomorrow, though. Be at your appointed time, 10:30 a.m." We leave for Ken's, tired and frustrated, ready to resume tomorrow.

My 10:30 a.m. treatment is delayed by 20 minutes, but it happens. Because it's Friday, we wait around for my meeting with Dr. Kahn. He keeps it brief; there are many patients waiting. The breakdown of the machine has thrown off everyone's schedule. Everyone is tense. He omits mentioning the number of treatments I must receive in a week. I received two this week—Monday and today. Before I leave the department I see Barbara and check with her. She assures me I've had enough treatments for the week. I'm doubtful, but I breathe a sigh of relief. It's the beginning of the Memorial Day weekend, and we are anxious to get out of the city and home before the explosion of people and summer visitors—a.k.a. tourists—take over the Cape for the week-end.

People travel to the Cape from as far north as Quebec and as far south as Florida. They travel from New Jersey, Connecticut, Rhode Island, and throughout the Northeast. On this weekend they travel on three- and four-lane highways that converge onto a two-lane highway, causing a choking congestion as they attempt to cross over one of the only two ways of getting onto the Cape Cod peninsula, the Bourne and Sagamore bridges.

After a quick bite to eat, we finally get out of the city and onto the expressway. My cell rings. It is Charles, one of the radiation therapists.

"Martie, you'll have to come back for a treatment. You didn't receive enough this week for it to be effective."

"What? I was told I could leave."

He ignores my response and continues. "We did a check on everyone and most of you have to come back over the weekend."

"Oh, no. Do I have a choice about which day?"

"Saturday or Sunday, you choose."

"I'll take Sunday."

"What was that all about?" Joe asks.

"I need another treatment for the week, I didn't have enough."

"I wondered about that."

"I even asked Barbara about it. You heard her; she said I received the right amount for the week. Arrrggghhh."

"Well, I'll take you up..."

"No." I cut Joe off. "You're tired and doing a lot already. I'm going to ask my brother."

"You've asked him before."

"Yes, but I know he'll do it if he can. Besides, you've done a lot of driving. I don't want you driving to Boston. This has been a tough week on you, too. I see how exhausted you are."

"OK. But only if he says yes. If not, then I'll drive."

"Deal."

We continue the ride in silence. We're both tired, and I'm sure Joe is processing the events of the week, as well as today's. We're making good time. All we want to do is get home, unpack, and take a nap. And we have one of Margo's meals to look forward to. Traffic is moving smoothly, we are cruising at 70 miles per hour. About 10 miles from the Sagamore Bridge, Joe switches WBZ News Radio's "Traffic on the 3s." News is first. We hear a driver with a boat on his trailer is stuck on the Sagamore Bridge, causing the traffic flow to decrease from two lanes to one. We both let out a cry in the car: "Oh, no!"

Access to the Sagamore Bridge was recently reconfigured from a rotary to a straight flyway in order to ease the flow of summer traffic. As Cape Codders, we endured the construction and inconvenience of using a one-lane bridge for about eight months. Here it's the first weekend of the summer and, once again, only one lane is open. We hear this jolting news in time to take the exit to the other bridge—the Bourne Bridge.

For us, we experience firsthand what summer folks do. The bumper-to-bumper sea of autos, the stop-and-go movement of the car, barely going three miles per hour, and the unspeakable frustration. It takes us one and one-half hours to travel five miles: a stretch of road leading to a rotary, once around that rotary, and across the Bourne Bridge to the highway that takes us home. Once home we find our respective favorite areas to nap. We are both so irritated we can't talk. Home feels especially good today. It's been a long week. We find it hard to believe we came home for a few days in the middle of the week and had lunch on the beach. Seems long ago.

However, Margo provides us with a renewal for our spirits. She delivers a sirloin tip roast, pink and medium rare. It's on a huge platter with smashed potatoes and squash. A salad of fresh crisp romaine lettuce is included with Paul Newman's raspberry and walnut vinaigrette.

"Margo, you're amazing! You're doing too much. After the week we've had, though this is so-o-o very special."

"That's why I'm doing this for you; it has to be hard."

I nod my head. "You're right. My humble thanks to you.

"See you next week. Will it be the last?"

"Not sure." I give her a brief version of the events of the week.

"How awful." She gives me a strong hug.

———

When Martie and I began our senior year of high school, we both fell for the same ploy. The teachers. Christian Brothers and Notre Dame nuns, claimed that if we wanted to get into college, we needed to have a list of extra-curricular activities on our application. Colleges were looking for well-rounded applicants. So we were told to join the many clubs and activities available. Other than being on the track team, I had no other activities. I needed to find something to make me appear "well rounded."

During my first two years of high school in the seminary, I had taken speech classes. I lost my fear of talking in front of a group. My high school didn't have a debating club but it was scheduled to put on a senior play. Dramatics would be a way to document my well-roundedness on my college applications. I joined.

The head of dramatics was Brother Michael—a young Christian Brother. He chose *Ten Little Indians* by Agatha Christie as our first-semester play. I tried out and won a part. I had one line but it was the first line of the play. I didn't know Martie at that time but she was picked to handle the props and to be a prompter when an actor forgot his or her lines. There were two to three rehearsals a week. We all got to know each other better. I knew the guys but in our school the boys and girls were on different sides of the building. So for the first time I was around girls my age on a regular basis. They got my attention.

At one of our rehearsals Brother Michael was called away for a phone call.

"Martie, you're in charge. I want everyone to continue rehearsing as if I were here." Off he went. We continued to rehearse for a while. As a bunch of 17-year-olds, we were easily distracted. I think the sound that started us down the wrong path was a fart. There was nothing funnier to a boy like me than a fart. We guys burst out laughing. The reaction from the girls was delayed but soon they joined in. We rehearsed our farting noises and rolled on the floor with laughter. It was impossible to stop. What fun, laughing uncontrollably with girls about farts!

From within this chaos I heard a raised voice: "Stop it! We are supposed to be responsible seniors. Brother Michael expects us to be grown-ups." None other than my future wife. A voice from my unconscious said, "That's the woman for me." Like throwing gasoline on a fire, all of my adolescent passions exploded.

After we performed the play twice to a packed auditorium, the school gave all the actors and crew a dinner and dancing at a local hotel. That night Martie and I danced, and I asked her to be my date at the Christmas Cotillion. About 50 years ago. I will never know if being in the Dramatics Club helped me get into college but it did provide the opportunity for me to meet my lifelong mate. All because we both fell for the ploy.

———

Martie and I are each ending a phase of our careers: she is terminating with her last few Natick clients and I am facing the final briefing on the Ajax project, which will be my last project at Bentley. On Tuesday morning we drive together off Cape. I drop her off in Natick then make my want to Bentley. A graduate intern, Beth, and I go over the PowerPoint slides one last time. The deck will serve as our final report. The project went well in my view. We collected data from customers and we have some useful recommendations based on our results. Over the past three weeks the slide deck has been back and forth between us and Ajax. They have been refining the message they want us to give to their managers. The negotiations over the slides have been professional and productive. They have an insider's knowledge about the politics of their organization and they know how far they can push on key issues. I know what our data shows and I want to make it speak to Ajax's business goals.

We focus on adding some pictures to the slides to illustrate points and make them more lively. I email the final version to Ajax so there are no surprises. We then load the slides onto my laptop and make a backup of the file on a thumb drive. The backup file may be needed if we use their computer to show the slides. I am ready to leave to pick up Martie to have dinner when I receive an email back saying that they have a few final changes they would like. I am not happy but this the way the high-tech world works these days. Clients have the expectation that you will be available via email or cell phone 24 hours a day. They think that because they are working late, you should be. To my relief Beth agrees to make the changes and bring the new file to Ajax tomorrow.

I pick up Martie and we load the last few items from her office into the car. We are alone as she walks around the room one last time. It has been a good setting for her. She built her own private practice against the odds and made it a success. Over the years we spent many hours talking over the challenges she faced with her clients. Her approach is to make a connection with each one hoping to gain their trust. Without trust, they will never open themselves to reflection. In my view, many of her clients had spent their adult lives avoiding connections and sabotaging relationships. Hearing about them I was often frustrated. They lie and hide key facts. What frustrates me the most is their lack of or extremely slow progress. Many don't or won't change.

Perhaps my frustration is really caused by seeing myself in them. I had my own therapy for several years. I know that there were topics I would not go near, such as my anger at my mother and Martie and what I was avoiding by working so hard. Even though I trusted my therapist, I did hide some things from her and progress was slow. But I received enough insight to feel more comfortable with myself and be happier. For that I am grateful to her. I never made it as far as I and my therapist wanted to go. For me, it was too frightening. In the end, we agreed that if I chose to dig deeper, I could come back. I am not so different from Martie's clients after all.

We check in at the Red Roof Inn. Martie's exhausted. She takes a nap and I go over my slides one more time. The next morning, we drive to

Ajax's headquarters and I ask my client if he has as place for Martie to stay while I do the briefing. He knows her and her condition. He finds a conference room and gets us some water. Beth arrives with the new slide deck and we go the auditorium to set up. The room is not too large, about 50 seats. I make sure that I know how to run the projector and I run through the presentation in my head.

I go back to the see how Martie is doing. She has attracted a crowd. There are several of my former Bentley students there who now work for Ajax. Everyone wants to know how she is doing and I can tell she is pleased. Amazing how she makes a connection with everyone there. The fact that these people would take time out of their day to visit is heartwarming. I suspect that they wanted to see for themselves if Martie had changed from her pre-tumor days. Except for the bald spot, she looks the same. There's lots of positive energy in the room.

Time for the presentation. Beth and I had agreed how we would split up the briefing. I begin with a project overview and try my best to project a sense of competence. Inside, I'm a bit nervous. I didn't have much time to think about the final changes and I'm anticipating some resistance to our findings and recommendations from some of the managers, especially from one who insisted on a design concept that the customers rejected. If he's defensive about his brain child, he might challenge my data. I try not to let my inner turmoil show, project confidence and a feeling that I understand their business goals. It goes well. The 60 minutes flies by and everyone leaves for their next meeting or to read their email. My Ajax contact thanks me for everything and I thank him for the positive working relationship. I believe I was correct in thinking that I was the right person to lead this project and to solidify the relationship with Ajax. I slayed another dragon and I feel good about myself.

Back in the conference room Martie is still holding court and I have a chance to catch up with my former students on their careers. Martie and I pack up and get on the road.

"No more Red Roof Inn," I rejoice."

"No more Ajax. We can spend the summer relaxing."

"And next month you can start driving again. That'll be another positive step." As soon as it comes out of my mouth I know I have stepped in it again. Driving is something else to worry about. I suspect that Martie is afraid to drive. I think she feels cared for when I drive. And we have an unspoken concern that another seizure could lead to an accident. But having to drive all of the time suffocates me. I don't have any time to myself. At home I take care of Martie's needs and I drive her most places she needs to go, including to her Yarmouth Port office to see clients and then back home again. I would like some time to myself. I don't see how that can happen any time soon.

Saying the wrong thing sometimes is part of the mine field that is caregiving. In any relationship there are events that provoke distress or anger. Married people come to know the topics that are likely to set their partner off. In our relationship, Martie and I tend to stay away from those topics. Occasionally, we do end up talking through a conflict. But most of the time we would rather avoid a confrontation. That may not be entirely healthy but it has worked for us most of the time. With me being the caregiver, I have a new set of taboos, issues to avoid and feelings to keep to myself. I cannot belittle or made light of Martie's limitations. Even though I don't want to say those things, sometimes words come out that could be interpreted as doing so. I may have said this before, but it takes Martie forever to get ready to leave the house. I know that this is a common issue with couples. Men throw on a coat and are ready to leave; women have to primp, make wardrobe choices, take that extra look in the mirror, etc. But Martie's cognitive and physical limitations add even more time to her preparation. It takes her longer to put on clothes and make decisions. And she worries more about being cold, locking doors, trying to remember what she wants to take with her. It's frustrating to me and I frequently start to get angry. I don't feel that I can express my feelings verbally, even with a sigh, or with my body language. So I try to relax and go outside into the yard and look at the health of the bushes or pick up debris. Eventually she is ready and we are off.

So by bringing up her driving, I have let out that I am tired of taking her everyplace. It puts pressure on her to start driving, something I did not intend but if she doesn't start she can't get back to it. I should have waited for the right moment instead of ruining her expectation of a relaxing summer. I decide not to apologize, just keep it to myself.

———

Radiation treatments are over. I had my last one this morning. I'm done. Cooked. Now what? I'm so tired. That's the fatigue from the after-burn of the radiation. That's the fatigue from beginning to say good-bye to some of my clients, and to my practice. That's the fatigue from all the scheduling and logistical maneuverings to make everything happen. I just want to sit down on the sidewalk here at Beverly's and cry. What am I doing? What have I just done? Why did I agree to these treatments? I'm so tired and irritable, and I have no answers. Nobody knows whether the radiation was effective. I don't want to wait until tonight when Joe gets here from work.

I have four weeks of client appointments to finish. Joe has Boot Camp at Bentley next week. And his final presentation for the Ajax is on the horizon. That must be a big project for him, as well as Bentley, because I've been hearing about it for the past few weeks. There's so much jumbling around in my head, but I glimpse a point of light. I remember my friend Joan. She had a gentle but emphatic tone to her voice when she called a few weeks ago. "If there's anything I can do for you, please let me know. I will come and get you and drive you anywhere."

"Joan, it's Martie. I'm in Dedham right now; my radiation treatments are done."

"Oh, I'm so glad they're over for you. What can I do for you?"

"A big favor. Would you come up here and drive me home? It's early in the day and I don't want to hang around until five waiting for Joe."

Joan is happy to make the drive. I gave her directions to Beverly's house, and I am home before lunch. As crabby as I felt earlier, I am happy and home.

My client calendar in Natick is filled, as is Joe's Bentley calendar. How will we manage getting me to Natick? Who will drive me to my practice? After all the friends I've asked favors from, somehow I feel immobilized and cannot ask anymore.

"Joe," I begin, "how will I get to my practice during June."

"I don't know." He goes back to reading the paper.

And here the conversation stops. Dead. That has an all too familiar rhythm to it. Anger joins the rising frustration. I'm not analyzing our situation here, not thinking about his needs, I'm thinking only of mine. I let out a puff of air. That's when I find myself yelling at him.

"Why do I always have to do it myself?" I kick the front screen door, acting like a five-year-old, but I can't take hold of my actions. It's like they have a life of their own. I barge out the door. "I am so angry...and pissed." I repeat these words over and over as I walk down the street, around the block, and around the block a second time. A second time because my anger hasn't dissipated yet. I realize Joe doesn't have the large pocket of people resources that I do. It will be up to me to sort out the ride situation.

"I guess I overreacted, huh?"

"Hmmm, at least we don't need a new screen door," Joe laughs.

Later we both look at our calendars and note that we will need to stay overnight only twice. I feel relieved. We can stay at the Red Roof Inn.

Some of my May clients are rescheduled in June. Some cancel, and some act out by not showing up at all. For the clients who do show up, it's a spiritual moment. I'm overwhelmed by the emotion each one evokes. It demonstrates the strong connection we shared over the years in our work together. I'm fascinated by the way each session plays itself out in a similar fashion. After the initial greeting and sharing of "so happy to see you" and "glad that you are OK," each client automatically drops into session mode with a current need. We work on that for a while. During that time, in my head, the words "we need to say good-bye" are rolling around. Just before the session ends, I introduce those awful words. We talk about it for a bit, how hard it is, and what the future will be for each of them. I offer a referral. Most refuse, but some will remain with the colleague who covered for me. Our good-byes are weepy. I cry after each one, after they leave, when the office door is closed.

I schedule my clients so I can nap in between or take a long break. It's the last week of June and I have a four-hour hiatus. After lunch and a nap I spend time sitting in Natick Common saying my good-bye to the town—the town I lived in for 30 years, the town in which my children grew up and learned about life. I feel misty-eyed as I look around.

There's the hardware store where I bought wallpaper. I papered all the rooms in my home myself. Across from it are the post office, our dentist's office, and the funeral home. We attended services for many friends there. Adjacent to that is the new town hall. What a difference from the old one. Across the street more tax dollars are reflected in the new library. Adjacent to the library is the old Congregational Church—established in 1631. It has a beautiful steeple. One year while watching the Boston Marathon runners come through town, we observed two runners look skyward and say to each other, "This must be Natick." It was years before I discovered they were looking at the steeple, which is a landmark along the race route for the 10-mile mark. Across the street from the church is Bakery on the Common—one of my favorite places. The sugar content is high, and the items containing that sugar are delicious. I've met many friends and colleagues there for breakfast and lunch. When I worked nights at my office, I would often grab a sandwich there for my evening meal in between clients. This is a poignant moment for me.

Out of the corner of my eye I notice a young father with his twin daughters, probably close to a year old. He's playing with them on this beautiful sunny June afternoon. Their big black dog accompanies them. That scenario looks like it could be my son, Tim, and I know how much he wants a family. He and his wife have been waiting so long to hear from China about adopting a little girl. I laugh with the young father, but at the same time I feel angry at the universe for not speeding things up for Tim. He will make a good father.

Back in the office waiting for my next client, my telephone rings.

"Mom, I have some news." It's Tim, from Montana. I'm wondering why he's calling me. "The agency called us this morning, and we're going to get our little girl from China!" We are both crying now.

"Oh, Tim, when will you go?"

"We don't know any of the details yet, just that she's almost two years old, and she will be ours." Tim reminds me I will be a grandmother.

"Where's dad? I want to tell him."

"Call him on his cell."

"OK."

"Congratulations, Tim, and to Joanna, too. So happy for you."

Joe and I have dinner at the Dolphin, a local restaurant. We celebrate our 43rd wedding anniversary and we celebrate grandparenthood. Surely the worst is over.

DISCOVERIES

I am depressed. Or I think I am. I've felt down for some time. Moody. Irritable. Sad. Not sure if my feelings, or symptoms, measure up to the DSM-IV. That's the statistical and clinical bible used as a reference by mental health professionals to determine a diagnosis of depression in a client. Hmmm, do I meet the two-week-or-more-duration of symptoms criteria? Probably. I've been crying a lot and feeling weepy and down since June 26, when I officially closed my practice of almost eight years, and said my final good-bye to my last client. I've been feeling low and blue and very fatigued since the radiation treatments ceased entering their beams into my brain on June 2.

I'm lying in bed after my nap thinking, thinking as I cry. I need to talk to someone...get my head out from under these bed covers. Who to talk to? What do I need? I need emotional nourishment, hugging, babying. I need: "There, there, Martie, what you've just been through was awful, terrible. Just be with me while I hold you and let you cry it out." I need that someone to rub my back while I cry, and to hold me, and tell me she loves me, and she will protect me, and she'll make sure it will never happen again. But who can make a promise like that? No one. Who can be supportive and protective and hold me like I want? My mother. We all want our mothers when we are hurt.

I realize I sound like a self-centered five-year-old little girl who has fallen off her new tricycle. She's crying because she's in pain. She's suffered road burn when she scraped her chin, knee, and elbow. She's also surprised by the fall. She'd been peddling fast, feeling the fun of the wind in her face and the freedom of peddling the bike on her own. She didn't expect the trike would hit a pebble and lose its balance and tip over with her on it.

My mother is not available. Today I miss her dearly. If she were here, she would take care of me the way I need, the way for which I am longing. I lost my mother when I was 30 years old—she was 53. She died in 1974 from colon cancer—a devastating death for me. I never expected her to die in that way or that young. We were just fashioning a new mother-daughter relationship. When she was initially stricken, I was living in Michigan (she in Massachusetts) with my two sick babies and couldn't get to be with her as she went through her initial diagnosis and surgeries. Three years later, I had moved closer to home and was with her when she died. Even though it was expected, I was devastated and overcome with terrible grief. That was the first time in my life that someone close to me, someone I loved dearly, died.

My grief was long and painful. I grieved and cried hard for two years. My grief then was like a trauma, similar to the trauma I am experiencing now. I told everyone I met about my mother. Over the years of grieving, I developed an awareness of and acute sensitivity to other people's feelings. I didn't realize at the time, but I was developing empathy for others. That was preparing me for my later career in social work.

While I was developing empathy, I was also becoming moody, bitchy, and angry at the world for not treating me well. Over time I was trying to advance myself in my career. I began at Boston Edison(now NSTAR), a computer company, and then at T.J. Maxx. I was not advancing. I was feeling sorry for myself. I felt misunderstood. I felt Joe didn't love me anymore. I couldn't look at myself to see that it was all *within me*. I was a self-righteous person. I knew all the answers. I was always right, so why would I listen to anybody else? I was impatient with others. I did everything myself. My perfectionism put a wedge in our relationship. I didn't let Joe do anything around the house because he couldn't do it right—couldn't do it *my way*. Why was I the first to be in the pack of lay-offs? Why wouldn't I get hired? Why wouldn't I get promoted? Why wouldn't you love me?

Over the years—it was about 13 of them—I became so low about myself that I eventually sought counseling. Me. The perfectionist. The know-it-all. I had to, I was having bad thoughts about myself and feeling like my life was out of control. Finally, I had to do something. And that something was asking a professional for help. I had twirled myself into a state of intense confusion from which I could not get untangled. I was surprised to discover from Liz, this warm and friendly and supportive psychologist, that I was still grieving—all those years later—the loss of my mother. Surprise and relief hit me at the same time. Because her words resonated strongly, I figured her to be right. She helped me take a look within and I realized how angry I had become; I was stuck in the anger stage of grief. How could I move on if I was stuck there? I continued grief work and slowly, slowly began to feel better.

Grief was the first feeling I identified in my vault of feelings. Over time I discovered I owned plenty: sadness, fear, joy, love, happiness, and the hardest one of all to acknowledge—anger. It's normal to have and to feel all these feelings. That took a great deal of time for me to sort out.

Through the years, as I worked on my feelings, I developed a better sense of myself. I felt better in my own skin, and I began to like myself. I felt more comfortable in my relationship with Joe, too. Career advancements were not coming in my job situation, and with the new clarity I gained for myself I realized I was in the wrong job. Personal effectiveness training became an opportunity where I discovered a crucial attribute about myself: I wanted to make a difference in people's lives. Then came exploration of other careers. I had considered occupational therapy but was concerned about my age and lifting people. By that time I was 46 years old. On Labor Day weekend our friend, who is a research psychologist teaching at a university, stayed with us while situating her daughter at Wellesley College. She knew of my plight and suggested psychiatric social work. That set off fireworks in my head and I thought, "That's it!"

When I began my schooling and clinical training for social work the feeling persisted that this is what I have been training for all my life. In 1994, at the age of 50, I walked down the aisle in my cap and gown and graduate hood with great pride. Joe and my sons were present to see me walk across the stage beaming, and they watched me accept the beautifully scripted paper declaring that I had been awarded a master of social work degree.

It was the development of my empathy toward others and the discovery of my feelings, those feelings I let out of the vault, that led me into the field of social work. Over the years I gained clinical experience to become a psychotherapist and move into a successful career as a clinical social worker with a private practice.

Now I'm sloshing back and forth with feelings that I can't unmask. I sit in my depressed funk a bit longer with a whirlpool of agitated motions swirling about me. Since I can't talk to my mother, I need another female nurturer.

My Aunt Mary comes to mind. She was a friend of my mother, and is one of my father's sisters. Over the years we've developed a loving relationship with a nurturing bond. I know I can reach out to her and talk about my feelings. When I call, I'm told that she's just traveled to Pennsylvania to be with her sister, Ann. My Aunt Ann, another of my father's sisters, is dying of cancer. I have a relationship with Ann, too. How wonderful, I think to myself. I can speak with both of them. I won't talk about me; I'll concentrate on Ann and her feelings. When I call however, I discover Ann's children have clever ways to field the phone calls, and I never manage to speak to Ann, or Mary.

Finally, I can no longer tolerate my own behavior. My feelings are sloshing around and squirting out, like from a water balloon with pin holes. And those pin holes are getting larger. In addition, I am uncommunicative with Joe and moody. I notice he works at hugging and loving me. I appreciate him for his extra efforts, but I need more, and he can't give it. No one can. I realize what I must do. My experience as a therapist is alerting me to significant signs. I am getting so low I am despondent, and I've got to stop. It's time to find a therapist for myself. I don't know enough about the few I know in the area. It's important to find someone who has a sense of the trauma I am experiencing. I call Amanda, the clinical social worker, at Spaulding.

With two names on my list I call the one that has a pull toward me. My first surprise occurs when I reach a live person and not an answering machine. At first I figure her to be the intake coordinator. My thought: this group hired an empathic and knowledgeable coordinator. When I made an appointment, I experience my second surprise. I had been talking to my new therapist.

Some people might believe that because I'm a therapist, I would size her up. By that I mean compare behaviors, words, and style, and critique her as we went along in therapy. Not so; that's too much work. The most important aspect is what I learned in graduate school and in clinical training: the ability to create a rapport and establish a relationship. Elle began that process on our long phone call. I remind myself: I am the client now. By the time I enter her office for my first appointment, I have a sense of empathy from her and a sense that a relationship is beginning—all from that intake/first phone call. We are off to a good start.

In the waiting room, however, I notice the environment and make observations and compare them to my former practice. I notice that this office consists of two people—Elle and her husband. There's hot water for tea and coffee for waiting clients, and music playing. I see books, an assortment of magazines scattered around, and plenty of places for clients to sit where they can have privacy and personal space as they wait. The space and its accoutrements remind me of the waiting space I had for my practice.

Elle is a middle-aged woman, probably four to five years younger than me, short in stature. Beautiful short grey hair with a bit of a wave frames her round face. That face holds hazel eyes and an eager smile. As soon as preliminaries are complete—the info dance—Elle provides a bit of her history. She and her husband, both clinical psychologists, have been practicing together for about 25 years. Then, "How can I be of help?" Tears flow, along with intense sobbing. I feel vulnerable, but comfortable enough to let it all go. Elle waits patiently, allows me to cry. Then, without my realizing it, the therapy begins. Supportive words. Words of comfort. I feel heard. I feel embraced. Released. Grounded. At ease. At peace. Then, education about trauma. Yes, that's just what it feels like. A trauma. I can't stop talking about what happened to me. It is very much out of the ordinary...huge...outside of my personal reality...I can't absorb it yet...can't fit it into my life…into myself. And it hurts, a lot, emotionally. Much like a trauma.

Elle and I talk about medication. Between the two of us (here's where two clinicians concur), we decide I am situationally and clinically depressed, and medication could provide some relief. But I refuse because of the powerful new medications I currently ingest, and we both know antidepressant medication can take up to six weeks to become effective. My appointments will be on a weekly basis, and I know how to monitor myself and report negative symptoms to her. She agrees to no meds for the present time. And I have what I wished for: a female nurturer. I leave with a real hug from Elle, an appointment for the following week, and a lighter feeling in my soul.

My low funk is slowly on the mend and lifting to higher spirits. I notice I am happier. Friends call for lunch dates. It feels good for a sense of normal to return to this part of my life. I notice on these occasions that when I gaze at the menu,

I am overwhelmed and feel indecisive; I don't know what to choose, a sense of panic emerges. This is new. Before I had not been indecisive. I feel tightness across the middle between my chest and stomach; I always need to know others' choices. Most of the time that doesn't help, it's a stalling technique I use. When the wait staff arrives to take my order, I blurt out something I've heard from somebody else. My choice is placed in front of me, and I wonder why I ordered it.

After one lunch outing I asked my friend to stop at the store, I needed to purchase some wine. I am still not driving—not until August. That's the date I chose even though I continue to announce, "I'm not driving ever again." I do not feel ready. I feel vulnerable and not safe enough to get behind the wheel of my own car. And today, the middle of July, I don't know if I ever will.

Our neighbors invited me to dinner that night, and my friend waits as I purchase the wine. Inside the store I stare at the wine section. It's not huge, but I am flummoxed by the selection. I don't know which wine to choose. There was a time when I knew my wines, but not now, not today. My cell phone is with me. I call Joe. He appears perplexed by my request. "You know your wines," he says. "Any wine you choose will be fine." That didn't help. He put the burden and the choice back on me. My head feels cloudy, light-headed. I put my hand on top of it, hoping to steady myself before I go into dizzy. That happens to my brain when I get confused. I finally pick a red wine because I like the look of the label. I ease my friend's perplexed look with an apology and an explanation of my recent difficulties with decision-making.

What's happening with my brain and decisions? In the past, that is, prior to brain surgery, I was a decisive, determined person who knew what I wanted and where I was going, and I went ahead and did it. (I admit I was not patient with those around me who procrastinated and couldn't make decisions.) Now those qualities have been shattered—like a mirror. On days before the tumor I looked into that mirror. Reflected back to me was a woman of physical and emotional strength. She possessed confidence about her life—she was living her dream: living with her husband of 43 years on beautiful Cape Cod, continuing to practice the work she loved—a psychotherapy practice in Natick and one in its nascent stage on the Cape. Yes, she became tired, but the yoga practice and the cardio and strength training at the health club revived and replenished her. In between times, she was initiating a social life. She was a happy and content woman—and still in love with her husband.

Without warning, one day the mirror falls from the wall. It shatters into hundreds of pieces. I look at the fragments on the floor, all those jagged and sharp edges, and cannot find myself. Where did I go? What do I do now? All those pieces of me. Do not sweep them up. Do not discard them. I need to find myself again.

Today I spy some pieces that look like me and have been glued together. I have full physical care of myself. Some brain patterns have been reworked and neurons awakened so that I am walking unassisted. But even by stooping closer to the floor, I can't seem to find other missing pieces, like decision-making. Re-creating the brain pattern for decision-making is full of frustration. That will take practice, too, like the jump-starting of my limbs. I think back to all those tedious exercises. With decision-making I'll have to work it over and over and over. It's frustrating. I feel like throwing those pieces against the wall, or discarding them, but that will cause more havoc. I must learn patience again—another quality I've lost.

It must be frustrating for Joe when I accompany him food shopping. He sends me to an aisle to obtain an item from our list. I become distracted by the other food items in the aisle. Several minutes elapse and I'm in the same spot he left me, and I don't have the article he sent me to get. And I can't remember what it was.

I also notice I'm subject to hyper stimulation. We were walking through the Sears store one morning. I have difficulty with the racks and racks of clothing. It felt like a never-ending maze. I can't find my way out of there, and I had difficulty keeping up with Joe. The lighting is very bright. Joe is talking to me and asking me a question. At that moment a loud speaker opens up with a sale announcement in another department, and it feels like the speaker is directly over my head. That's when I announce to Joe, "I'm out of here!" I run out of the store and head for the car.

Social get-togethers with a small group of people are becoming difficult. Going out to lunch with my Aunt Mary and her daughters was always a treat, but now I find it daunting. Getting my body into a chair, or a booth. Choosing from the menu. Keeping track of the conversation. Telling my story. I notice I have this urgent need to tell my story. Part of this is the trauma, and part of it is a defense; if I talk I won't have to keep track of the conversation. All these things are tiring and overwhelming, but at the same time I'm a social butterfly, and I don't want to miss out on any fun. I take a long nap after those lunches.

Sometimes at larger social gatherings where there is a crowd of people—20 or more—I'm learning to take a break from the group. My head feels extremely light and dizzy. I am fearful of passing out or of having another seizure. That's my brain's signal to my body to go visit the coats. Usually there's no one to be found in the room where the coats are tossed together. I can sit there for 10 to 20 minutes, do some breathing exercises, close my eyes, and then return to the crowd. Sometimes the break works, and sometimes it doesn't. The break is a way to give my brain a rest from the stimulation of so many people at one time: their energy, talking, laughing, noise. I'm amazed at what my brain requires and am happy to oblige soothing it because it's endured much abuse up to this time, and it's up to me to care for it.

I continue to enjoy my sessions with Elle. She is kind, supportive, and knowledgeable. We laugh a lot, which is good for my soul. I have learned that what I have gone through, and continue to endure as I recover, is indeed a trauma. It's satisfying to have a label for how I've been feeling. And she says, "It's no surprise you're feeling all this intense emotion now. You didn't have time to feel any of that while in the hospital or rehab. Your job then was to heal your body." Hearing those words makes a huge impact on me. And, of course I cry. It's like Elle gives me permission to cry more.

As the sessions continue, I learn more. It's important to talk about this trauma with her. She understands the trauma and connects with me in each aspect of it. I feel I need to get it—all I've been through with my brain surgery—out of my system. I wonder if I ever will. I talk about it all the time to everyone I see.

As Martie recovers, we begin to go to gatherings of family and friends. These events are not fun for me. I find myself emotionally isolated. I watch Martie to make sure she is not getting overwhelmed. She is the center of attention. Everyone wants to talk with her to see how she is doing and to hear details about the surgery and recovery. Her admirers don't realize how taxing it is for her to interact socially. She tells me that she can't filter out the crosstalk going on in the room. She has a hard time focusing on her conversation. She loves seeing everyone but quickly hits her limit.

Am I jealous at all the attention? No. Do I feel left out? Yes. I get scant praise for being the dutiful caretaker. It's ironic. Being a good provider was never recognized—it was my role as the husband in the family. Now, being a caretaker is not recognized—it's what I am supposed to do. I am not whining. It's just the way it is.

At these events, I search out Martie regularly so I can assess her state. I don't want to be the hovering, controlling husband who keeps his wife in an emotional birdcage so she can't fly. I want her to have a normal life. She should be able to enjoy the attention she gets. She loves talking with anyone, especially the people with whom she has been close. I want her to get the nurturing that comes from those interactions. But once her focus shuts down, the consequences are severe. She loses the thread of conversation, and she looks like she is not paying attention, which she isn't. I watch for the look.

I also assess the emotional load on Martie from the person with whom she is talking. The people I think of as "nurturing" give off positive energy. They fill her up with it. Consequently she likes to be with them and feels their energy. She gains from the interaction. Some other people are the opposite; they emit negative energy. She has to work to have a conversation with them. The conversation is mostly about them and their issues. Unless she actively resists, she takes in their negative energy. They are high maintenance. And sometimes they just won't go away.

Watching Martie talk with people, I make a judgment about how nurturing they are. I don't claim my judgment is perfect but I have a pretty good idea which side of the energy spectrum the candidates are on. I look at Martie's eyes and her complexion for signs of fatigue, the glazed look, the flushed cheeks. If I suspect she is getting tired, I join the conversation and look her in the eyes. Usually they will tell me if she needs a rest or if we need to go. If they don't, I wander off. If I suspect that she is in trouble, I probe, "How are you doing?"

What is frustrating to me is how distracting this vigilance is and how it fits so neatly into my instinctual reaction at gatherings. Early in my teenage years I decided that I wanted to be a priest in the Catholic church. By chance, a priest from the Carmelite Order came to my school recruiting candidates for the seminary. That seminary took in boys who were starting high school. So at age 14 I left home to live at the seminary with 100 or so other guys of high-school age. In many ways it was a lot of fun. I learned how to study and that men can be both learned and manly. Without that experience, I don't think I would have made it into college. After two years I left because I didn't feel that being a priest was the life for me.

While I was prepared academically, it was difficult, at 16, to integrate myself back into the local high school. The guys had grouped themselves into cliques around sports or other activities. I liked sports, but I was not good enough to gain anyone's attention. I did join the track team, with limited success.

The girls didn't know what to think about me but a failed priest-to-be wasn't high on their list of dreamboats. My strategy for getting some attention was to act out. I tried to be a bit wild to counter perceptions that I was a saint. I played hockey late at night. I drank beer as often as I could get any. I went with guys who took risks driving and drinking. Over the last two years of high school I managed to remake my image from priest to cowboy without ever feeling included in any group. My guess is that I was not very different from other teens my age.

My many cousins still saw me as a seminarian and an oddity. They had been hearing all their lives from my mother that I was near perfect. One of my cousins loved to refer to me as "Mr. Shreve, Crump, and Lowe." It was her way of saying that I wanted to be upper-middle-class and above her and my other cousins. She might have been correct. She was the only cousin who would openly express her perception of me, which I appreciated.

Earning a PhD didn't enhance my image in my extended family, especially being in psychology. Most people assumed that I must be a clinical psychologist or some kind of psychiatrist. So how does a guy whose extended family contains no one with even a college degree decide to go for a PhD? The answer is "I didn't plan it that way." My two years in the seminary moved me toward more intellectual interests. I began reading books all of the time. Psychology was of interest. I read about child psychology and a biography of Freud. During my senior year in high school, when I applied to colleges they forced me to choose a major on the application. At that time, I became interested in an afternoon TV show about family therapy. From what I remember the half-hour show presented a family in conflict over five episodes a week. On Friday the conflict was resolved by the all-knowing therapist. I was interested. Wouldn't it be cool to know enough to put a fractured family back together? Be a hero? That role was very appealing to a former seminarian. So I wrote "Psychology" down as my major.

It didn't take long for me to learn that psychology was a scientific discipline as well as a therapeutic one. The faculty at Boston College was heavily focused on psychology as a science. And I soon learned that to practice it, I would need a PhD. Eight-years later I earned one. Those were by far the longest and most stressful of my early adult years. By my senior year at Boston College I was prepared to apply to graduate school. It was the mid-1960s and education in America was oozing money. My grades and references were good enough to give me a chance at being accepted. In the end, I decided to go the SUNY Buffalo, an up and coming university well-funded by Governor Rockefeller. The year before, Martie and I were married and our son Ken was borne three days after I graduated from BC.

It was a great opportunity. Martie and I were both ambitious and wanted to make our way on our own. We charged ahead, made the move to Buffalo, and found an apartment at $85 a month. Then the reality hit. My assistantship paid $105 twice a month. Martie had to get a job typing radiology reports in the evening while I put Ken to bed and studied. We had no savings. Still we considered ourselves lucky to be on this adventure.

When you go to graduate school, you are under constant observation by the faculty and your fellow students or at least you think you are. The most important quality they are looking for is whether you are smart enough to be let into the club of PhD hood. There are also other factors, such as your dedication to the profession and to the faculty you are apprenticed to. But being viewed as smart enough is the key. Being constantly evaluated is stressful for all grad students. For me, with no family history of academic success and my failure to achieve even average grades in my middle school years put doubts into my head. The monkey on my back would periodically whisper that I would fail. What would failure mean? To me, it would mean that I was intellectually deficient. Could I look myself in the mirror if I failed? Don't think so. Could I expect my wife and other family members to respect me if I failed? Wouldn't they be saying, "He thought he was smarter than everybody else. But he could not make it as a priest or a doctor." I could only manage my thoughts about those imagined put downs, and the anxiety they produced, by working as hard and long as I could.

I needed to make A's in my courses, write papers that were better than my fellow students', and show the faculty for whom I was a research assistant that I could help them conduct studies that would be published in journals. I had to be attentive and engaged during classes and find ways to demonstrate that I was smart. Every conversation with a faculty member or a fellow student was an opportunity to show what I knew but without seeming to be overly ambitious. I had to dig deeper into the research literature than my fellow students in order to show my dedication.

At the end of my second year I took four exams that together are called "prelims." If I passed, I would be allowed to work toward a PhD. If I failed, I would be awarded what was called a "terminal Master's" degree A terminal Master's is a kind of consolation prize. You can't go to a university and teach with it or join a research lab. Another term that is sometimes used to describe people who don't complete a dissertation is "ABD" – All But Dissertation, a term of dishonor. But you have only wasted two years of your life and you have a graduate degree.

The exams were scheduled the week after my final exams for the courses I took that semester. I managed to get the highest score in two of those exams. Each prelim exam was 2.5 hours followed a few days later by an oral exam by the four faculty members who wrote and corrected the exams. I did pass and came close to passing "with honors." The initial pressure was off. I was smart enough.

By that point I had spent six years studying and conducting research for faculty members. The success I achieved came at a price that I was only dimly aware of. Fear of failure is a full-time occupation. One way to muffle the anxiety is to work continuously. I couldn't risk asking myself how I was doing or what the future might bring. I just moved ahead. While this calmed the anxiety, it made it nearly impossible to relax. I was not fun to be with. To Martie and Ken I was mostly an absentee husband and father. I needed their support but I couldn't give them any. I isolated myself emotionally. In some ways, I was following in my father's footsteps. But he had no choice about working six days a week. And his work as a heavy equipment operator had resulted in a hearing deficiency, which made it difficult for him to hold a conversation. I had no such excuses. When you get married at 20 and have a child at 21 you repeat the patterns of your parents, the only role models you have.

As I said before in Chapter 3, thirteen years of group therapy taught me that I had been emotionally comfortable staying on the sidelines. I avoided making an emotional connection with people in groups. It felt safe. Others didn't know how to interpret my silence. My group therapy colleagues saw this behavior as aloof and a sign that I was probably feeling superior, that I wouldn't lower myself to their level. That isn't what I was feeling—I was often trying to figure out what to say. But by remaining silent, I was choosing to let others decide what they thought of me. I also was missing out on the energy that emotional connections bring. My colleagues in the group forced me to grow because they cared.

My caretaking of Martie takes me back to my old habit of staying on the sidelines. Never having been great at small talk, I feel myself reverting to being a wallflower.

———

What I've discovered about the brain, post-surgery and post-radiation, is that it requires a long time to heal, along with a great amount of rest. Fortunately, I am in tune with my body. By that I mean I am aware of and listen to signals I receive from different parts of it. When my brain feels light-headed, cloudy and slightly dizzy, I look at the environment and learn to take my brain out of it. Then rest. Through trial and error, I've discovered that rest is the key. My chest often feels tight along with a swelling feeling when I am, as I call it, *"beyond tired."* That also means my stamina level indicator is pointing to low, and I'm often irritable. When that happens I need days—sometimes as many as five—of rest and sleep before I feel ready to take on my life again.

My stamina is a part of me I could always count on and took for granted. Now I find myself tripping over it, running ahead of it, and becoming acquainted with it in a new way. It's another fragment of the mirror I have retrieved. In getting to know my stamina I have had bouts of irritability and crying because I've pushed myself beyond my limits. I'm trying too hard. A familiar theme. To do what? Find me? Become my old self? Get my life back on track? I need to shed the idea of the old me. No one who has gone through a traumatic, life-changing event like mine can be the same person. I need to shift and continue to piece together the new me. The pieces slipping together so far are pleasing to me. I like the woman I am becoming. I am embracing new pieces.

Diminished stamina is a new piece. To manage the diminished stamina, I must rest, and if it takes five days, I will do just that. Sometimes I watch TV—shows I've recorded ahead of time. I feel like a slug, but I am not only resting but feeding my stamina to regain my strength. After so many trials, I have found the remedy. Five days of rest provides a return to a stronger stamina and a feeling of being back to normal. I can live my life again.

Joe constantly reminds me how to keep from entering that diminished stamina state. He often asks: "You burning that candle of yours at both ends again?" He's the person who looks out for me, and he's right. Reminds me of the time when I closed my practice and, in my overzealousness, I scheduled too many clients in a day. I must be watchful as I schedule my social life each week. I believe I am, but I swear, I am surprised again and again when my energy indicator shows I'm running on empty. Again I look back to see how I went off course. Most of the time I can't see what I did, but then...if I take a closer look. And I try again—until the next time. The fatigue versus stamina struggle goes on and on and on. I am learning to pace myself. That's another part of my recovery, and my new life.

———————

Joe's always been a guy who enjoys cooking. When we lived in Michigan, he announced on my 28th birthday that he was preparing a surprise gourmet meal for me. I was thrilled. It seemed as though he cooked all day, but he was referring to the cookbook and the meat needed to cook for a few hours. The meal—boeuf bourguignon using Julia Child's famous recipe—was superb and the table setting included candles and linens. I loved it. That birthday celebration marked the beginning of two things: Joe entering into the cooking arena and the two of us cooking together on Saturday nights, which evolved into a special night of togetherness for us.

Today, I am grateful that Joe can cook and cook well. As the years went on, he taught our sons how to cook. We both joked, "They will each make a good catch." Joe and I cooked together during the week when we were home together. Our lives changed as the boys grew older, especially when they left our nest to be on their own. Often we were not home in the early evening. I met with clients two evenings a week. Joe had professional meetings, group therapy, and stayed late at the office to complete proposals for his work. We were often getting something on the fly. Since we've moved to the Cape we're back to cooking together more often—until now.

It's August 16, a lovely warm sunny day on the Cape. Joe and I are going for a walk. I am walking for longer periods, my left side is stronger, and my stamina is cooperating, too. Today is significant because after our walk, when we return to the parking lot where we left the car—my car, I will drive for the first time since January 16, seven months ago.

I had a good talk with myself and decided it was time to start driving. I'm beginning to feel isolated. All my friends are eager and happy to drive for me, but I'm feeling the dependency on others, especially Joe, for transportation. And it is time for me to get behind the wheel. I have this nice black Toyota Camry that handles beautifully. Why not drive it?

With anxiety, I approach the driver's side door and get in. After adjusting the seat and mirror, I start the ignition. I back out of the parking space and drive in the empty parking lot. It feels good—like getting back on a bicycle, one never forgets. And like riding a bicycle, driving makes me feel a certain freedom. I drive the route we previously walked, then home. Anxiety has dissipated. That's enough for today. I did it. I am back driving.

Route 6A is a fairly busy route because it's summer and the tourist are here, and they drive me crazy. I am careful to watch out for them. My hands grip the steering wheel, and I feel intense. I don't want to cause an accident. I feel the heaviness of the medication I take. In addition to the tourists, I wonder about the other people who live on the Cape, others, like me, who are under medication, maybe heavier medication than mine. How are they driving? Are they being as careful as I am? I feel vigilant and super alert. That's also how I feel as a passenger when Joe drives. At busy intersections I often stop our conversation because I have to be sure we can get through it unscathed. It is as if my not talking and my hyper vigilance are protecting the car and making our journey safe. All the time my hand is riveted to the arm rest. Tourists in town or not, it's always a challenge taking a left onto 6A. There again, I do not talk until Joe makes the left turn safely. To myself, I breathe a sigh of relief.

Now I'm alone driving and waiting to take a left onto 6A. I hear my father's words when he taught me how to drive: "Take your time, there's always a break in the line of traffic." It takes a bit longer in the summer but hearing his words in my head helps me relax. Eventually there's a break, and I make the left turn. I drive along intensely focused, watching all the cars, when another phrase of my father's springs to mind: "Always, always, look out for the guy behind you, in front of you, and around you." Well, I'm doing that. Oops, I'm glad I stopped in time. Someone just pulled out in front of me.

When I drive there's a constant dialogue running in my head. I focus on the road, try to stay on my side of it, and check my mirrors. Uh-oh, I'm coming to an intersection, must slow down. Look both ways, watch that car, he's taking a left. OK we can go, now. Oh, thank god she stopped, that was scary. Road's clear now, we're OK for a bit. Watch that curve, can be tricky. Oh, here comes a truck. Don't worry he's on the other side. He knows his lane. He won't hit you. Whew, he's gone. Traffic light up ahead, prepare to slow down. I sound like a driver's ed teacher, but my conversation helps keep me focused and lessens my anxiety.

It took months for me to venture out onto the highway—Route 6. The posted speed limit is 55 miles per hour, but some travelers go as fast as 80. I am on an incline—the entrance ramp at Exit 8. I move slowly. I feel scared to death as I approach this highway. I peek ahead and view cars speeding along, and I know I must join them. There's no turning back. Holding my breath, I accelerate and merge onto the highway, even though the sign says Yield. (Who yields?) Instantly, I am among a swarm of cars and trucks. I glance in the rear-view mirror, and the left-side mirror, hit my left blinker to signal. I need to move out of this merging lane that will end in a few feet. I feel as if no one will let me out, so I daringly slide on over, holding my breath again. That's when I notice I never exhaled from the first time. Aaaah, I did it! Now my job is to keep up—not at 80 miles per hour, but at least 60.

One day Joe suggests, and I agree, that I prepare supper on my own. After all, for over three decades I prepared supper without any help. When I was a young mother, most days I was visiting with a friend who had kids the same ages as my sons. The purpose: the kids could play and we adults could talk. Those were the days before mothers worked, and mothers craved talking to another adult. Today we call these arranged "play dates." When it came time to leave, around supper time, I was known as the fastest cook in the East. I could get the boys washed up, the table set, and supper started in about 20 minutes, and it wasn't a frozen meal.

Here before me is another meal to prepare: boneless chicken breasts with fresh green beans, noodles, and a salad. Joe is in the living room watching his favorite sports commentary show, *Pardon the Interruption.* He's my safety net if I need him. I am happy to prepare this meal, and I'm not feeling anxious.

I begin by seasoning the chicken—basil, oregano, salt, pepper, and a little paprika—place it on the aluminum tray, and slide it into a hot oven. I'm using the cane now as I move back and forth between oven, fridge, and countertop. I yell out to Joe, "How long does the chicken take, 18 minutes?" I hear a yup from the living room. I set the timer for 18 minutes.

I let out a sigh and look around me. What's next? The beans. I reach for the fresh beans in the fridge, pull the pan and its cover, from the wall. I snap off the ends of the beans, cut them on the diagonal, then into thirds. My right hand scoops them into the pan, and my left hand fills the pan with water. I place the pan, with the cover slightly ajar, over the burner, but do not turn it on. I'll wait until the timer for the chicken reads seven minutes to go. The noodles won't take long. I can put that burner on when there's three minutes to go. I work on the salads.

Joe has taken down the salad bowls ahead of time. I tear off the lettuce, and my mind starts to race. We eat complicated salads. Joe wants celery. I need to cut some. He eats bacon bits, I do not. Then there are the two kinds of nuts, and the craisins. I like them, he does not. I use salad dressing. He does not. Which kind do I want tonight?

There's a murmur of a pain beginning in my stomach. I wonder how much time is left for the chicken. I look over at the timer. It still reads 18 minutes. I never pressed the start button! I haven't even filled the saucepan for the noodle water to begin boiling. Oh my God! Arrrggghhh. I can't do this. My brain freezes up, I feel dizzy, light-headed. My stomach pain is getting worse. I can't even speak...I haven't even...I hold onto the counter to steady myself.

Joe enters the kitchen and sees me staring out the window. "Need some help?"

"Aaahh, can't think."

"Why don't you sit down, take your cane."

"All right." I am too stunned to cry. I tap myself along with the cane into the living room and sit down. I close my eyes and don't think of or feel anything.

After a few minutes, my mind wanders back to what has just occurred. Was it the timer? Was it forgetting the water for the noodles? Was it trying to keep the salads straight? I have no answers. When I report this incident to my friends, their first defense is, "You're getting older." That's true, but something else is going on, something they're not wrestling with. Their brains are not rockin' and rollin' around like mine trying to find itself. I don't tell them that. It's of no consequence to them. I sit with it by myself. But I know that those are tasks I could do before my brain surgery. Why did my brain jam up? That's what it felt like. And then my body became immobilized. I felt stuck, I felt paralyzed, I just physically could not move. This is hard to bear. Will this get better with time? I'd like to know: what the hell really happened!

Joe comes into the room and finds me crying. I always hate to have him see me like that because I feel like a failure. I talk to him through my tears. "I so wanted to be able to do this."

"I know." He is rubbing my arm. We sit in the living room quietly for a few minutes. He shuts off the TV. After a few minutes, I take a breath and release a huge sigh, signaling my tears have ceased. Joe in his upbeat manner gives me a broad smile, and says, "I'm hungry. Everything's ready. Let's eat."

During the period between rehab and radiation, Martie and I began to realize that she had some cognitive deficits that we had no idea would occur. But even cooking dinner is a multi-tasking activity. Over the years, I had cooked more and more. In the early days of our marriage, we had a typical cooking arrangement for couples in the 1960s: she

cooked and I cleaned. During the 1970s, I took an interest in cooking. I would cook "something special" on Saturday nights. When Martie started working full time, I often prepared dinner for the four of us. I was used to cooking.

As Martie regained her physical strength, she began to cook more. Before the surgery, she could cook a dinner and talk on the phone at the same time. But no more. One night she was preparing dinner and all of a sudden, she stopped, stared ahead and said, "I can't talk. My brain is shutting down." I was stunned.

Turns out that making dinner involves preparing each of the courses in parallel and timing it so that they all are ready more or less at the same time. It's like doing five things at once. For most of us, this is a skill we do easily, but Martie could not any more. Talking while she cooked made the confusion worse.

At first we attributed this difficulty to fatigue. I had her sit down and rest while I finished preparing the meal. But on subsequent nights she would forget a course or a step. It gradually became clear that the cause of the difficulty was not fatigue or only fatigue. Doing more than one thing at once seemed to be the problem. No doctor had even hinted that this might occur.

Some days later we were in a store and Martie was looking for something, I don't remember what. I wandered over to another department while she decided. When I came back, she was standing in the middle of the aisle staring straight ahead. She said, "I have to get out of here. My brain's shut down." She had been trying to make a decision about what to buy. A clerk came by to ask if she could help. And people were walking down the aisle, requiring Martie to move her body to let them pass. All of these together were too much.

From my study of cognitive psychology, I know that the inability to multitask or to filter out extraneous sounds are not uncommon in people who have brain damage or have had brain surgery. We were not told by any of her doctors that it was a possibility. Looking at the literature, it seems that not everyone has this deficit, and those who do have it to different degrees. But that is no excuse for not talking about it at all as a risk. Of course, Martie would have had the surgery anyway. But how can a side

effect with such a big impact on the quality of life get so little emphasis during the treatment?

———

Elle applauds me for the work I am doing. Sometimes she reminds me of the type of clinical work I have done with my clients. And speaking of my clients, I have picked up some referrals, which feels like I am building my practice in Yarmouth Port. I am lucky to have found this space not far from home. It's new and professional looking, having a different character from my space in Natick. In addition, an EAP—Employee Assistance Program—has contacted me and asked if I would partner with them. That would be new for me. In Natick I did long-term work, working with clients for years.

Large companies engage EAPs to provide a benefit for their employees. The purpose of the EAP is to help the employer by assisting its employees who have personal problems that might impact their work performance. These personal problems are on a continuum from minor to major. For example: work relationships, financial problems, family issues, health-care concerns, major life events like births, deaths, and accidents; emotional distress; alcohol and drug abuse; and gambling. The EAP company offers short-term counseling to the employee to assist them in their dilemma and then referral for further services, if needed.

For me, partnering with an EAP would mean fewer sessions, usually six per client, but I would get a chance to meet lots of people. I accept.

Elle and I continue my trauma work. She says it's hard work and that the trauma is still external, that is, outside of me. And that's OK. The major piece to trauma work, and what makes the work so arduous, is internalizing it. That means making it—the trauma—a part of me. When she said that it scared me. Make all that I've been through, and what I am continuing to plow through, a part of me. My first reaction is: "No way!" I calm down, talk about it with her, and think about it a bit. I remember from the clinical work with my clients—that's the treatment. It was always difficult for them, and in some cases, impossible to do. I am experiencing, firsthand, why.

Elle talks me through every step I have taken, as if she were there by my side. That says to me that she listens to me and gets my feelings. Seems like a long time ago since I woke up with that seizure. A lot has happened to me, to us, since that awful night. Whenever I think of it, or talk about it, especially in her office, I sob hard, right down to my toes. It was and is so hard to endure. At the same time, I am lucky. Lucky because I am alive, and I don't have cancer. The trauma and the luck are my constant companions. It's like I have fallen off a 500-foot cliff—and merely walked away like the Road Runner cartoon character. I survived.

———

It's September 12 and my next MRI. I will find out the results of the radiation today. During the radiation treatments, I remember asking Dr. Kahn if I would have an MRI to see how the treatment was going. I know it happens with some cancer treatments. He said, "No, we wait for three months after." But I don't remember his reason.

"The tumor has melted," claims Dr. Kahn. "This is good news."

"Yes, it is," Joe and I agree together.

"Now we could go three or six months before the next MRI," he muses. He sits a moment and thinks.

My thought is, let's not fool around with this; let's make it three months. I'm always trying to work calculations in my brain, and quickly arrive at December 12.

At that moment Dr. Kahn comes back with, "Six months. There's no reason to do three, everything up there looks clean. Let's set up the next MRI for March. Otherwise, tell me how are you doing?"

"Fine. I get fatigued a lot, and I rest to take care of it. But I struggle a bit with my left foot."

He nods his head, then says. "Well then, very good. We'll see you in six months. Craig will set that up for you." He stands up, signaling that our visit is over.

———

Thank-you notes.. In my office at home there are stacks and stacks of cards that people sent me while I was in the hospital and rehab. They have been accumulating ever since I've been home.. There are cards associated with flowers and plants. In addition there are games, candy, clothes, and playthings. I was on the receiving end of a great deal of love, and it's all represented in the stacked cards in the corner of my office. I look at it and feel that love. I want to write thank-you notes. In preparation for that writing task, I called Joe's sister, Grace, who works with greeting cards in her job at the drug store in Natick. I asked her to pick out all the thank-you cards she has and send them to me. In addition I requested packets of thank-you notes. And here they rest in a soft blue bag waiting to be opened. I can't begin to write those notes. Some days, as I fall asleep taking a nap, I draw up a plan in my mind as to how I will begin. But I can't do it. Not yet. I'm not sure why. I know within myself that I am not ready.

At my next session, Elle and I talk about the thank-you notes and their troublesome effect on me. Elle has a theory. It seems the writing of those notes is bringing back the trauma work we are doing, and they might bring forth some pain. If I write them now the trauma I am processing may move in too close. My heart reverberates strongly when she says these words and tears fall. She is right. I know when I write those notes I will place myself back in the hospital, rehab, etc., where I will recall my feelings when I received each gift. More feelings than I can handle. That's why I can't attempt it right now.

We talk further about the thank-you notes in a lighter tone. Elle suggests, "If etiquette dictates one has a full year to write thank-you notes for a wedding gift, why not one year, or more, for gifts received after surviving brain surgery?" I laugh and agree: "Sounds good to me."

I know you are wondering about the sex. Don't worry, I'll leave out the intimate details. I'll start with the baseline, what it was like before the brain surgery. We had been married for 43 years and were dating when we were 17. Our sex life had undergone several phases, some good, some not so good. Probably not unusual for people of our generation and the length of our relationship.

During the 10 years or so before the surgery, the sex had become quite satisfying to me and, from what Martie told me, for her as well. I don't have any doubts that she was being honest, though like people of our generation we don't talk frequently about such matters. As long as there doesn't seem to be a crisis, our sex life continues in a predictable manner.

Needless to say Martie's month in hospitals recovering from surgery and rehabbing resulted in a period of abstinence. Sorry, no late-night sex in the hospital bathroom! When Martie came home, we slept in separate beds for a while so she could use a cushion to keep herself from falling.

I am not sure how long it was before the idea of having sex occurred to us, about two to three weeks after she returned from rehab, I think. I had been waiting for Martie's lead. I wanted to be sure she still had the desire. One day we kissed and looked at each other in a way that told us both we were thinking the same thing. So we talked. We both had the desire, and we were uncertain how the sex would evolve.

I am happy to say that it worked out well. We resumed our sexual pattern. I am enjoying it more than ever, and I believe Martie is also. During the remaining months of that year, our sex was the best it had ever been. We worked around Martie's left-side weakness and did not miss a beat. When I look back, I am still amazed at how well it went. I know that I am thankful the trauma had not changed quite everything. We could still enjoy each other's bodies and the comfort of physical closeness.

The holidays are coming: Thanksgiving in two weeks, and then Christmas. I pause to reflect back, not just at what I have come through, but also at how far I have traveled in my recovery. I see the changes in Joe and me, the ones we have made separately and with each other—our new roles. I've ceased stooping to look and pick at fragments of that old mirror, the one that fell from the wall. I've finally discarded the remaining fragments. They don't fit me anymore. I'm now looking in a new mirror.

The new reflections are changes that are pleasing to me. I like what I see: a smiling face, beautiful blue eyes, and hair that has grown in for the second time, only this time it's very curly. I see a sense of pride in that face for the work I have accomplished in bringing myself back from a severe medical trauma. I walk on my own quite well after 11 months, becoming stronger each day. I also drive here and there to local places. I maintain a small private practice, and I assist with meal preparations. Also, I've reclaimed my desire for sex and enjoy intimate times with Joe.

I continue to have trouble thinking of more than one thing at a time and get confused easily, especially under stress. I notice my movements are slow, especially when performing tasks, for example, folding clothes, slicing cheese, cutting beans, preparing gravy, carving meat.

I consider myself lucky: as devastating as that meningioma was, no cancer was present. I have many friends and neighbors who support me. Also, I can depend on Joe for almost everything and am discovering he's quite proficient at his caregiving skills. I'm learning to trust him. I also realize that depending on Joe doesn't mean I'm losing myself. And I continue to reweave my dream on the Cape.

My strong determination continues as I push myself to improve my physical and emotional strengths, and to increase cognitive awareness. But, underneath it all there is a subtle layer of shakiness and vulnerability, like a kitten that has been neglected. If the doctors didn't tell us about the cognitive deficits, what else are they hiding? Is there collateral damage from the radiation that may surface? Will the tumor grow back?

I have been wounded once and fear it may happen again.

LIGHTNING STRIKES TWICE

It's going on seven o'clock, Thursday evening, December 13. Joe and I are sitting on the couch after supper waiting for the movie, *The Hunt for Red October*. Several times I've tried to catch it in its entirety, only to be interrupted. I read the book a few years ago and enjoyed it. I move my left hand to the back of the couch to retrieve an afghan—I'm feeling cold—when I notice I have no control of my left arm. It feels like a dead weight. In a nanosecond the fingers on my left hand meld together and cannot be pried apart. That's when my left arm goes into a spasm and begins to shake. I know what's taking place. Joe does not.

"What the hell are you doing?" he asks, mystified.

"I'm having a fuckin' seizure!" I shoot back at him. I am perplexed myself. Up to this point, before the surgery and throughout my recovery, Joe has not witnessed any of my seizures. Now he is frozen in place. I mirror him in my own shock. At the same time I cannot feel the left side of my body, even though I'm aware it's shaking. I am conscious. I wait to see if I will lose consciousness like I did in the ER last January. The shaking seems to go on forever. It's frightening, terrifying. When will it stop?

When the tremors finally end, I am crying. I hear Joe on the phone, calling 911. He informs the dispatcher, "My wife's just had a seizure. Can you help me about what to do?"

He returns to me. "I've never seen you have a seizure. I didn't know what to do."

237

"I didn't want you to see me like that," I sob, my head in my hands. "It seemed to go on for so long." Now I'm rubbing my arm, grateful to feel the sensation of it and my leg, too. "Can you tell how long it lasted?"

"No, I was concerned about you. But I guess it was no more than 30 to 40 seconds."

"It felt like it wasn't going to stop. That was the scariest part. So many scary parts. I felt like I had no left side of my body, to me there was nothing there — gone. And there wasn't anything I could do about the shaking; I couldn't control it." I cry some more.

"It's OK," says Joe in a soothing tone.

"What are we going to do? This isn't supposed to happen."

Flashing lights outside the window interrupt our conversation. The EMTs are at the front door in an instant. A strange sense of eeriness and déjà vu swarm over us. The stretcher arrives in the living room just like last January. Was it just 11 months ago? This time I am fully clothed, I have on my shoes and retrieve my warm jacket, and I am not in a fog. The EMTs quickly assess my condition, strap me into the stretcher, and put me into the ambulance in one swift movement. Joe is again warned not to follow the ambulance. We are pros now, we know the drill.

One item not in the drill from last January, however, is snow—three inches of it, with a thin layer of ice created by a drop in the temperature a few hours ago. That ice impedes the ambulance moving out of the driveway. On the first try the ambulance skids into our outdoor lamp post. It falls to the ground like a felled tree. Several more tries, more skidding. We're not going anywhere. "Let's try a transfer," suggests the driver. Calls are put out for another ambulance. All ambulances accounted for in the area are out—many accidents tonight. Finally, after several more calls—this time to towing companies (they are busy, too)—a wrecker comes to our rescue and pulls the ambulance out of the driveway. We advance to the highway, lights flashing.

━━━━━━

When Martie has the seizure, my sense of equilibrium changes. After six quiet months and a clean MRI in September, I believed that the worst

was over and that Martie's progress would continue to be positive—a smooth upward trend into the indefinite future.

It's hard to express the complex of feelings watching a seizure evokes. It takes a few seconds of watching her shake uncontrollably before I recognize it's a seizure. My adrenaline propels me into action. I stand up beside the couch to keep her from falling off, but there is nothing else I can do. I'm helpless. Martie is making sounds of distress. I can't tell if she's in pain. Her arm shakes, then her whole body. She is looking at her hand, but I can't tell what she is seeing. The sounds make it seem like she's conscious, but I am not sure, and I don't know whether that's good or not. I'm not sure she'll hear me if I say anything. I stroke her other arm just to make some physical contact.

Then it's over. It seems a long time, but I figure it at about 45 seconds. Once she stops shaking she sobs, looks away, and makes sounds in her throat that seem to say, "I never wanted you to see me that way." She lays back and begins to massage her hand.

Thoughts rush in: Why a seizure? Why now? The tumor must be growing again. Maybe there is swelling or bleeding. Whatever it is, it's not good. There is no explanation that doesn't point to disaster.

"I'm afraid it'll start again," she whispers.

"I'm calling 911."

I call and then I sit and hold her.

As an adult man, I have seldom experienced fear. I am not afraid of physical harm. Walking in a strange neighborhood doesn't bother me. I don't fear for my health. It's not something I worry about. Even when I had a melanoma on my back in 2000, I never feared it would spread. It just wouldn't happen to me. But the seizure starts a reaction that's hard to shake. I feel like the electrical activity was running through my body and I have no control over it. I'm scared.

Once again my assumption that today would be another day about like yesterday is refuted. For me, the seizure is more traumatic than the events of that night when the tumor first made itself know. There were signs that preceded the discovery, although I didn't know how to interpret them. There is nothing, however, unusual that happened before this seizure. Watching it is torture. My best friend is in distress, and all I can do is watch.

I am not sure I will ever lose the feeling that a disaster is waiting to happen. Adding this latest trauma on top of the first one makes it harder to deal with. I haven't worked through the emotions from the tumor yet. I block out any thoughts about tonight's seizure. I put a wall around the questions with no answers, about why this is happening. I have feelings of terror and lots of anxiety. I can't stop them. But I can wall off the thoughts. No analysis please!

———

The ER has a cold feel to it, a haunting familiarity. I'm scared, filled with dread. Memories of last January's visit envelop me, especially that seizure where I blacked out. It's hard to concentrate on the surroundings. My mind is busy with all kinds of chatter, mostly negative. I've learned during this past year that seizures—those abnormal electrical discharges of activity darting around in my brain—are harmful. What kind of damage is happening to my brain? I have dutifully taken my medication to stave them off and have had my blood drawn to check the Dilantin levels. I've worked hard on my rehab exercises and am walking again. What's happening? What have I done wrong? I have been faithful to all the treatment plans, and now a seizure. Something is out of control and very wrong.

An IV with saline is inserted and blood is drawn. My temperature and blood pressure are checked. I want to scream, "Is this really telling anybody anything? I want to know why I'm having a seizure!" I'm wheeled over to Radiology for a CAT scan. It comes back negative. Good news. No tumor. But the Dilantin level from the blood screening registers 9.11. The reading is only slightly out of range, the therapeutic range is between 10.0 and 20.0. That's perplexing. I should not have had a seizure at that level. I want answers.

I am sent home with no explanation, but with the following instructions: no driving for six months. "It's a state requirement," says the ER doc. (The doctor is partially correct. It's six months if you lose consciousness, which I did not.) Notify Dr. Anderson about the seizure incident. Increase my Dilantin dosage from 300 milligrams a day to 400 milligrams a day. Get another Dilantin level blood test.

I feel relief just being at home. Maybe not enough Dilantin in my blood is the answer, but I'm dubious.

Two days later while relaxing in my recliner, my fingers cramp together and cannot be pried apart. I know instantly what's about to occur. I yell for Joe.

"Rub my arm," I shout. My left side has disappeared again, but it is shaking violently, more so than two days ago. I am frightened.

"I am," he says in a calm, soothing voice I feel he's not understanding me. I scream a little louder, "My other arm!"

I sense he's rubbing my right arm. I scream as loud as I can, "No! My left arm!"

Tenderly and gently, Joe says over and over, "I *am* rubbing your left arm. Stay with me, just stay with me."

I want to lie down but I can't. I hear what can only be described as my muscles knocking together, sounding like blocks of wood, in a rhythmic motion. Freaky. I don't know or understand my own body. I keep calling out, "Rub my left arm!"

Afterwards I'm confused, disoriented, and very anxious. My stomach is tight, I have no appetite. When I stand I feel wobbly, my knees almost give out, and I experience difficulty with my balance. I fear walking on my own, that I will bring on another seizure. Must hold on to Joe as I move from one room to the next, or one object to another. Joe is wise, he finds some Valium—left over from my radiation treatments—and gives me five milligrams. The effects start quickly, and I regain some peace. I close my eyes, but I'm afraid to go to sleep.

Joe places a call to Dr. Anderson's office. He's already begun his holiday vacation, but the on-call doctor knows about me and my condition. He advises us not to go to the ER, but to increase the dosage of Dilantin by 100 milligrams—to 500 milligrams. He reports to Joe the results of my blood test—a level 15.0. That's a therapeutic level. Why am I having seizures? Maybe there hasn't been enough time for the extra dosage to become absorbed into my blood. That was a hell of a seizure I just endured. Don't want another like that.

Dr. Anderson called me the day after the first ER visit to check on me before he left for his vacation. I appreciated that gesture. During that phone call he suggested it was time to seek a neurologist to follow me. A good idea. But it seems like I could have benefitted from that specialty earlier. Why not sooner with that referral?

At bedtime I require Joe's assistance in undressing and dressing. I am fearful that too much motor activity will bring on another seizure. When I wake in the night to use the bathroom I hold onto objects in the room along the way. My balance is compromised.

The next day, Sunday, I feel stronger, my balance is restored, and I walk with ease. I use muscles on the left side without thinking and without worry. Later in the day while answering emails the fingers on my left hand began migrating together. Immediately I stop the emails—fearful of another seizure. I discover that if I rub and massage my fingers there is relief and they rest in their normal position. I continue to rub them compulsively.

By Monday, I notice muscle weakness. I need help with my coat, and I cannot squeeze out the toothpaste with my left hand. The following day, while reading and alone at home in the afternoon, I suffer two more seizures within three hours. Without Joe here with me I feel isolated and very frightened. When he returns from his errands we go immediately to the ER on our own. That was a mistake. Folks who arrive at the ER via ambulance take priority over those in the waiting room. We wait a long time.

Once I am in a bed, I experience what I call an "aura of distress," much like what I experienced that day last January when I cancelled my afternoon clients and came home. That aura is difficult to describe. It feels like a hand is clutching my stomach in a very tight grip and twisting it, and I feel slightly outside of my body. In addition, I know something is very wrong. I alert the medical staff to the cramping of my fingers and its significance. Immediately Valium is administered through my IV and instant relief swells throughout my body. The cramping ceases and the aura of distress disappears. Another seizure averted.

My blood work reveals two interesting items: a Dilantin level of 23.0, which is out of bounds on the high end, and an elevated LFT—liver function test. The elevated LFT triggers a memory from my physical exam in August with my new primary care doctor. She made a comment about it when she read the results of my blood work. At that time, I wondered why she didn't pursue other avenues, or provide an explanation. Now it appears the medication, Dilantin, may not be effective because it is absorbed by my liver. An hour later, the pre-seizure conditions—the aura of distress and finger cramping—revisit. Valium administered again with the same quick relief and same result—no seizure. I am relieved, but still scared.

Approximately seven hours later, at 2 a.m., a decision is made for hospital admission. No one informs me, or Joe, of the treatment plan, but my guess is that I am there for three reasons: one: observation (will I have another seizure?), two: medication change, and three: an MRI. They, and I, want to know what's going on in my brain.

My hospital stay lasts three days and is not pleasant. I am admitted to the old section of the hospital, not the new wing I had previously been in when it first opened last January. To begin with, the bathroom is not in my room; it's down the hall. My room is a double, I have a roommate. My room is located at the end of a long corridor. It is dark and dreary with dim light. Few of the medical staff roam by to check on me. If I have a seizure, how would they know? By the time I press a button and somebody arrives at my bed, the seizure will have passed. And when I request a Valium because I feel the pre-symptoms of a seizure, I am told curtly, "Here on the floor we can't do that." Why not? What happened to patient comfort? I spend 40 minutes rubbing my fingers and separating them along with deep relaxation breaths in an attempt to avoid a seizure. I succeed, but with great anxiety. I feel as if I have been shut away from everyone.

Much discussion occurs around the medication. I'm taking 500 milligrams of Dilantin a day, and it registers out of bounds in my blood at 23.0, while at home I continued to have seizures. It seems at this high dosage it's also affecting my liver. I feel like I am falling through the cracks. Does anybody care? I can get Valium when I need it in the ER, but not when admitted! None of this makes sense. Is anyone paying attention here?

I'm frustrated and confused. This is crazy-making. Are my doctors watching me closely? Do they know what they are doing? Do they care? Are they bothering to talk to each other? Is it because I'm in my sixties that they don't pay attention? Would I be better served in Boston? What I've endured this past year was pretty damn serious. Don't abandon me!

A neurologist, Dr. Murray, visits. He seems a bit eccentric but bright. I don't understand why, but he couldn't get the Valium for me, but encouraged me to massage my fingers, especially since that worked.

"You know," says Joe, "the reason the medical staff isn't willing to give you Valium is because they are waiting for you to have a seizure!"

Hmmm, I think to myself, why didn't I think of that? And why is Joe telling me, and not the nursing staff?

Finally a new medication, Neurontin, is chosen. I start on 300 milligrams three times a day, 900 milligrams total. And I have an MRI. An interesting note here. It's standard practice at this hospital to electronically send the MRI to have it read by a radiologist from Brigham and Women's Hospital. In the report, there is a "suggestion of swelling," but the Impression section, at the end of the report, states: "Findings worrisome for recurrent neoplasm," which suggests there might be another tumor.

That thought, that notion, does not register. The cognitive part of my brain, right now, resembles a telephone answering machine that only contains a limited amount of message space. At a certain point more information cannot be inserted: *Message box full.*

Because I had no seizure and I appear to tolerate the new med, Neurontin, the medical staff decides to send me home. It's the Friday before Christmas. Upon discharge, the attending physician, whom I am meeting for the first time and is known as a hospitalist, notices weakness as I walk. Where has he been? That's not a new development. I want desperately to go home so I minimize the weakness. He becomes more serious and walks the corridor with me observing how I walk and trying to detect any further weakness. I feel like a kid who does not want to stay after school. I want to go home and be there for Christmas. Today is Friday, December 21. The hospitalist and I reach an agreement: I will use a walker at home, and call the hospital if the weakness progresses.

———

"Joe, I'm having another seizure." I am home just about a half an hour and sitting down. Joe runs to my side.

"Stay with me, stay with me." My body is shaking violently. After what seems like an eternity the seizure ends. I'm limp, but not weepy. I feel secure with Joe around.

"You OK?" His arm encircles my body, soothing me.

"Yes, but I'm so discouraged. That's my fifth seizure in eight days! What's this all about? If only I could have had one while in the hospital. Where's it going to end?"

Joe phones the neurosurgeon doc-on-call. He claims it is safe to double the dosage of Neurontin, bringing the total daily dosage to 1,800 milligrams.

Life is rolling along...out of control. I'm having difficulty keeping up with everything. It reminds me of an avalanche when it creaks and starts to move away from the mountain cliffs. Joe and I are walking along when that avalanche breaks. He grabs my hand. We run as fast as we can, trying to beat the snow as it gains momentum. It gathers clumps of debris as it rolls its way down hill. With a feeling of relief we reach the bottom of the mountain, but I look back and point, showing Joe, "Look, there's more coming at us, we have to hurry." We run some more. We can't outrun it. Suddenly we are hit from behind by a huge clump and find ourselves buried. With much effort Joe pushes his way out. He uses his hands and body to pull me out and up. That's when I discover I can barely walk.

Joe and I decide that I will not return to the hospital. That's a mighty big decision, especially when I made an agreement with the hospitalist, on discharge, to call if the weakness worsened. It has. My left side is becoming weaker.

We are known for making mighty big decisions in our lives. We pride ourselves on being fiercely independent. Our independence first sprouted when we decided to marry—at the end of Joe's junior year of college. The people we shocked the most were our parents, of course, and our respective aunts and uncles—the older generation. "You're too young." "He's still in school." "Why don't you wait until he graduates?" "What if she gets pregnant?" "He doesn't have a job!" "He still has years of schooling." And on and on and on. We did it anyway.

When Joe was in graduate school in Buffalo and our first son, Kenneth, was approaching the age of two, we decided it was the right time to have our second child—even though we were poor. Joe was a student, I worked nights, but completing our family—that was important to us. Some of our peers, most of whom did not have children, thought we were crazy. We did it anyway.

Joe was teaching in Rochester, Michigan, and feeling he needed to stretch his career legs, venture out in his field and explore. He was waiting on a decision of tenure. Receiving tenure from a university was like receiving the golden key to a city. One can stay forever. Joe decided it was time to leave. Together we felt the tug to return home to Massachusetts, where our families lived. We had been away nine years and our boys, now almost six and nine years old, needed to be reunited with them. We shocked our peers by announcing we were moving back to Massachusetts—"job or no job." We had money saved for a down payment on a house. That money would go toward the down payment or moving expenses to get us home. Joe did receive tenure at the university. And he landed a job in Cambridge, which as an added benefit paid our moving expenses.

For over 20 years Cape Cod provided a vacation destination for us. While there we always dreamed of living on the Cape, probably when we retired. Probably never, I thought. In 2000, Joe had a medical scare with a melanoma. He was lucky—stage 0, caught in time. Around that same time a friend of ours in his fifties died of a heart attack.

Joe was working hard in his consulting job. It was exciting work—at the New York Stock Exchange—but it required travel every week. My practice in Natick was quite successful (that would be hard to close). Both sons were content and on their own. Timmy had married Joanna a few years earlier. Ken moved into his dream—a condo in Brookline. We weren't old enough to retire, but it was time to begin the dialogue.

"How can you pack up and leave the family homestead?" "Where will your kids land when they want to come home for the holidays or special occasions?" "What about all those memories from living in a place, a town, for 30 years?" "You're not ready to retire yet." "What will you do for money?" "How will you live?" Questions sound familiar? Those were the questions shot at us by folks who did not understand our move to the Cape. We did it anyway.

Now it's the Christmas holiday weekend of 2007, and we've agreed to another major decision. We both feel dubious about the care I would receive in the hospital, what with holiday shifts, skeleton crew, etc. We inform the VNA nurse who arrives for her assessment of me, and she concurs.

My left side is becoming weaker. Joe needs to lift me when I need to use the bathroom. I teach Joe how to handle me as I get up, and I use my right side in the manner I was taught at rehab.

"Grab me under my left arm, but from my right side."

"Up we go."

"Yeah, that's it. I didn't know you were so strong."

"Oh, I still have surprises left you don't know about," Joe says, with a wide grin.

"Is that right!"

"Hey, can you lift your left leg a bit?"

"I'll try." It's hard, but I manage. Together we slide along the floor with my left foot thumping up, then down.

As the weekend drags on, my left side becomes weaker and weaker. At first I am able to lift my left foot up and help Joe as he assists me, up and off the couch and into the bathroom. Now my foot is like a dead log that I'm pushing ahead of me. I can't even will it to move.

I am dismayed. What about all those exercises to train my brain, create new pathways, new networks of neurons? Are they all dead? I'm frustrated. At the same time I am overcome with love. Joe is caring in a way I have never in all our years together experienced. He needs to help me dress. He puts the sweatshirt or sweater over my head, my arms into sleeves, legs into jeans, socks on, then shoes, ties laces. He places the toothpaste on my brush, lifts me so I can sit on the toilet, gives me the privacy I need. He performs these activities naturally. I sense no resentment. How does he do that? These are intimate moments for us. This is what "in sickness and in health" means.

———

After Martie is released from Cape Cod Hospital on the Friday before Christmas, she comes home to another seizure. We decide to stay together at home and try to make it until the day after Christmas, the following Wednesday, five days away. All of the specialists she has been seeing are gone for the weekend. Lying in a bed in the hospital with minimal nursing care for five days isn't an appealing option. I am prepared to handle her care myself as long as I can.

We feel that the health care network has abandoned us. Only doctors on call for her specialists are available, and their repetitive response is to take more seizure medication. The most difficult part of the medical crisis is not knowing its cause. Why the seizures? Why the returning paralysis? Is there a new tumor? Bleeding? The doctors on the Cape disagree on a cause. Whatever the cause is, it will not be good.

In spite of the return of Martie's paralysis, there is a cozy feeling about the weekend. We have time to be with each other and enjoy the holiday. We sleep in the guest room, avoiding the stairs. There is a closeness between us. We will get through this.

Martie's left side becomes weaker. She can't use the walker because she can't grip it with her left hand. To help her walk, I put my arm around her waist as she moves her feet slowly. We make trips to the bathroom and back and to bed and back, but little else. I prepare the meals. I am afraid to leave the house for any length of time because of the threat of another seizure.

By Monday the paralysis is so bad that Martie can't plant her left foot as I lift her off the couch. Previously that move had worked because she had been able to move her weight forward as I lifted. But now her left foot slides when she tries to plant it. It's dead weight. I have to move her foot into a position below her knee so she can keep the leg from sliding. We actually laugh at what this move might look like. (I was thinking about a Seinfeld episode called "The Move.")

I do begin to question my own motives and my sanity. I can't expect Martie to make decisions. Her feelings about the seizures and what they mean are on autopilot. She needs to keep her emotions in check to get through these days.

Is it my need to be in control of my life and hers that makes staying at home attractive? Am I being foolish? Will I be to blame if something bad happens? Probably. Am I putting Martie at risk of who knows what? Maybe. Should I get someone else's opinion? Who? Who would know the situation better? I imagine calling someone and saying, "Martie is almost completely paralyzed on her left side and it's getting worse, she has had five seizures in the past two weeks. I am having difficulty lifting her. Should I take her to the hospital?" Would any sane person say no? Still, I believe that staying at home is best for her—unless the situation deteriorates further. I do not want to hear any other opinions. Call me "stubborn" call me "brave" call me "foolhardy" call me "determined." Just don't say, "He wasn't thinking."

———

During the weekend, Joe and I discuss what's happening to me, and we devise a plan about what to do next.

"We should call Dr. Kahn on Wednesday," I begin. "He needs to know what's been happening."

"Yeah, I think you're right. And what about that neurologist at the hospital, what's his name? Dr. Murray? Didn't he say to give him a call when you got home?"

"Yes, him, too. We've got to start somewhere. Maybe he could prescribe a steroid." During my hospitalization I was on steroid medication. With the medical knowledge we both gained the past year, we wondered: had I been discharged on a steroid would I now be paralyzed?

We celebrate Christmas by ourselves. It is meaningful. Christmas has been just the two of us for several years and that's OK. Tim is in Montana with his wife, and Ken likes to be with his wife on that day; they come down around New Year's Day. Phone calls and Christmas wishes come later in the day, and we inform our sons of my medical status. We exchange gifts and Joe prepares dinner. He has to cut my meat just as he did last January when I was recovering from surgery.

Wednesday, the day after Christmas, we begin our plan. I call Dr. Murray for an appointment. He has a cancellation; can we be there at 10:30 a.m.? The next piece is notifying Dr. Kahn. I leave a brief message on voice mail that I would like to talk to him—nothing more.

———

Dr. Murray's office is in Hyannis, a 20-minute ride away. I get Martie dressed. I am always impressed by how much she learned at rehab about how to dress. She knows which sleeve goes in which arm and which arm to do first. It's a struggle to get her sock and shoe on her left foot because it and her leg are dead weight. With her winter coat on, we inch toward the car. She can't lift her left foot, so she drags it along. I open the car door and stop, not sure what to do.

"Hold on, I know how to do this," she says.

"What do you want me to do?"

"I need to pivot my body so that I can sit down sideways on the seat." Easier said than done. I use the door as a way to hold her up and put my arms around her. I try to pivot her body so that her backside is facing the seat. It takes four or five small moves.

"Use your right arm to hold onto the center post of the car and gradually lower yourself into the seat."

She holds on, then falls with a thump into the seat. I guess it's not so easy to lower yourself with no strength on one side.

"Lift my left leg into the car while I move my body." I lift while she shifts, then she swings her right leg in. Mission accomplished. I grab the seat belt strap and click it in place.

When we get to the doctor's parking lot, I realize that I won't be able to get her into the office without help. I have her wait, while I go in. I open the door and I'm greeted by the raucous barking of a tiny mechanical dog on the secretary's desk. She seems not to hear the barking. I spot a wheelchair in the corner.

"I need this to get my wife in." Her face indicates that she heard me but there is no other response. I grab the wheelchair. At the car door, we reverse our moves for getting Martie into the seat. I am glad that I have the strength to move her into the wheelchair.

Back at the office door, the dog greets us. He barks at any movement in the room. I have a fantasy about picking him up and filing him in a draw and shutting it. Fortunately, we don't have to wait long for the doctor.

The doctor asks what insurance we have.

"Tufts"

"I don't work with them," he says. A great beginning.

He goes through an exam of Martie's strength. "The increasing paralysis is not something that we should let continue without some additional tests. And I suggest you go to wherever you had the radiation treatment. They need to see the MRI."

"I can go to the Brigham, but how do I get the MRI results there?" asks Martie.

"You can get the disk and report at Cape Cod Hospital. I will call, and you can get it now. Going to the Brigham is a good move. I don't have any contacts there, but they have the people who can deal with a case like this."

He calls the hospital and tells us where to get the MRI disk and report and wishes us well. I'm encouraged about moving to the Brigham, and I'm grateful for his help in getting us the MRI. As we leave, the dog barks good-bye.

———

By the time we return home there's a message from Dr. Kahn's assistant. When I return the call and explain my situation, he requests that I fax the MRI report and FedEx the disc to him, providing me with the Brigham's special charge number. He informs me Dr. Kahn will call.

Joe and I are not waiting around for Dr. Kahn to call. I fear another seizure, and my situation is becoming worse, about as bad as we can handle. Tomorrow, Thursday, we will head off Cape to the Brigham to see Dr. Kahn and/or get me admitted. That's the next piece of our plan.

———

With great effort Joe manages to get me situated in the car.

"You ready?" He asks.

"Let's go."

Traveling off Cape with the cell phone in my right hand and phone numbers on my lap, I call Dr. Kahn's office first, and inform him on voice mail (because I can't reach him in person), "I am on my way to Boston right now hoping to see you when I get there. There have been some changes in my brain, and my life, you need to know about. Craig should have the copy of the MRI by now and its corresponding report." My strategy is that he will get the message early in the day and make a decision by the time I arrive at the hospital. That's part of the plan. As far as the end result, that's not in our hands.

I call my primary care doctor, Dr. Peterson. I'm not able to speak to her in person either, but leave a message on her voice mail informing her of our plan.

Next I call Pearl Ryan, the social worker who befriended us during my radiation treatments. I leave a message about our plan on her answering system. I wait for return calls. Dr. Peterson calls first. She agrees with our plan and strongly encourages our trip to the Brigham. She adds that while she has no hospital privileges there, she will call Dr. Kahn and speak with him about me and the medical consequences to date. I give her my thanks.

Pearl Ryan calls and says, "Of course, I remember you." She spends a great deal of time listening to my ordeal. She, too, supports our plan. "Call me the minute you step foot in the ER, and I will come by to see you."

Dr. Peterson calls again to report Dr. Kahn is on vacation, but she has spoken to another doctor on his team, Dr. Nelson, who is aware of what's happening to me. Dr. Nelson asks if I am taking steroids. I tell Dr. Peterson—No! She relates the message from Dr. Nelson that I get a "fresh neurological evaluation," and that folks in the Radiology Department await me. That's when I learn the Radiology Department cannot admit people to the hospital, but Dr. Peterson urges me to continue on with my trip to the ER. My primary care doc, Dr. Peterson, is new to me, and I appreciate her special effort in my case.

I report the information to Joe as we drive. He smiles often and lets out a sigh of relief. We both feel encouraged and pushed in the right direction, like some validation from the universe, like we are back in control. Not!

When we arrive at the Brigham, Joe foregoes valet parking and heads for the tiny emergency room entrance. It is tucked away in a corner adjacent to the hospital's main entrance, hidden. No wonder I never noticed it. Joe parks the car, grabs a wheelchair (from where?), moves me into it, and through the ER doors in a swift, but smooth, movement like he's always done it. How does he know this? He approaches the desk. I hear him say, "My wife's having seizures." He nods his head toward to me in the wheelchair. "Where do you want us to wait?" Immediately we are ushered into the ER hall of waiting. Part one of our plan is complete.

———

I find myself on a gurney in a small cubicle. An IV is attached to my arm, saline moving through. Blood pressure checked. Temperature taken. Phew. I've passed the initial tests. I am allowed to stay here. For now. After a period of time, residents from the Radiology Department arrive one by one to perform neurological tests. I know I pass the ones where I follow their light with my eyes.

"Can you shrug your left shoulder for me?" Uh-uh.

"How about your fingers...can you move your thumb?" No movement. I stare at my lifeless left hand.

"And your left foot, can you wiggle it...lift your leg?" No to those requests.

Time passes, another resident comes through to assess again. Dr. Nelson, covering for Dr. Kahn, visits. She performs her own neurological tests. Other residents visit my cubicle. They think their tests will be successful. I flunk them

252

all. The entire radiology team agrees I need to be admitted. But they are not allowed to admit patients, and I have no doc sponsoring me who is affiliated with the hospital. Joe and I feel our spirits lift when Pearl Ryan visits. She spends time talking and assessing the situation. She calls the Radiology Department and talks to them. More time passes.

The first time I meet with the doctor-in-charge at the Emergency Medicine unit I announce, "I'm transferring my care from Cape Cod Hospital to the Brigham." She looks back at me in surprise. I get the sense that she thinks that I am taking advantage of her and the Brigham, trying to talk my way in. We are here on our own with no doctor to back us up. I guess that was a brazen thing to say, but where else can I turn? Dr. Kahn is my link; he is treating me through follow-up visits after the radiation treatments. That has to count for something. When she returns a little while later she lightly broaches the idea of sending me home with physical and occupational therapy services, or to a rehab. I think to myself: how preposterous. I can't move. What is it she's missing?

The volcano within is smoldering. I have spent almost a year recovering from a serious brain tumor. Months of determination, effort, and hours of arduous rehabilitation prevailed in order for me to walk again. Now I find myself paralyzed. Again. I don't know why. And, there isn't one medical person, who is following me, who can answer that question. My anger has been held in so long it is bursting at the seams ready to explode in judgment. Was anyone paying attention to my care? I'm not going home until I get answers, or a resolution to my problem. Unlike Dorothy in *The Wizard of Oz,* who cries throughout that she wants to go home, I want to stay here in Emerald City. I know they can fix me—even if it's with steroids.

Joe's pacing around wondering what's going to take place. I like it when he leaves the cubicle. It gives him a break. He spends time talking with Pearl Ryan. That gives me time to reflect and review what's happening.

So what happened? Where did things go awry? When did the safety net fail? A balancing act on a trapeze, I mustered my strength and balance for months only to have my net ripped away for reasons no one can ascertain. And when I fell, there was no soft cushion on which to land. Were my doctors not attentive? Could it have been the nurses? What happened to the blood draws? Was my Dilantin level to be tested on a routine basis? Those elevated liver function tests—weren't they a red flag? Did I need more tests of my liver function to be performed? Why, when I'm in the throes of seizure after seizure, was it then recommended I get a neurologist? That was not a soothing idea, nor timely. It seemed overdue. And my specialists happen to be on vacation when I'm in crisis!

I'm a nice lady and I'm not supposed to blame people or point the finger. I'm not supposed to yell. Or get angry. But I *am* angry. I want *answers* and I want *action*.

But I must turn down the heat of my smoldering volcanic fire, dump some water onto the hot coals. My anger exists, but it has grounded me and given me purpose. It allows me to speak from my core.

The EM chief approaches me again. I'm beginning to understand she's the gatekeeper, and she's trying to keep me out! It's her job. "We cannot keep you here, or admit you to the hospital. You are not medically appropriate for admission. So we are thinking it's best to discharge you to a rehab. Do you have one you prefer?"

The position of the gurney allows me to be face to face with her. I look directly into her brown eyes. She is a young Middle Eastern woman of average height exuding the confidence that doctors gain from their training. My anger fuels my confidence, and it matches hers.

I begin in a strong but grounded manner. "Let me explain something to you, doctor. Sending me off to a rehab is not the optimum thing to do—for me or the hospital. I'll be back in the ER within a day. You see, a rehab hospital demands that a patient work at least three to four hours a day. I cannot move one muscle on my left side, and it is getting worse." Oh, how I wanted to shout and scream at her. But that wouldn't do. I douse more water on my fiery embers, ground myself some more, and continue. "Think about it a minute. How can I do the work at rehab if I cannot lift myself up off this gurney, get down from it, and move across that hall to use the bathroom. I can't even walk."

Her response is steadfast. "I don't believe we can admit you." By now she looks exasperated.

"Please," I plead. "Talk to whomever you need to and make this work for both of us."

I wait. I notice the radiology docs, along with Pearl Ryan, in a huddle. I hear murmurs and a word here and there but I cannot make out what they are saying. Another hour passes. I doze.

I meet the young resident from Radiology again, only this time he's not alone. He has a neurologist with him. Together they perform their neurological tests on me. Again, I fail—all of them.

"I can't understand why the paralysis is increasing," this neurologist exclaims. "There's something going on."

Finally! Did somebody give him the correct lines to read in this play? I may get some action. At this point I discover that the technicians in the Radiology Department are unable to read the MRI disc from Cape Cod Hospital—different technologies. At the same time Joe and I spy the neurologist approaching the EM chief. It looks like he is telling her I am to be admitted. Turns out a neurologist has admitting privileges. And kudos to the entire the Radiology staff for working as tenaciously as they did for me.

Part II of our plan is not only complete, but a success. I am to be admitted. There is hope I will recover and walk again!

———

Once the Brigham agrees to admit Martie, her care changes dramatically for the better. Within minutes they inject steroids, and later that night she begins to see four doctors. The difference between her care at Cape Cod Hospital and at the Brigham is significant in its results but a bit hard to explain in process. One case history does not qualify as evidence of a trend. I can only say that in her case, the care between the two hospitals differed.

All of the doctors at both hospitals seem to be very competent at their specialties. When I look up their credentials and reputations on the Internet, they seem first rate in my layman's view. They also are all committed to Martie's care. I never doubted that.

But at the Brigham, the doctors know each other and often appear together in her room at the same time. It's as if they are all from the same neighborhood. They talk with each other and act like a team. When they need a new specialty, they know whom to call. As they interact in front of us, they seem egoless. Not one sign of grandstanding or one-upmanship. I am sure that they do have egos and that they do clash. But in front of us they're a united team, and that makes me feel confident that Martie is getting good care.

At Cape Cod Hospital, we never saw two doctors in Martie's hospital room at the same time. In fact, for the visit following her seizures, it was not clear who was in charge. She was admitted through the emergency room. She was seen by a neurosurgeon, a neurologist, and the hospitalist. The three doctors seemed to disagree on the cause of Martie's seizures and said so openly. It's as if they were visiting from different neighborhoods. Though they were always professional, they did not present themselves as a team, and we often felt we had to tell them what the other doctors had said to us.

The disheartening issue we faced during the five days we spent dealing with Martie's seizures and creeping paralysis at home was being abandoned by all of her specialists on the Cape at the same time. Don't get sick on a major holiday weekend! None of her doctors were available. I don't begrudge them their time off. But when they don't see themselves as a team, they can feel free to leave at the same time. They do leave doctors to cover for them, but those doctors take a very conservative approach. They don't know the details. In Martie's case, the only advice we were repeatedly given was to take a higher dose of the antiseizure medication. When Martie was at the Brigham over the New Year's holiday weekend, some of her specialists were always available. I believe that this was a function of the doctors feeling that they were a team. It's only one example, but I believe that it is one of the reasons why the care at the Brigham was superior for us.

One other point about this issue. The doctors at the Brigham and the doctors at Cape Cod Hospital don't know each other. Several people, including two of our Cape Cod Hospital doctors, urged us to go the Brigham because of the complexity and risk of Martie's condition. But they couldn't give us a referral. Because our main contact at the Brigham was on vacation, Martie had no clear path to being admitted there. And radiation doctors don't have admitting privileges because their patients are treated on an outpatient basis. This is a weakness in our health care system, not just at Cape Cod Hospital.

I can only speculate about what would have happened if the social worker, Pearl, had not befriended us during the radiation treatments. She stayed with our case all day. She took the initiative to intervene on our behalf. Interesting that social workers have low power in the hospital hierarchy but can make things happen in their own way.

Once my admission has been approved, a steroid is immediately administered through my IV. I am relieved on both accounts. I am worried though. Not about the steroids, I want them—it's the seizures. I've just suffered five of them in eight days, and I'm concerned about the damage to my body and to me, emotionally. I'm not medically equipped to understand all the ramifications, but I sense they are not good. For now I push those worrisome thoughts aside and concentrate on my wellness.

I wait in the hall of the emergency room until my room is ready. My cubicle is used for another ailing patient. Joe leaves, now that he knows I will be taken care of. He will stay with our Ken and his wife close by, in Brookline.

It's dark by the time I arrive in my room. It's a double room, but unlike Cape Cod Hospital, the bathroom is part of the room. Not that it is a benefit to me. I will need personal assistance this time, unlike last week (was it just last week?) at Cape Cod Hospital, when I could walk. The nurses are ever present and kind. I teach the nursing aides how to grasp hold of me in order to help them when I need to use the bathroom, or to sit up in bed or a chair to eat. My roommate is friendly. She's here because of an anesthesia reaction. That's scary to ponder. Time to move my thoughts from there.

I've missed the supper meal, but an aide says she will happily bring one to me. She presents the choices, then whisks away to get me a meal. That's a nice welcome. Sleep comes easy tonight.

The following day, Friday, I meet early with a team of young doctors headed by a chief resident, Dr. Evans. Dr. Evans takes on a teaching role, but lets the other residents—about three of them—and any visiting doctors who happen to be around at that moment and want to join—do the work. There are more neurological tests. As before I pass their light test. Thankfully my vision is not affected. The muscles continue to be weak, except I can move my thumb a bit. Steroids are doing their part; however, I cannot shrug my shoulder.

There's much discussion about medication. Why can't I take the first line anti-seizure medication, Keppra? I'm allergic to it. Other medications are dismissed for various reasons. Finally, there is talk of Topamax I can't keep up with their chatter. Topamax is the only med that stands out. A radiology technician manages to get a reading of Cape Cod's recent MRI of my brain. Again much discussion. First: the doctors don't know why I'm in the state I'm in. And they are not afraid to say it. Second: they have two theories. One, a radiation treatment effect triggered the seizures that caused the swelling. Two, an emerging tumor. They do not mention the lack of effectiveness of Dilantin. Their theories have no resolution. It's such a relief to be here, among these doctors who are participating in my treatment.

What do I think of their theories? I can't believe it's a tumor. I guess I don't want to believe it. I rationalize: it's too soon. From an emotional standpoint, I'm too scared to think about a tumor. On the other hand, the radiation treatments were completed six months ago. Is this fallout from radiation treatments? Swelling of the brain? Seizures? I just want to be able to walk again. Resume my life. That's where my thought process is.

It's Friday afternoon, and I've been here one and a half days. I hear talk of discharge—not from any doctors—but from Isabel, the discharge planning social worker. I was in that position at one time and understand the need for a discharge plan, but this seems early. I'm barely beginning to move some muscles. Isabel works hard with my insurance company to get me back to Spaulding, where I was last February. I tell her discharge to a nursing home rehab program is not desirable. Spaulding has a bed. She has success and is pleased with herself. I can see it in her smile. I will be discharged tomorrow, Saturday, December 29.

But early Friday evening I am visited by Dr. Evans. He informs me I will not be going to a rehab yet. "You're not ready," he says. I'm relieved. "I'm hoping to see you experience more motor improvement."

On Saturday morning, I am visited again by the team of doctors lead by Dr. Evans. I sense this is hospital rounds, but I didn't expect it on the weekend. I am happy to see them because I can show some improvements. "Look," I begin, "I can move my thumb and my toes."

"Can you lift your leg up?" asks one of the residents.

"No, but I can move it back and forth in the bed." I don't want to disappoint him. I consider myself a team player.

"Good, shows progress."

"Yes." I am pleased with myself.

The team congregates around me and talks about my progress, possibly a discharge to a rehab, and another MRI. Dr. Evans writes the order for an MRI. "I'm not sure when it will happen," he says. "This is a big hospital."

A big hospital indeed. It is made up of many buildings and circuitous corridors and connections, hallways, and elevator banks to those connections. Connections are to other buildings of the other hospitals that make up this large medical teaching facility. This is an old hospital. Brigham and Women's Hospital is the product of a merger in 1980 of three Harvard University–affiliated teaching hospitals: the Peter Bent Brigham Hospital, the Robert Breck Brigham Hospital, and the Boston Hospital for Women. Today it is one of the largest teaching hospitals in the world.

I don't know how anybody finds their way around here. Traipsing to the lower level for my radiation treatments every day was easy compared to finding one's way to the patient floors. Scheduling a diagnostic test must be a logistical whisker away from gridlock. All those tests, all those patients. There must be a computer model that technicians and the medical staff rely on for the scheduling.

My MRI occurs early Sunday morning at 1:40 a.m. I ask the time when I am awakened. With the number of patients in the hospital at any given time, servicing them at 1:40 a.m., 2 a.m., or 3 a.m. seems inevitable. We take two elevator banks before getting to L—the Lower Level—where the diagnostic radiation equipment is located. This is one level above LL, where my radiation treatments occurred.

The radiation therapist asks, "Are you claustrophobic? Do you need a Valium?"

"No, I am not," I answer sleepily. Not anymore. Not after 27 radiation treatments with a mask so close to my face it nearly took the hairs off. The MRI mask is about four inches away from my face. It's made of Plexiglas and I can see through it. The radiation therapist slides the cage-like protective barrier over my face and my body glides into the machine's long tube.

By now I know what to expect. I take a few breaths as I wait for the test to begin. There it is. Those first two loud blasts—short ones—that herald the beginning. They remind me of trumpeters from King Arthur's day alerting the crowd: "The King is coming, the King is coming." In my case, 45 minutes of loud noises are coming. There's a pause. Now a loud, sustained medium-to-low-pitch sound. It's loud and seems to go on and on and on. I try to divert my mind elsewhere, and just when I think that noise will drive me mad, it stops. Another pause. Rat-a-tat-tat, rat-a-tat-tat, rat-a-tat-tat, rat-a-tat-tat, rat-a-tat-tat. How could I forget that sound driving into my skull? It's like a machine gun shooting at a mob of thugs, or a jackhammer drilling into concrete. In the background of the rat-a-tat-tat, I hear another sound that keeps a steady beat, like a grandfather clock, but the sound is extraordinarily loud. It's not the tick, tock one typically hears, it's enormously loud with a pounding sensation, GLICK, GLOCK! That's the ensemble of noises bouncing off the magnets of the MRI machine and into my ears. After the many times I've found myself in this tube, I visualize the noises as music. It's a way to cope through the exam. I know that's a stretch, but it keeps my mind occupied. When I listen carefully, I hear a rhythm among the noises...or do I conjure up a rhythm?

With an ensemble of music and rhythm there must be a conductor. I visualize a small thin man who wears wire-rimmed glasses and tries to manage these extraordinarily loud sounds; a true conductor wouldn't go near them. My little conductor is approximately three feet nine inches tall, 49 years old with straight hair the color of straw. He's quite thin due to conducting these noise orchestrations on an hourly basis. As you can guess, he exudes energy conducting the racing sounds. He dresses in a two-piece pinstripe grey suit with double vents in the back of the jacket. And, yes he unbuttons his jacket as he begins. He gets quite a workout.

I'm getting a workout, too. All these sounds/noises are colliding with one another. They persevere in one-, three-, and five-minute sequences. There is a pause after each sequence. That's when I take a breath and visualize the little conductor wiping his brow. Instantly he lifts his baton and readies himself for the next onslaught of sounds.

Finally, we are into the last movement. There is a cacophony of sounds, all in contrapuntal action with each other. There is that long sustaining sound underneath with the rat-a-tat-tat bouncing off the trumpets. The GLICK GLOCK is racing loud and fast against...what? I've lost track. And so has the little conductor. Each sound is racing and roaring loudly, especially the trumpet blasts, toward a finale. Racing and roaring, loud and fast, racing and roaring, loud and fast, then silence. The little conductor has fallen flat on his face. All his blonde hairs are projecting out from his head as if he stuck his hand into an open electrical socket. I breathe a sigh of relief.

The MRI is over.

———

The following day is Sunday. Dr. Evans and his team arrive. I am pleased because I have something to show them. "Look what I can do." I raise my left leg and left arm together with pride. All the doctors, especially Dr. Evans, are pleased.

Joe arrives after breakfast. Today's the day Ken and Danielle are coming, not just to visit, but to celebrate our Christmas. We always celebrate Christmas with them the weekend after the holiday. They usually drive to the Cape.

Ken walks in with bags of presents and a look on his face that I've never seen. It's free of defenses, and I see...what? Is it concern? Worry? It must be love. I appreciate seeing that. He walks over to me and hugs me. Next he places a Santa cap on my head and says, "Hi, Mom, Merry Christmas." The son taking care of his mother. This is new. I'm not sure how I feel—a bit old. I am feeling the love. I pull my hospital gown around me more, I am cold. My body's way of reacting to new feelings—from myself, and from my son.

Danielle is here, too. She gives me a hug as well. Joe pulls the curtain around to claim a boundary for our own little rounds. We have our Christmas—Joe, Ken, Danielle, and me—right there in my part of the hospital room. We exchange presents with ooohs and aaahs and laughs like we were in our living room at home. Lots of nice presents and good fun. The best part is that we are all together. It's quite memorable.

———

I wouldn't have believed that celebrating Christmas in a hospital room would be so much fun. Martie is recovering her mobility quickly, and we expect she will be transferring to rehab in a day or two. Ken and Danielle bring their gifts for us to Martie's room, and I bring our gifts for them. It's

such a joyous day. One of our family traditions is to create funny tags to put on presents. On a tag for Martie, I write, "To: The social worker, From: The consultant." I often identify my son as "Map Man," a nickname he gets from his work as a cartographer. Ken and Danielle have taken up the tradition in their tags to us and each other.

The day when Martie was finally admitted to the Brigham I had called Ken and asked to stay for the night. We had stayed so many nights during the radiation treatments that it felt comfortable staying with them. It's only a 10-minute drive from the hospital. Each night thereafter we would talk over the day's events, and Ken and Danielle were always encouraging. It made for a comfortable end to the day.

I find it rewarding to have a close relationship with my son as an adult. When he was born I was 21, and it was just three days after my college graduation and three months before we would head to Buffalo for my graduate school training. That long, dry summer I was working at a golf course as a greens keeper. There were opportunities for overtime, watering the course. I was grateful for the work because we only had a few hundred dollars saved. I worked seven days a week, and an August drought brought overtime pay after 40 hours. One week I made two weeks' pay with all of the hours. Martie had a hard time breast-feeding Ken, so he was up several times each night. But when you are 21 and about to head off to graduate school, you deal with the sleep loss and life is good.

Once Martie decided to switch to bottle-feeding, I helped with Ken's care a bit. But he and I did not have many hours together when he was awake. Once we moved to Buffalo, I was at the university most of the time. I was consumed by the challenge of taking courses and working with faculty on research projects. During that first year I was not sure I could survive in graduate school. I almost was kept back in seventh grade. I was a late bloomer, very late. It never occurred to me that I was making a choice to put my achieving ahead of my fathering and my husbanding. I was determined to be the good provider that my parents expected of me. That meant doing well in courses and being visible to the faculty. I must not fail. So again I did not make much time for Ken. He was a great baby. Once he started sleeping through the night, he would sleep from 7 p.m. to

7 a.m. When he woke in the morning, he would play in his crib and babble to himself.

A decade later I began to regret how little time I had spent with Ken. In high school, he became interested in making movies, and I enjoyed his creativity. One of our projects together was picking out the best college to nurture his interest in film. We went to college nights at local high schools and to the library to look at college catalogues. He ended up picking Syracuse's Newhouse School of Communication following a weekend visit by the whole family. It was gratifying to see him pick a college that would be good for him rather than pick the opposite, which some teenagers do.

Ken is a very gregarious man, loves to talk. With his Santa hat and sense of fun, he acts as the leader of the present swap. Our little area inside the curtain is an oasis of family togetherness. A wonderful break in the tension of the past two weeks.

———

Later in the day, Dr. Evans comes by while Joe is still here. Speaking to both of us, he says, "You've made progress in a short time, since we administered the Decadron. I am pleased with that."

"Yes," says Joe. "We've had quite a scare. Any news from her MRI, doctor?"

"The results of the MRI done here at the Brigham are ambiguous—just like the Cape's MRI. There's still swelling on the brain, and we're still unsure of the cause. Could be the seizures, could be effects of the radiation. I am encouraged by Ms. Dumas' progress with her mobility though, and feel she's ready to continue her progress at a rehab."

"I hope Isabel can find another bed at Spaulding."

"I'll leave a note in her box so she can arrange it for tomorrow. Be sure and tell her of your preferences."

Later that day one of Dr. Evans' residents arrives at my room. I'm surprised to see him so late.

"Dr. Kahn will return from vacation on January 2 and would like to see you at 1:30 on that day."

"Oh." I am surprised by this. That's one day after I arrive there. He hands me an appointment card. "Thank you."

Before Joe returns to Brookline, we talk a bit. I open our discussion with, "So, what just happened?"

"What do you mean?"

"To us, to me. Where are we headed?"

"I know where we have been but not where we are going."

"It seems like that seizure in the middle of the night happened so long ago. It's almost a year, isn't it? We were just getting our lives back together, and this thing happened again. Don't have a name for it, do you?"

"Life? Reality redux? What if it happens a third time?"

I can't think of "what if", as in "what if my brain seizes or a what if I never walk right again?" There isn't room in my head for that conversation. I **will** walk again, and I **will** walk out of that rehab hospital. I'll get myself back to where I was before these catastrophic events, the radiation effects and the antiseizure medication be damned!

Our discussion tires me out. I look over at Joe. He looks done too. Tired and all talked out. He takes a breath and looks stonily serious. "I don't think I can handle another relapse."

I have no words, no response, or an obvious retort.

It's over. Our discussion.

———

I surprise myself when I say, "I don't think I can handle another relapse." The words just came out. Part of me is protecting itself from another shock. I know I haven't worked through the emotional toll from the events of the past year. The thought of another trauma makes me nauseous and sick to my stomach. When I fantasize about it, my reaction to another relapse is to opt out, run away. Just get in the car, go the bank for some money, and keep driving. Put it all behind. Just like Richard Kimble of the television series The Fugitive. Go from town to town hiding who I am. Have adventures.

I know that times have changed and the one-armed man would find me quickly. And people would dump on me for abandoning Martie. I don't

care what they say. I don't care if other people have survived more than I have. They are not in my shoes.

———

The following day, there is more motor improvement on my left side. My team seems as excited as am I. My discharge is in place. An ambulance is arranged, and I will travel to Spaulding in Sandwich to continue my recovery. Dr. Evans approaches.

"I will follow you as your neurologist. I understand you have an appointment with Dr. Kahn tomorrow."

"Yes, but Spaulding doesn't know it yet."

"Meet me in Neurology afterwards, my appointments will be in step with his."

"Thank you, doctor."

A nurse peeks in my room and announces, "The EMTs are here."

SECOND TIME 'ROUND

The day Martie is to be released from the Brigham, I call the rehab hospital on the Cape where she will be going. I ask how she will be transported and find out that they will send an ambulance. I ask if I can ride along and they agree. I bring some clothes for Martie to wear during her rehab.

The ride to Boston is uneventful. I talk with the EMTs about their job and they want to know about Martie. We get a VIP parking space at the hospital and go up to her room with a wheelchair. She is more than ready. On the way back, it is after 3 p.m. so I expect the EMTs to take the HOV lane, the express lane for cars with two or more people in them, potentially saving 30 minutes.

"We can't use the HOV lane," one of them explains. "It's company policy. We can't take the chance of getting stuck in there if there's an accident."

Seems like a rare event to me, but then I think about what it would be like if Martie had a seizure stuck inside the HOV lane. Two rare events make a catastrophe.

———

Here again. Same place. Not the same room, but it looks identical. I have the window again, for which I am thankful. But that's about all. I hate being here. Again. I know it's a good thing that I am here. They will help me walk and help

266

me dress myself, again. It feels shaming. There's the old whiteboard with my name on it, and down at the bottom, names of the folks taking care of me. Soon the board will fill up with all kinds of symbols informing whomever of what I can and cannot do, and what I must do. My goals. In response to all the work to be accomplished, I blow out a puff of air. I don't like it that I find myself here. I don't want to do this again, but I have to. Feels somewhat like failing, having to do it all over again.

I meet all the therapists: occupational, physical, recreational. It's like old home week. They're the same young women and men with whom I worked last February, almost a year ago. Can't seem to wrap my arms around the date. Today is New Year's Day, January 1, 2008. Another new year.

Dr. Davidson is on vacation until tomorrow. I seem to enter his life when he's on vacation. The last time I was here, he was off on the first of my two weeks. There will be someone covering, a Dr. Van Hooven. My ears are sensitive to words in a conversation. My radar is back. Two people are talking. I hear something like, "why discharge?...have to go back...makes no sense." They must be talking about me and my discharge yesterday and my need to return tomorrow. Probably has to do with the insurance company.

When I meet with her I mention my appointment. "Dr. Van Hooven," I begin, "I need to inform you I have an appointment with Dr. Kahn back at the Brigham tomorrow at 1 p.m."

"Really?" she says in surprise. "How can you be serious about your work here in rehab, if you can't start on the first day?"

Why is she talking to me like this? "I expect I'll manage it, but right now his appointment is a priority for me."

Our discussion prompts her to peruse my chart. After several minutes she looks up me and smiles. She proceeds to perform a strength test on my left arm and leg.

"I see by your record that you've had many radiation treatments since you left us last February."

"Yes, I have."

"That appointment with Dr. Kahn is important, then. We'll arrange an ambulance to get you there in plenty of time."

"Thank you. I have a small request. Can my husband accompany me in the ambulance? He goes to all my appointments with me."

"I don't see why that can't happen. We can send both of you in a wheelchair transport van."

"Thank you, doctor."

Ah, that's settled. I'll see Dr. Kahn tomorrow and Joe can come with me in the van. I'll call him and tell him.

———

This time when I meet with Dr. Kahn I am in a wheelchair, different from when we first met last March when I walked with a cane to meet him. My visit with him has surprises. He tells me he is glad I found my way back to the Brigham "Although on vacation, I was at home. I was receiving emails from my residents about you and what was occurring each day. Tell me, no more seizures?"

"No, thankfully."

"Any other symptoms: headaches, dizziness, nausea, vomiting?"

"No, none of those either."

Next he performs the familiar neurological exam with his light, the muscle strength test, and the eyes-closed arms-open test.

"What do you think's happening?" asks Joe.

Dr. Kahn looks pensive and is quiet for a few seconds, as if he is in deep thought. Finally he says, "We are in a state of uncertainty. This could be a treatment effect—as in side effect—of the radiation treatments last spring."

"It takes this amount of time to just show up?" I ask.

"Yes. This can happen five to six months after those treatments are completed. Your brain is still moving slowly back to the position it had resided in before the tumor pushed it aside. Another treatment effect is a vascular bleed, but that's not what I'm seeing here." I am grateful for that; I don't know what it is, but it sounds awful. Dr. Kahn continues. "The swelling in your brain is in the area where the radiation occurred, and is also where the seizures occurred."

I'm feeling perplexed and a bit angry. Was this "treatment effect," as he is calling it, on that sheet of paper? The one with the penciled star on it that listed all the things that may go awry during radiation treatment? I wish I had a copy of that paper. And treatment effect? Isn't that a fancy word for side effect? I'm feeling tired and frustrated.

"I want to watch you very closely for the next few months. I'll schedule the next MRI in three weeks." He looks at a calendar. "January 24, and then another in March." He turns toward Joe and me for a response. We look at each other and nod our heads in agreement. "I understand Dr. Evans will follow you as your neurologist."

"Yes, he will."

"Ah, this is good. And you will see him after, or before, your appointment with me?"

"That's the plan."

I am satisfied that I have a neurologist on my team. It feels complete: a neurosurgeon, a radio-oncologist, and a neurologist. Three specialists will follow me. It makes me feel important, almost regal. The queen has three important doctors with whom she consults. Although having many doctors didn't keep her from sitting in this wheelchair again—*Off with their heads!*

Dr. Kahn talks about the muscle strength tests he just performed. "They are good. I think you will make good progress in rehab, probably faster than last time."

"That would be nice."

"On discharge from the Brigham you were given instructions to taper off the steroid Decadron, yes?"

I nod my head.

"I'm going to rewrite that taper into a much longer one, one that will take you through to and after your discharge from Spaulding. Will you give it to your attending doctor there?"

"Yes, no problem."

———

Our limo—a.k.a. wheelchair car—awaits and whisks us back to Spaulding. We are both exhausted. Joe returns to home and I to my room to sleep.

The next day I begin my routines in earnest. Have to demonstrate I am serious after taking a day off. Routines, exercises, and all the attendants are familiar to me, plus the disappointment and frustration of being here again.

Dee Dee, one of the aides, remembers me. She is assisting me in the shower when she notices my tears.

"Hey, you crying?"

"Yes, I thought it'd be a good place to hide them, what with all this water."

"You're going to be fine, you're doing so good already."

"It's hard being back here."

"I know, but you're in the best place, and you have the best assistant working with you." She is laughing now, and I laugh with her. She's right. I will work hard and get myself out of here and back home.

Things happen fast. In no time I am dressing myself, showering and washing my hair without assistance, moving from wheelchair to walker. The next step: walking with a cane. By Friday of the first week, which is day five, Dr. Davidson, back from vacation, approaches me. "How do you feel about going home, say Sunday or Monday?"

"Wow, could I? Do you think I'm ready?"

"The team thinks you are. You think about it, and let me know if *you* think you are."

He surprises me and gives me a lot to ponder. I review my progress. It has been fast, I would love to get home, get out of here. I have an appointment with a client on Monday. Perhaps I could see her and not have to cancel, even though I certainly have a good excuse and she would understand. It's that old shame surfacing again, telling me that I must not let anybody down.

It seems like I don't have to work that hard at all. Muscle memory is kicking in, and my muscle strength keeps improving. By Saturday I am getting out of bed and walking to the bathroom myself, with a cane. My body almost feels as if I could do it without a cane, but I am cautioned against it. I comply with the rules. I am good at that. I admit I do feel a bit shaky, but I want to go home.

Sunday I'm being discharged. Joe arrives. We are both happy I am coming home. With him in the room I practice walking solo. I feel a bit guarded, but I like doing it, it feels like getting back to normal, for the second time. We wait for the nurse. We know the drill. She needs to go over the discharge in a proper manner. That's the procedure. Then we can leave. I sign the discharge papers and am ready to go. She says she will return with a wheelchair to take me out. It takes her a long time. Joe leaves to bring the car close to the door and returns to my room. Still no wheelchair.

"I'm going," I say, and start walking out of the room. That's when sparks fly. An attendant notices me walking down the hall.

"Wait," she says. "You need a wheelchair." I think it was her wording that caught me, because I don't *need* a wheelchair. I keep walking toward the elevator, Joe keeping pace with me.

Someone finally finds a wheelchair. "It's hospital policy that you leave in a wheelchair," she said. That's when I get in and sit down. Down the elevator, into my car, onto Route 6, and home.

AFTERMATH

I cannot get out of bed. It's been several days now, and I continue to have this difficulty. It's not that I can't for a physical reason; it's just that I don't *want* to get out of bed. It's warm. It's cozy, and I feel safe here. Besides there's nothing for me outside of these covers.

These days Joe is up before me eating his breakfast and reading the paper. There was a time when that alone would be a motivator to move me out of bed. But not these days. I am spent. I feel like the stuffing has been taken out of me, like the Scarecrow in the *Wizard of Oz*. In the movie he wanted a brain. But I remember a scene when the wicked witch saw to it that he lost most of his straw—his stuffing. I watched as Dorothy and the Tin Man fiercely stuffed the straw back into him to help the Scarecrow regain his shape. That's how I feel. How did that happen? Oh. I remember now. All those seizures.

It's the middle of January 2008, I saw my last client two weeks ago. I need referrals. It's been a few weeks since I've heard from the EAP I am associated with, but they'll call again. My network of colleagues is building, but currently there's a dry spell. That happens in psychotherapy, especially building a new practice. I'm impatient. I remind myself I am healing from the aftermath of multiple seizures and left-sided paralysis for the second time. A good dose of healthy self-talk is required, "Slow down, Martie. Take a breath...relax...take the time to heal." That's what I would tell my clients or my friends. I need to listen to my own advice.

Finally I rise from bed and begin my day. Most of my days begin in the same manner—reluctantly. I guess I'm depressed. I make a mental note to call

Elle for an appointment. It's time for us to start talking and resume *my* personal psychotherapy.

"Ah, the queen is up," declares Joe with a smile that spreads across his face. I smile back, he is so dear. He doesn't give me a hard time for sleeping in.

With the walker I make my way to the kitchen for breakfast. My brazen act of walking out of rehab was just that—brazen. Since I've been home, I've been prudent in using the walker and the cane. I don't intend to injure myself.

"Did you get a chance to practice *Stardust*?" I sense Joe nudging carefully, not wanting to push too much, but trying to keep me on target—a tough balancing act.

"I have time." I muse. I'm working on my daily puzzle. I don't want to engage in conversation (that's not like me), and Joe must be picking up on this, too. I'm sure he's noticing my behavior, but he's not calling me on it—yet.

Twice a week I meet with a physical therapist and an occupational therapist. Again. I embrace the exercises. Thankfully, they are very different from last year's. My deficits are also. I have two exercises that are my favorites: the *drunk driving walk*, which speaks for itself, and the *dancing ladies walk*. The dancing ladies walk requires me to stand facing the counter, place my left foot (the weak one) behind the right foot, move the right foot to the side, repeat the left foot behind the right again. Continue moving along the floor to the end of the counter. Repeat, but initiating with the right foot behind the left foot. In the beginning, it's hard with the left foot being so weak. But as with most exercises, it gets easier, and my left foot becomes stronger the more I practice. The goal: perform this exercise without holding on to the edge of the counter.

Jonathon is my new occupational therapist. He is very quiet, but manages to ask the right questions. The right question, in my case, concerns my piano playing.

"I know nothing about playing the piano or even about music," Jon says. "But how about we do this. Why don't you practice one page of that last piece you were playing before your brain tumor. What was it called?"

"*Stardust*."

"OK, *Stardust*. Practice that and play it for me when I return next time. How does that sound?"

"Sounds great." I am excited about his idea. That's what I need. Someone to give me an extra push, a reason to practice. Jonathan closes his files, stands up to leave, but hesitates a brief second. "What?" I ask. From the look on his face he has one more thing to say.

He stops short then asks, "How did you get your name?"

I laugh a bit, feeling confused, then understand. "Oh, you mean, how did I get the name, Martie?"

"Yes."

"I was 12. Back then we 12 year-old girls watched the *new* show on TV: Walt Disney's, *The Mickey Mouse Club*. (Today my granddaughter watches her updated version.) Each day there was a 10 minute segment of a serial called, *Spin and Marty*. And we 12 year-olds loved those boys."

One day I asked my mother, "Where does the name Marty come from? Is it a nickname?"

"Yes," she replied. "It's a nickname for Martin." She continued. "It's a nickname for Martha, too."

My face lit up. "Really!" It's not that I hated my name, it's just that at 12 years old it didn't fit me. Who wants to date a girl named, Martha, when my aunts and my mother's friends all had the same reply. "Martha is an old-fashioned name." Then they would add, as if they realized what they said had upset me, "it's such a beautiful name."

"What if I changed my name to Marty?" I asked my mother.

"You could do that," she said. "I'd suggest spelling it with an 'i-e' on the end. It's the feminine version."

"And," I offered. "When you push the letters of Martha and Marie together you get Martie. Taking out the 'h', of course."

My mother laughed. "Yes, you do."

Changing my name would work for both of us. In my extended family (my father was the oldest of nine and seven of his siblings were married and producing many children), I was one of many, many cousins and known as Martha Marie. By the time I was 12, I was called 'little Martha' to distinguish me from my mother. My mother, who was 35 to 40 pounds overweight at the time, was called 'big Martha'. I imagine she was very sensitive about both – her weight and that moniker.

In my thirties we moved back east to be closer to our families. One of my nieces, whose middle name is Martha, and named for my deceased mother, said. "You know, Aunt Martie, Martha is such a beautiful name. (Another generation calling . . .). Why don't you change it back? She asked me enough times to cause me to think about doing it. But first a *test run*. I went on a five-day business trip to Washington, D.C. and did not disclose my name to be, Martie. I spent the entire week with lots of people in my research area – demography. Whenever anyone hailed me or called out my name, there was a slight hesitation from me, an *oh-I-think-that's-me* before I responded. I couldn't get used to being called, Martha.

I agree: Martha is a beautiful name, but it doesn't fit me. I'm glad my niece provoked me and I tried it out. Martie fits. It's who I am. It's who I've become.

———

It's January 24th, three weeks since my last MRI, and we travel to Boston for the next one. I will meet with Drs. Kahn and Evans. This time I walk with a cane. Dr. Kahn views the MRI outside of our waiting room. Then he joins us.

"I'm still not certain," he begins, "There is some swelling, but it's reduced slightly from the last image."

"Probably from slowly tapering off the steroid?" Asks Joe.

"Yes." Turning toward me Dr. Kahn asks, "How did the taper work for you?"

"It was hard." I answer. "Especially where sleep was concerned. I slept two hours a night, got up and read for four hours, then tried to go back to sleep again."

"And now?"

"Much better. Now I'm at the other end, sleeping too much." At this comment he laughs, but has nothing to add.

"We'll schedule another MRI for March, and then we'll have more scans for comparison. I don't have enough information yet to determine if there's a reemergence of a tumor."

"So, I guess we're still in a wait-and-see mode, huh doctor?" asks Joe.

"Yes, for now, wait and see."

My appointment with Dr. Evans is next. We follow the directions to the Neurology Department: take the stairs, travel across something called "The Pike," and keep walking until we find Neurology on the left. Reminds me again of the complexity of this huge facility. With my cane, I'm able to manage the stairs and travel down the long, busy Pike corridor. There are people—doctors, medical personnel, families—coming at us, burrowing behind us, and passing us at an alarming rate. I am aware that I am a slowpoke.

Our first time here. We are given steps to a different information dance.

"Do you have a blue card?" the receptionist asks. It's like being asked if I know the password to be here.

"Yes." I grope frantically through my purse to produce it. I obtained one before I began the radiation treatments.

"Fill out these forms," she instructs. I balance my pocketbook, my cane, and the clipboard with three double-sided pages. Thankfully Joe is by my side to assist.

These pages are different from those I've completed in other doctors' offices. After writing in the addresses of the doctors who treat me and need to receive information, there are many ratings to complete. These are to be answered: always, sometimes, or never? And the questions concern neurological symptoms. Are you fearful of having another seizure? Do you suffer from dizzy spells? How often do you feel that way? What times of the day? And I must list my medications at the end.

"Ah, Ms. Dumas, hello, come right this way," welcomes Dr. Evans. I'm surprised he greets me himself from the waiting room. There is no *little* waiting room here. His office resembles most physicians' offices. It is small, stark, and clean.

"I understand you just came from Dr. Kahn."

"Yes," Joe and I answer in unison. I'm surprised he knows already. I guess that's a benefit from practicing in the same hospital complex.

"It's good news that your MRI is unchanged."

"But we still have no answers," I say.

Dr. Evans performs the familiar neurological and strength tests. I know my left limbs are still weak. I walk for him, with the cane. He is pleased with the progress I've made in three weeks.

"I'll see you in March after the next MRI and your appointment with Dr. Kahn."

I understand these meningiomas are slow growing, otherwise I'd be filled with anxiety over these enigmatic phrases: "Hmmm," "wait and see," "not certain." Time to return home and continue my rehab. I need to practice the piano.

In February I receive a referral to my practice—a man in his fifties, a divorced father of two sons, and new to therapy. He is a fiercely independent thinker who usually does things himself, but now he is having trouble with his business partner. For the first time in his life he is scared. When I sit with him I notice a struggle within me—not unusual, because as a clinician I have learned how to sit across from a client, sense their emotional state, identify it, and feel it. Sometimes I hold onto that emotion, and sometimes I reflect it back.

Today I'm having trouble and wonder about the discomfort I'm feeling. Is it his or is it mine? Something is different. For the present I attribute it to my client's anxiety over his first time in therapy. Over the next few weeks that struggle persists inside of me—I can't seem to pay attention—plus something else in me is *not right*. I feel out of synch. What does that mean, I ask myself? Synch is short for "synchronous," which means happening or existing at precisely the same time. We—my client and I—are not doing that. He needs particular words reflected back to him, and I'm not providing them. These words, some are feelings, some universal ideas, some clinically oriented. I cannot retrieve them. My brain fails me. Something is missing. What's going on? I know I'm not tired. I took a nap earlier so I could be rested, present, and able to sit with him. We have several more sessions, then he abruptly decides to cease therapy. Unlike most clients, he wants to talk about his decision with me over the phone.

During our phone discussion—which lasts as long as a session—I discover that a friend "forced" him to call someone for help and gave him my name. This client went on to say he "liked me well enough," but our therapy together wasn't working for him. When I pressed him further, asking why, he answered, "it wasn't what I was looking for" and "I wasn't getting anything out of it."

That stung. Despite my own feelings, I was sure we were making progress. We agreed to part, but not before I gave him a recommendation for therapy, even though I felt his reluctance to do so. I extended my thanks for his candor.

I spend days ruminating over our parting conversation. I scrutinize our whole therapy together. I interpret the therapeutic picture from different perspectives. It would be easy to say the client and I were not a good fit. That does happen. But no, I can't leave it at that—too easy. My gut tells me something critical was happening. Not sure what it was. Another sense I have is that he may have made up his mind about his course of action—the problem with his business partner.

He had a solution in mind and needed to talk it out loud with someone. Once he did that he was prepared to go forward with his desired action and no longer needed therapy.

Then there's the information he divulged about his friend forcing him to report back once the initial appointment was made. Those clients usually don't stick; they are not invested in therapy and not motivated to do the work because the decision was not theirs. It's like pleading with a loved one who has an alcohol problem: "Go to rehab for your mother, you'll make her happy." Any gains from the rehab program will be temporary.

I feel this client wasn't ready for therapy if a friend coaxed him in such a forceful way. In the end we probably weren't a good fit, but I feel something else is going on. Within me.

I ponder further and wonder. Maybe my client is not the only one not ready for therapy. Perhaps I'm not either. Not ready to practice psychotherapy. Wow! That's an enormous statement for me to admit. If I'm not ready to practice psychotherapy, then why? My anxiety level is shooting upward to the sky. Practicing psychotherapy is the work I love. I believe that and that's what I tell everyone. It's my *dream job*. Practicing psychotherapy is an enormous part of my identity.

When I discovered this corner of social work where I could expand my career and make a difference in peoples' lives in a one-on-one and direct fashion, I felt like I had finally landed. Everything I had done previously in my life—my marriage, raising two sons, my corporate career in finance and computers—had prepared me for this career. Not only did I love it, but I was good at it. Just like that adage: "Find something you love, and you'll be successful."

Here come the questions to myself—why am I good at it? I never thought about it before, never picked apart what was once an inherent gift. I look at data and results. Being married to a scientist all these years, I have learned from him to think critically.

I had lots of success. How did I measure that success? I have no numbers, as Joe has, but I have clients who entered therapy with me, made the choice to stay, and spent the time working on life issues. Many of my clients made changes in their lives; they felt better about themselves; they learned things about themselves, their peers, their families. Often they came back for another go-around of issues when needed. More important, they referred others to me. Sure, I had some that were not a good fit, but the percentage was low—about 7 percent.

Not all my clients were happy people when they entered therapy, but they chose to continue and work on issues. They needed someone to talk with and someone to listen. Why would a client stay if their issues were not clear? Because I treated everyone who walked through my door with respect. I offered them hope and a chance to make changes in their lives and to feel better. They made a connection with me right away. Why? I provided them with a safety net of respect and confidentiality. Clients responded to that. How can I not practice anymore?

I puzzle over my struggle and realize my empathy is compromised. I once had an enormous amount of it—about the size of Texas. Now it's been reduced to the state of Rhode Island. My empathy has always been inherent, second nature, and on the front line. Before I never had to think about that type of inter-action—compassion and empathy for another person—it automatically occurred and poured from me. That doesn't mean I don't care now, it's just I cannot get a sufficient arousal out of the *care* part of me. It's as though there is a false bottom to my empathy, and I can't get through to what I once had. I need empathy in order to hold onto the emotion in a session, to create synchronicity in the session, so I can instigate challenges needed within a session.

The stuffing has been taken out of me. It feels as though I've lost a piece of myself, of who I am. I wonder if all this is related: losing a piece of myself, feeling like the stuffing has been removed, and now my struggles with practicing psychotherapy. I'm scared. I didn't have these emotional debilitating deficits after my surgery, after rehab—the first time. Even after those fatigue-ridden radiation treatments, I was able to find my empathy and establish a warm blanket of safety and confidentiality, which allowed my clients to confide their inner thoughts What happened during...after...the relapse to make all this happen?

I dwell on these emotional deficits that are intertwined with my brain and wonder about the attributes that once graced me and allowed me to be a good therapist. It's not a process susceptible to explanation. What I do is not scripted; it differs for each client. Never did I have to parcel out and define these attributes because they were part of me. They defined me.

As I write about these struggles, I feel I am expressing myself poorly. It's as if I am reconstructing me again. Not in the same way when I picked up the pieces after my first time in rehab. Those pieces were all about my physical doing and strength. While recovering at home I added more pieces, trying to bring forth my

279

spirituality and shape a new sense of self. At the same time I discarded old pieces that didn't work in my new life. During, and especially after, the radiation treatments, I had felt confident and pleased with the construction of the new normal and the new Martie. This time it's radically different.

My deficits and losses—physical and emotional—seem to be in the mix with that *stuffing* I've lost, that straw. Intermingled in that straw of mine was a level of stamina I no longer possess, that I've lost. Empathy was there, too. As I mentioned, I've lost my ability to synchronize my thinking, and responses, with what my clients are presenting. I'm not sure how well I'm expressing myself on this predicament, but that also shows the difficulty. The only way I can put into words the inherent gift I once had in order to practice psychotherapy is a certain presence. It was the presence I possessed that strongly resonated with a client and allowed me to make an instant and deep connection. And in that deep connection was the privilege of connecting with clients in order to help them. I sense these moments with clients are gone.

A more important question remains. Will I get my gift back?

———

I am stunned when Martie starts talking about not seeing clients any more. They are the main focus of her work life and have been for a decade or so. Her identity as a psychotherapist seems strong. I know that she is proud of her ability to help her clients and that they stay with her, which is as good a measure as I know of her skill. I assumed that she would continue working once she fully recovered.

So I ask why, and then don't let her tell me. I interrupt with, "Is it the fatigue?" I know that that was an issue when she was closing her Natick practice.

"No."

"Can you tell me why, then"

"I just don't have empathy anymore. I have trouble connecting."

"Wait a minute. You mean that you don't care about them? Is it because you have been through so much that their problems seem trivial?"

"No, that's not it."

"So it's not a lack of empathy. I didn't think so."

"When I sit there with them, something is missing in me. I am not sure what it is."

"So let's talk about it some. What's it feel like"

"Before, even after the surgery, I could project a presence to my clients that connected us. Without even trying. It was just part of me. They trusted me and it allowed them to dig into their issues, even if only a little at first. I could listen to what they were saying, and they knew I was with them. Now I can't do that."

"So you don't trust them?"

"No, I do trust them, but I can't project my trust, that I am with them and won't hurt them. You know how there are some people that you just trust implicitly? It's hard to say how that trust gets communicated, but it's there, and I don't believe that they are consciously trying to make you trust them. It's more intuitive. In fact, you can't project it if it is not there to begin with."

"How could that just disappear? I don't get it."

"I don't know, but since the relapse, the seizures, it's gone. And it makes me ineffective as a therapist. The foundation on which talk therapy depends is no longer in me. I am wasting my clients' time. I won't do that anymore."

"But it will come back. It may just take more time."

"Maybe, but I don't think it's a gradual thing. It's there or it isn't."

This situation is hard for me to accept. I have to believe in her perception of what is happening. But I don't get it. Over the time she has been a therapist, I acted as her supervisor and we have talked for endless hours about her practice. I was fascinated how Martie could stay with them emotionally. Listening to her, I know that I would not have the patience to wait for insight or progress no matter how long it took. And she could forgive them when they lied and they relapsed.

The March MRI. Dr. Kahn spends many moments looking at the report in front of him. Joe and I wait patiently like two schoolchildren called to the principal's office, not knowing what to expect. Will we be punished for our mischievous deeds? But in our case there are no deeds, just the results of my recent scan.

"There's some swelling, but not as before," he begins. "I've compared this scan with the others—the two from December and January, and now today's."

"And...?" I ask.

"What do you think?" asks Joe.

"I'm ready to say with certainty the swelling is from a treatment effect of the radiation. There is no evidence of a tumor emerging."

Joe and I look at each other and together we heave a sigh of relief. A few tears grace my eyelids. Joe grabs my hand.

"Dr. Kahn," I begin, "Our son has just adopted a little girl, our first grandchild. Is it OK for me to fly? I'm anxious to meet her?"

"Yes, yes. Where is she from?"

"China, but she's now living in Bozeman, Montana, with her new parents, our son and his wife."

"Oh yes, you can fly. No problems there, go and enjoy." Then he continues with, "I'd like to schedule the next MRI for three months"

"That will be June."

"Yes, then every six months after that."

Hmmm. I wonder if we shouldn't play the caution card and go every three months, given what has just occurred.

The visit with Dr. Evans runs smoothly. It's on time and short. He notices progress in my strength. Again my next visit will coincide with Dr. Kahn's. Dr. Evans wishes us a safe trip to Montana.

—————

I remember what it was like going to the Registry of Motor Vehicles to apply for my license when I was 16. It felt like a rite of passage into adulthood. If I failed, I was not an adult yet. If I passed, I could ask my father if I could have the car tonight. There was the verbal test on the Motor Vehicle Handbook, during which a Registry officer asked me questions, the answers to which I had memorized. That was easy. Then there was the driving test. I had been told by my friends that the Registry liked to fail

boys the first time they apply. Teach us a lesson in how superior the police were. I was about as nervous as I had ever been. The anticipation leading up to that day was unbearable. I knew that a failure would be very public. My father would know because he would be there, and the other kids applying would know because the officer would just leave the car and move on to the next applicant instead of doing the paperwork for my license. Of course I failed the first time, passed on the second.

Hearing the results of Martie's latest MRI is a bit like applying for a license. Each time I expect the worst. A new tumor, swelling, bleeding. This adventure has been full of surprises. Surely there must be more. I think about what has happened to her over the past couple of months. Martie being especially tired, or stumbling. That might indicate a relapse that would be confirmed by the MRI. What would I do if the news were bad? I would probably shut down my emotions and put one foot in front of another. That is how I've made it this far.

But the MRIs continue to show only progress. No signs of a tumor or swelling, and Martie's brain is slowly moving back into its normal shape after being pushed aside by the tumor. Each time I hear the good news, I take a breath and push aside my fear. It will grow again as we approach the next MRI.

———

Bozeman, Montana, has a small airport. It is so small that one can park a car close to the gate for incoming passengers. That is unlike Boston's Logan Airport. We disembark from our plane. It is the second plane on which we have traveled today to reach our destination. One cannot get from Boston to Bozeman on a direct flight.

We had our choice of connecting cities: Chicago, Denver, Salt Lake, Minneapolis and, I think, San Jose (but I don't see the logic of overshooting the mark). Today we flew to Denver first. Once we landed in Denver—a much larger airport than Boston's—at Gate B 33 we had to walk to Gate B 88 for our connecting flight to Bozeman. That's a lot of gates and a lot of walking.

Walking is slow and arduous for me. I tire easily. And those moving sidewalks! My anxiety is high every time I approach and step off one. But they move me faster than I can walk, and we are in a hurry to get to our gate. Oh-oh, here's another. I hitch my carry-on up over my shoulder, grab onto the rail, hold my breath, and step on with my right foot, drag my left. Then I must get myself ready to walk off. I ready myself with my right foot first, then left, and finally steady my body on the floor that does not move. Twenty minutes later, and not a minute to spare, we arrive at our gate for the boarding call.

We arrive in Bozeman. I spy Tim right away. He's not hard to miss. He's tall, thin, and wiry. Joanna is standing next to him—all smiles, the proud mom. Immediately I spot the little handful in Tim's arms. What we know about her is that she is a little over two years old and that she made a connection right away with Tim and Joanna. When they first met her, she took their outstretched hands and didn't let go. That was a great relief to them. Her name is Nina Mei. Tim and Joanna were able to name her. Originally they planned on spelling her middle name "M-a-y", but when they learned the orphanage papers had a middle name spelled "M-e-i," they decided to keep it that way.

I see a pink snowsuit with a hood hanging down her back. I have a little stuffed animal—a soft white furry bunny—peeking out from my carry-on bag. I pull it out farther in the hope she will notice it.

"Hi Mom, hi Dad." Nina looks around at us puzzled and curious. We give Tim a hug. "This is my daughter, Nina!" Tim is filled with pride. Joanna is beaming as she hugs us in welcome.

"Hi Nina," we both reply. Nina whips her head back around, away from us, and buries herself in her dad's shoulder. She is shy. Who are we? She doesn't know us...yet.

She is beautiful. She has big brown soulful eyes, the shape of dark almonds, light olive skin, a clear face, and I just want to kiss her and hug her to pieces...but not yet. She needs some time. I pull the bunny out even more.

"Look Nina, I brought a present, a little bunny, just for you." Slowly she peeks out from Tim's shoulder to investigate. I push my carry-on bag a big closer, like a peace offering, and quick as a wink, she grabs the little stuffed animal, buries herself back in her dad's shoulder, and holds it close to her cheek. A victory of sorts, I think.

"Hi Nina," says Joe. He is trying on his grandpa voice—a soft, higher-pitch sound—and his grandpa charm. It works. He gets a smile.

We begin two weeks of getting to know our granddaughter and the fun and joy of bathing her and eating, talking, walking, playing, and laughing together. When she goes to bed at night, the four of us talk. Tim and Joanna take us on their 10-day journey to China. They detail the adoption process, the foster parents, the revisit to the orphanage, and how Nina held tightly to their hands. Joanna recorded all of it with a picture album. It is magnificent. It includes papers in Chinese from the orphanage as well as from the local newspaper. That album will be memorable for Nina when she gets older. To my surprise and delight, Joanna made an album for me, too. Over and over, Tim and Joanna refer to Nina as their "treasure."

My stamina is challenged while I'm here. I take many naps, sometimes in the middle of play, like "row, row, row your boat," with Nina. When this happens I feel badly, she looks up in surprise, but there is always another adult to take my place. We also have the two-hour time difference to wrestle with, and the first few days Joe and I are napping and early to bed. The altitude of almost 5,000 feet poses another challenge. I am not bothered as much as Joe. In the beginning it appears to sap his strength, but then he gets his air legs.

Nina stakes a permanent place in our hearts, and it is difficult to leave at the end of two weeks. They live so far away. I vow to myself that this little girl, Nina Mei, will get to know us and learn how much we love her, even though she lives across the country. We will visit at least once a year, if not more. When Tim and Joanna earn back more vacation days, they will visit us on the Cape. There will be phone calls, maybe even Skype when she gets older. My mind twirls through ideas as I sit behind my tears and the plane zooms down the runway and up, up into the air to take us home.

When the plane stabilizes and steadies itself at 35,000 feet my tears taper off, and I make mental promises to myself. When I return home: I will call Elle and resume my personal therapy. I need to get myself out of this down feeling. I will call Amanda at Spaulding for information on support groups for people like me. There must be one somewhere. And, I need a step-down aerobics class.

Before my brain tumor, I belonged to a health club on the Cape that had strength-training equipment identical to ones I used when I lived in Natick. I attended yoga classes and developed a cardio fitness program for myself. Today my body will not allow me to keep up with that type of yoga. I lack the endurance required and cannot get myself down or up off the floor. After the brain tumor but before the relapse, I could. In fact I was practicing yoga at home in August (before the relapse), and I had no trouble getting up and down from my yoga mat or with any of the postures. Another reminder of the destruction caused by this relapse. As for strength training, my body is not ready for that yet, but a step-down aerobics class, I think I could do. But where would I find one? I know there is a place called Mayflower—a nursing home—I think. I know they have the same strength-training equipment as my old gym in Natick. Somehow the idea of calling a nursing home...But if I want to make improvements on or in my body, I will call them when I return home and investigate. Perhaps they have a step-down aerobics class.

It's time to get on with my life.

———

I call April the "door month." With a heavy heart I make the decision to close my practice in Yarmouth Port. After all my soul scanning, it feels like the right thing to do for me. After closing that door, two other doors open.

I contact Mayflower Place and discover it is a retirement community. People live there—in apartments. There have areas for assisted living, rehab, and "continuing care"—the twenty-first century term for nursing home. At one end of their buildings sits an in-ground heated swimming pool and a small gym. It is there I find my step-down aerobics—in the pool. Did I mention I'm wary of the water? But I promised myself I would give it a try. The men and women in the pool—which is 89 to 90 degrees Fahrenheit and very inviting—all have their own disabilities. One woman is recovering from a stroke, two men suffer symptoms of Parkinson's disease, another man is in remission from cancer. Others have back problems, knee problems, or suffer from arthritis. They are a welcoming crowd; instantly I feel at home.

Amanda from Spaulding points me toward my other door. There is a Mild Brain-Injury Support Group that meets at the rehab hospital once a month. I start attending those meetings and enjoy being part of that group. The people who comprise the group are diverse—men and women, caretakers and those with a brain injury who are disabled, like me. Two women have experienced the trauma of an aneurysm, and two men have suffered brain injuries from falls. Another woman has several aneurysms in her brain; some have been clipped off, the others are being monitored. Another group member is there for support for her brother, another receives support of her grandson. From time to time a prospective new member comes to visit. I notice that only a few return and stay the course with us.

Elizabeth, our leader, is a registered nurse. She is very knowledgeable about brain injuries. Until I joined the group, I never considered myself as brain-injured or disabled. At first it felt strange and weird—those labels—but I realized that, on a continuum, I am somewhat disabled and I have damage to my brain, what with the surgery and the radiation, and then all those seizures. I know the labels provide a bit of comfort, a place in which to put myself, and it's not that bad after all.

———

The change that drove Martie to end her practice after the relapse, her sense that it "knocked the stuffing out of me," also affected her sexual response. The desire is still there, but her body doesn't respond in the same way. I mentioned earlier that the sex we had after her recovery from the surgery was the most satisfying of our long relationship. We both assumed that that experience would return after she recovered from her cluster of seizures and second paralysis.

But it did not, and it was not because of a lack of desire or effort. For a few weeks, she could not achieve her same sexual response. Though we did not talk about it at the time, we both knew it was happening. While the desire was still there and we kept trying, the internal voice in my head couldn't help but keep track of the difference. It was frustrating. After a few weeks, Martie began to have short, muted responses. I hoped that this was the beginning of a return to her normal responsiveness and pleasure. But it was not. Eventually we did talk about what was happening and agreed to just enjoy what we have together. It's part of our new relationship. We still enjoy each other and the physical closeness we have.

———

Happy New Year!—It's 2009. We are on our way to an historic event. For the first time in our history the American people elected a black president, and we are driving to Falls Church, Virginia, to stay with my cousin, Ginny, and her husband, Jim. We'll stay there for a few days and go to the inauguration. Yes, we will be one of the one-point-something-or-other million people on the Washington Mall watching the inaugural ceremony. I'm so excited I can hardly contain myself. Right after the election, I felt moved to attend and asked Joe if he wanted to go. He agreed. And here we are on January 20, 2009, standing chest-to-chest, all of us touching with our jackets of down (it's a cold day), singing, dancing, and swaying with almost two million jubilant people. When the moment comes and he says, "I, Barack Hussein Obama, do solemnly swear…,"I feel happiness and tears in my eyes just to be here, right now.

My friends and family, in particular my cousin and host, Ginny, worried about me making this trip. Later Ginny tells me she waited with anxiety for a phone call requesting that she come and get me. Over these past two years, my friends and family members have watched and learned how my stamina travels on a ghost roller coaster. It, my stamina, never knows when it will be up…or down. And given the endurance needed to travel two days to get here, my problems with hyper excitability, and crowds, I have no idea where my stamina lies at this moment. My adrenalin is driving me.

Back home I bask in the glory of that historic moment. The following evening I experience unusual sensations. The fingers on my left hand begin to jump around in involuntary movements. They also move back and forth in slow motion, as if they are looking for something. I watch these movements in awe, but then a shiver of fear travels through my body. Are these movements a precursor to a seizure? My fear is that I have pushed my body during the past week: I took my antiseizure meds at different times each day due to parties and other festivities. I arose very early on Inauguration Day and took my meds earlier than usual. Other nights with visitors at Ginny's, I lost track of the time and took them very late. The antiseizure meds were not going into my body in a timely and consistent manner. What will that do in the long run? Then there's my fatigue, which is crashing in on my body now. I am exhausted. I realize I pushed my body too far (it was worth it, but not for a seizure, it wasn't). I'm resting now. I plan to stay on the couch until my stamina starts its ascent.

I alert Joe. He soothes me by rubbing my arm and talking with me about what to do. He reminds me of our recent conversation with Dr. Kahn who recommended I take half an Ativan—0.25 milligrams—and place it under my tongue. In that way the medicine will get into my body faster than Valium. I feel better immediately and the involuntary movement in my fingers cease. Phew! What a relief. Plus my anxiety has decreased (it is an antianxiety med). No more seizures. That's my new mantra.

At my appointment with Dr. Evans days later he informs me that the movement of my fingers represented partial seizures. That was scary to hear. He also said I did the best thing by taking the Ativan.

———

Since the seizures, the only beach we can walk on is the one with the paved parking lot. Martie holds on to my arm as we walk so she can keep up. The sandy beaches are too difficult for her. Because she has no feedback from her left foot and lower leg, she needs to look at them when she is on an uneven surface. If she can't see her foot, she doesn't know where it is. She can't walk while holding a large object in her hands that blocks her view of her left foot. Carrying the laundry basket down a flight of stairs is impossible. I carry it down to the cellar where our washer and dryer are, and carry it back up with the clean clothes.

After her surgery, but before the second set of seizures, her walking was much better. We were able to do our beach walks. I assumed that once she recovered from her second paralysis, she would return to the capabilities she had before December. I was encouraged by her rapid recovery of functioning this time. She had been almost completely paralyzed on her left side for only a few days. Her muscles did not stay inert for long, so a few days in rehab were enough. But she has not returned to where she had been before the five seizures. She holds on to my arm all of the time. She is more unsteady, especially on uneven surfaces. And she is hesitant. If we are walking along and she see an uneven surface ahead, Martie stops, looks for an alternative path, and then at her left foot as she shuffles slowly along. It makes it impossible for her to walk on soft sand.

But, depending on our mood, Martie and I can choose a beach with a long, paved parking lot with views south toward Martha's Vineyard or a beach with a hard, sandy stretch with views of Cape Cod Bay. On a clear day, we may see the tower in Provincetown, all the way across the bay. Those walks remind us why we moved here.

———

Another piece of me was stolen: my sexual response. A topic people have trouble talking about, but it's important to mention here. Lovemaking with Joe has always been important. Since the relapse, my desire for intimacy with Joe persists, but my body will not, cannot, respond with the same bursting and sustained wild fireworks. Today the response is there, but it's more like a sparkler. Another cruel joke from Mother Nature.

———

"Joe," I holler, "where are all those cards and gifts?"

"Right next to the piano...in the corner...by the window."

"Found them."

Up to now I've been avoiding writing thank-you notes to all the people who were kind and generous with their love, presents, time, and cards. It's April 2009, a little over two years since my surgery, and the subsequent fallout from its aftermath. I can avoid it no longer. I am a writer of notes—be they thank-you's, memorial card acknowledgments, or friendly ones. Jane Austen and I would have made for a good friendship, perhaps rivals with our writings—hopefully peers. Today's the day, I tell myself, to tackle this "incomplete." That's what I call a project that needs to be done. Whether it be large, like changing winter clothes over for spring clothes, or small, like picking up the pile of newspapers, it's an incomplete.

There's a royal blue healing shawl sitting on top of two bags. Eyeing the shawl makes me pause. A year after surgery my chiropractor in Natick mailed it to me when she heard about my brain tumor. I sit a moment in reverie feeling her love and thoughtfulness bubble up. I open the first bag. It's filled with stuffed animals. Most came with flowers. The small white dog was from my son,

Ken. I remember Joe telling me those flowers were on the top of my car in the garage when he came home from the hospital one day. I spy the large brown bear. He's sporting two red boxing gloves and wearing a royal blue cape with a hood trimmed in red. He resembles a prize fighter. Tears bulge in one eye. The note states, "Martie's going to fight this and get better." I read further and see it's from Joe's colleagues in California.

I haven't come to the bag that has the cards and notes yet, and tears are slowly inching down my cheeks. How am I going to do this—write these notes? It's bringing back the pain, but just a little. More than that, it's bringing back the overwhelming love. I *can* do this.

The bag in which the notes are held captive is 8 inches high and 5 inches wide. When I look in, the first bundle I see is the acknowledgement cards for my father's death—two years ago. I never sent any of them to folks who were kind in their expression of sympathy to me. I can't send them now—it's too late. I will acknowledge those folks when I write my thank-yous.

As I dig further, I discover Joe has collected the cards and put them into bunches by category: his family, my family, his colleagues at work, my colleagues, my friends, our friends, etc. What a guy! That's something I would do. Now I pour over these cards. Time consuming. Lots of tears. The pain of that time returns, but the love helps heal that pain. I guess I needed a dose of that love. The crying doesn't bother or hurt; it soothes.

I place the cards in piles and begin writing. Each note is personal. I take myself back to the moment in time when I received a gift or card. Sometimes, if I feel moved to do so, I write a poem as part of my thank-you. My notes are long. They need to be. I return the love that was once given to me. I pace myself—I write four a day.

And then there's Margo. I think of those sumptuous meals we looked forward to after the end of each grueling week of radiation treatments. A special idea for her pops into my head. I remember each meal she presented to us with its accompaniments. I write my thank-you note in the form of a restaurant critique—with glowing reviews, of course. I detail every item she served us—salads, desserts, and the main meal. I have fun with my creative sense. When I finally give Margo my thanks in person and offer to do something for her, she takes my hand in hers and simply asks me to "pass it along." That's Margo.

I have a list—in my head—of the folks who drove me here and there for appointments when I couldn't drive. They receive a note from me. I write notes to the friends off Cape who hosted us in their homes while I was undergoing radiation treatments. We give gifts to people in return for their generosity and graciousness. It doesn't seem enough, but…. We vow to remember others in their time of need—with a ride, a meal, or whatever will help. Just as Margo requested.

While I was in the hospital and in rehab, Joe and I talked of making a meal for the firefighters in our town of Yarmouth Port. They had been summoned to our home twice and provided assistance. Our need to give back is strong. Joe calls the department today to inform them of our intention. The chief tells him the optimum time to arrive is late afternoon after shift change, right in time for the supper meal. We spend all day in the kitchen, and have fun preparing our special version of lasagna. That entrée is accompanied with a salad, garlic bread, and my special homemade brownies. It's a labor of love, our special thank-you. Later we present it to the chief with a note of thanks to the others for their quick response, their helpfulness, their compassion, and their courtesy. Our meal is well received.

My Uncle Mac has died. He was the youngest and last surviving brother of my father's family; my Aunt Mary is the only sibling remaining. I was close to Mac. He and his wife, Marie, took me and my brother and sisters under their wing when they realized my father rejected us. Aunt Marie was the one who called to check in with me to see how I was doing, and to tell me about the goings-on in the extended family. Mac's death, coming a little over two years after my father's, hit me hard. It is said by the experts in grief and loss that the present loss brings up memories and emotions of the most recent loss. For me, that would be my father's death while I was in the rehab hospital and physically unable to be present at his services.

Feelings of sadness and loss that I didn't know I had for my father are awakened and rising to the surface during Mac's services. It's a healing time for me. I am surrounded by my siblings and many cousins. These are all the folks who had been at my father's services, the ones I missed. I am surrounded by love, and hugs, which allow my tears to flow easily. The tears and the support from my cousins are healing. I feel a release in being able to grieve for my father today as I do for

Uncle Mac. Embedded in my grief is my love and, despite his hurtful actions over the years, I find forgiveness in my grief. I'll never know, or understand, why he turned his back on me, but I am letting go of that pain. In its place I hold on to his love, especially the love he expressed to me in the last two years of his life.

Uncle Mac was in the armed forces during World War II, just like my father. Before Mac's burial, there is the solemn ceremonial folding of the flag—part of the military honors. Young representatives of today's soldiers are present to perform this ritual. I find their demonstration of precision, the step-by-step folding, and the soft marching of the their boots moving. I cry from the depths of my heart at each skillful fold of the flag. I cry again as they present the completely folded flag to my Aunt Marie. Later I ask my brother, "Who got Daddy's flag?" "The flag," he said, "goes to the surviving spouse or the oldest child." Billy gave me my father's flag in its own flag case. It resides in my sitting room.

2009 is also the year I declare I'm going to get out and become social. I've spent the last two years inside my house rehabbing. I'm a social butterfly and am ready to spread my wings again. Joe reminds me "not to burn my candle at both ends." He's ever watchful and knows how quickly my stamina level can plummet. I do, too. But it's time.

I go to water aerobics three times a week. It gets me out of bed—a push I need. In a couple of months I'm hoping to begin working in the gym for cardio and strength training. My body is almost ready.

I've been meeting with the Mild Brain-Injury Support Group for about a year. About eight to ten regulars attend most of the meetings. I am getting to know them and feeling comfortable with them. But most important, they are getting to know me, and they like me. I enjoy learning about myself and the symptoms I endure, and that I'm not alone. We talk about things no one else can truly understand. We all talk about looking OK on the outside, but it's inside where our demons and deficits reside. We must deal with them. We talk freely about them in the group.

The group is also a place to talk about our day-to-day problems, concerns, and situations that arise. Before the meeting, even before Elizabeth our leader, arrives, we all check in with each other, thus start the meeting on our own. By the time Elizabeth gets to the table the meeting is in full force. She typically has an agenda. Her role is to keep us on topic, but we are quite skillful in not staying there.

During one meeting I casually talk about the length of time it took me to change the fabric on a deck chair. Before my brain surgery it took no more than an afternoon, now it has taken me three weeks, but in hourly increments. I talk about my brain feeling frustrated, but that I was not. Elizabeth provides incredible new information.

"Cooking and sewing are two of the hardest things to do after a brain injury."

"Really!" I am astonished.

"Yes," she continues, "it's all about sequencing. It takes time for the brain to relearn the multitude of steps required in those two distinct activities. Most people don't realize the number of steps—hence the sequencing—it takes to perform those actions."

"Well. That explains why I have trouble putting a meal together. The multi-tasking, the preparing of many items together at the same time."

In the two-plus years we dealt with the crisis, our doctors told us only half of the story about what the tumor, surgery, and radiation might bring. They told us about what I see as the straight medical issues. Martie would need to recover from the surgery, she would get tired and lose her hair from the radiation. She would need to take antiseizure medication for the rest of her life. The risks of other, serious medical consequences would be small.

But the quality-of-life issues that were likely, although not certain, to happen were never mentioned. The fact that Martie would have difficulty doing more than one thing at a time, filtering out ambient sounds, performing tasks that require sequencing. In short, skills that are a key part of our cognitive processes. Why the silence? Were the doctors afraid that we would not agree to have the medical procedures? We learned through Martie's brain injury support group that the loss of those skills is common for people with brain injuries and brain surgery. It would have made our discovery of those deficits easier to handle if we had known that they were a strong possibility, that they were normal after a brain trauma.

And the emotional issues that arise after brain trauma? Never discussed. I guess those issues are someone else's responsibility, not a surgeon's or a radiologist's. The fact that the patient will have to deal with a new normal and likely never be the same. The fact that I would become a caretaker for the rest of our lives together. Those issues were deemed not important enough to put on the table as we made decisions about what we would let the doctors do. We were left to discover them ourselves, as if they were secrets.

I believe that most of the surprises we encountered after the surgery, especially after the radiation and the cluster of seizures that occurred almost a year later, could have been prevented. All that was needed was an interdisciplinary team approach to Martie's care from the first few days that the tumor was discovered. "Interdisciplinary" means that the team has members from different disciplines and *especially* that they interact and make decisions in consultation with each other. If at least a social worker and a neurologist had been part of the team who worked together from the beginning of treatment, we would not have been completely surprised by all of the cognitive and emotional deficits that surfaced, and we would have had someone to normalize what we were experiencing as a couple. Furthermore, a neurologist would have monitored the levels of antiseizure medication that might have prevented the seizures and the second paralysis, which has had the biggest impact on Martie's life—as she says, "it took the stuffing out of me."

The concept of an interdisciplinary approach to clinical care is more than 20 years old. (See http://www.asha.org/uploadedFiles/aud/TeamApproaches.pdf). It's not a new idea. I conclude that the failure of the medical community to practice it everywhere is an indictment of their will, not their knowledge.

———

As of 2012, there is no evidence of a recurrence of the old tumor or of a new one. Martie is now going nine months between MRIs. They show some swelling on her motor cortex that probably will never diminish. But the good news is that her brain has gradually expanded into the extra space provided by the removal of the tumor. We know that—statistically—the radiation is likely to cause additional tumors someday. But there is a 10- to 20-year delay between radiation of the brain and tumor recurrence. Right now, that seems a long way off.

Martie's mobility is a constant struggle. She has been seeing a physical therapist to help her walking. She started the physical therapy because she fell several times. Fortunately, she was not hurt. Because she favors her strong right side, her left hip has weakened and she has a torn rotator cuff in her right shoulder. She also had gotten into the habit of walking toe first rather than heel first. She hoped that the physical therapy might allow her to ditch the cane. But that has not happened and likely won't. She persists with the daily exercises and, most of the time, is OK with her limitations. Her persistence and positive approach to life are amazing.

Our relationship has reached a new steady state. I continue to be the caretaker. We shared the writing of the book together. It was a daily topic of conversation and kept us emotionally and intellectually connected. We wrote our sections independently and then shared them. We discussed how our words fit with our goals for the book. On the whole, it has been fulfilling, collaborative work. I don't know what we will share now that the book is done. But I am confident something will arise.

We also share our time and enthusiasm with our sons and our grand-daughter, Nina. She and Tim and Joanna have moved back to the Boston area from Montana, which has allowed us to see much more of them and for all of us, including Ken and Danielle, to get together.

The support group is not only a safe haven for me, but a place of knowledge. I need it. I cherish the support of the folks with whom I've become acquainted. One woman lives not far from me, and each month we travel together to the meetings. The group also is instrumental in helping me embrace an important life concept—acceptance of who I am today and how far I've come in my mobility. I continue to have deficits on my left side, especially my left foot. Those will remain with me, no matter how many exercises I do. My son, Ken, reminds me,

"Mom, your foot is the furthest away from your brain and the signals have farther to travel." He's right.

Acceptance is a hard concept to master. I've spent a lifetime working on that—loving and being happy with myself and whatever is going on in my life at the present moment. I am grateful I can walk, even if my walking is hesitant and slow. No 5K races for me. My balance is compromised—I'm afraid of falling.

At a family function I watched my sister leave the table. As she walked away, I noticed her natural feminine sway and the way she walked with such ease. I thought to myself, I will never walk that way again—hips swaying, arms moving back and forth. I cried a lot afterwards. That's how I develop my layers of acceptance, through many bouts of crying. It helps.

My tears prod me, and that's when I remember another important life concept: gratitude. Gratitude reminds me how far I have come. It's like standing on top of a mountain. I remember a crisp fall day—a long time ago in 1993—Joe and I climbed to the top of Mount Monadnock in New Hampshire. It was a tough climb. I thought it would be a dirt trail to the top, but the route surprised me. It comprised of twisted trails with a multitude of rocks and huge boulders. The boulders served as steps and were difficult for me to climb. After a couple of hours we reached the top to behold a magnificent view. We could see Boston, about 60 miles away, as well as parts of Vermont, New Hampshire, and Massachusetts. While at the summit, I looked back to see how far we had climbed. It was a long, tortuous, difficult trail. It made the view more meaningful.

———

I am in my late sixties and in transition. Unlike Miss Jean Brodie, I am *past* my prime. I am slowly making the transition to professional retirement. I still work as a consultant three days a week and keep up with my professional network. But I know that it's time to think about giving that up.

My profession has been very important to me, especially to my self-image. When I was in my thirties, I looked ahead at where my life was heading. I wanted to be sure that at the end of my career I would be proud

of what I had accomplished. Just bringing home a paycheck for 40-plus years would not be enough.

I have written three books, many book chapters, and articles. I have developed a network of friends and colleagues. At Bentley University, I taught over 200 master's degree candidates who went on to become members of the profession. I helped several of them get jobs. I also have had the privilege of mentoring a half-dozen people as they were evolving in their careers. In 2012, I was awarded the "Lifetime Achievement Award" from the User Experience Professionals Association, an honor that makes me feel that I have become successful. It is hard to give all of that up. I have a strong need to be needed. How will I nurture that need without a profession?

I am volunteering at a food pantry one morning a week, stacking cans on shelves—a reflection of my first job as a 16 year old working at a local supermarket. I intend to do more at the pantry. There is something about providing people with food that appeals to my sense of altruism.

My body is feeling its age. More aches and pains. I can't eat as many spicy foods as I used to. Still, I am lucky to be as healthy as I am.

These transitions would be difficult enough to navigate without the traumas I have experienced by being part of Martie's journey.

I have changed since the discovery of the tumor. Some of it might have happened anyway. I can't help thinking that my aging has been accelerated. Here are the ways I feel different, in no particular order.

I am more patient. In spite of my external demeanor, I have been restless throughout my life. I have to have something to do every day. When I am ready to leave the house, I leave. I know men and women leave the house in different ways. Most women have to primp, put on lipstick, have the right shoes for the occasion, and so forth. All that takes time. But Martie is especially slow. Her pace is very deliberate. Her movements are calculated. It takes a very long time for her to get into the car. She has to use her arm to lift her left leg and carry it into the seat.

It took me a while to learn to be patient with her pace. Making myself angry was a waste of energy. If I couldn't be calm, my agitation would show, and the result would be constant bickering. So when we are preparing to leave the house, I get ready and then I walk outside in the yard and find something with which to busy myself. I pick up brush, stones that have strayed onto the driveway, dead leaves that appear on our rhododendrons, and so forth. It actually has a calming effect. There are other times when the pace is slowed, such as when we cook together. I try to just go with it. I know that she knows she is slow. If it made me angry all of the time, it would make her anxious and she would be slower. This is what "in sickness and in health" means.

I worry less about money. Being a child of Depression-era parents, family finances have always been a worry to me. We saved prudently during the years when we were both working and met with a financial planner to make sure we were preparing for retirement. The 1990s were very good years to be investing; the first decade of the twenty-first century not so good. For many years I had a dream that I would retire at 55. When I was about 53, I computed how much I would need to accomplish that dream. What a shock! I would have to keep working. But after the emotional upheaval of Martie's illness, I stopped worrying about finances. Money just doesn't seem to matter that much anymore. I look at the tables that predict our life expectancy into our nineties. I don't see that happening. So why not spend it now?

I am fearful of the future. I have always been a macho kind of guy. I don't fear for my physical safety. I don't lock my car or house doors because I refuse to live my life in fear that someone will steal my possessions. Theft is very unlikely. If it occurs, I hope to catch the thieves so I can beat them up. (Yes, I know that is not realistic, but we are talking fantasy here.) I climb on the roof to clean the gutters. Falling is not an option. I love to swim in the cold ocean off Cape Cod.

For the first time, I am concerned about my own health. I have kept myself in decent physical shape over my adult life. I ride my bike when the weather allows it. My yearly physicals don't reveal any serious conditions evolving. My father had colon cancer. It was diagnosed when he was 70. But it was well advanced. I am concerned, but my colonoscopies have been clean. All of those health fears seem normal for my age.

And yet, there is this sense of doom that persists. Not that I will be physically harmed, but that a disease or illness is waiting to grab Martie and/or me. I have no idea what the future will bring. I know it might look quite different from today. That fear sits in the background, behind all of the good things I have now. The return of her seizures out of the blue has made me forever wary. All that radiation seems likely to make her susceptible to more tumors. The radiation, the seizures, and the blockage of a major blood vessel in her brain has to put pressure on other vessels, which, in my internal calculations, makes her more likely to have a stroke. Her lack of balance makes falling a probability. I worry about all of those conditions.

A couple of years into my recovery, my Aunt Mary told me a beautiful story about my mother's treatments for cancer. My mother died of colon cancer at the age of 53. She's been gone almost 38 years. Mary told me of a time when she and my mother were discussing the cancer. Mary asked her, "Martha, do you ever ask yourself, 'why me?'" My mother's reply astounded me. She said, "Mary, I say to myself, 'why not me?'"

I felt a stirring in my soul when I heard that story. It was a part of my mother I never got to know, a profound part, a wise part. To this day I feel her loss because I missed knowing that deep personal part of her. On the other hand, maybe I carry that piece of her around with me. Throughout my recovery I've had people ask me the same question. "Martie, do you ever ask yourself, 'why me?'" Or sometimes they ask about anger. "Aren't you angry about what has happened?"

I pause before answering. "No, there is no anger. Not about the brain tumor." I feel, perhaps like my mother, that it could have happened to anyone. However, the relapse I suffered 11 months later carries a different feeling. I *am* angry about that. The principle reason is that the medical specialists put in charge of my care let me down.

Surely, the brain tumor changed my life. The insult of the radiation and the relapse left lasting effects—they stole core pieces of me.

But I've worked hard to achieve progress. I've traveled a long distance from the vulnerable waif of a woman in the bed who couldn't get out of it by herself. During that time my friends feared I couldn't...wouldn't...make it. Whatever that meant. Today I live with Joe, gaining more independence each day. I am walking on my own, but I need him, too.

People who know me—friends and family—tell me I look great and sound great, thus proclaiming I am back to the "old Martie." But I am not. My physical deficits are obvious, and affect the movement of my body. I wear a brace on my left foot for stability and balance, and I use a cane when I'm out in public.

With all my progress—and I am proud of all I have accomplished—I rely on Joe for some things. For instance, when we take our walks, some days my stamina is strong and I feel grounded. Those are the days I can walk beside him. Other days I can't find my center of gravity and must slip my arm through his and hold on to him as we walk.

I wish I were not so dependent on Joe, but I am. I worry about him being my caregiver...still. We frequently talk about this. Recently I tried to be the independent woman I once was. Why? *Because*. It seems I am balancing denial of the injuries to my body with "what is." My limitations continue to show me I can never be that independent woman I was before the brain tumor. Another level of acceptance I'm learning to embrace.

Sometimes I look down this road of disability to see where it ends. It does not. My disability is a set of attributes, like my blue eyes, the greying of my hair, and the lines around my eyes and mouth. It's here to stay. That disability road is continuous. It is my life now—my new normal.

Aging enters the picture, too. Joe's a bit slower than he used to be, he tires like he hasn't in the past. Joe's a strong macho guy and fears nothing. He doesn't like to admit to the "A word." He likes to say that when he looks in the mirror, he sees his hair is brown. Recently his granddaughter, who is six years old, informed him his hair is white.

When I look back and see how far I have traveled through this awful medical ordeal. I could not have managed it without Joe's love and strong support. I reflect back to when I was 17, waiting at the bus stop with him and talking about our future. That's the time I first felt a strong tug from my soul to his. I knew then he would be there for the challenges in life for the two of us, and I wanted to spend my life with him. How is it that I knew such a thing back then?

Our love has changed, been transformed. It began as teen love of early togetherness and grew into a rock-solid, loving marriage. Married life established itself with graduate schooling, then children. As time went on, love suffered as it has to in order to grow. It suffered and grew through childrearing, more schooling, and career building while we both searched for our separate identities. Love remained steadfast as we evolved and sailed back to each other. Love turned a corner with our empty nest and blossomed once more, sprouting tendrils of contentment. Our love endures. I slip my arm through Joe's and continue forward, one foot in front of the other.

AFTERWARD

For the Cape, it's an unseasonably warm May day. A day that features warm breezes off the water and makes you think of sand in your toes and a sip of wine on the beach. It's 76 degrees at four o'clock.

"Hey, Joe," I call to him out in the yard. "How about a sunset supper on the beach?" He looks up in surprise from the multitude of impatiens he is planting, thinks about it, then smiles. "Yeah, let's do it. Let me finish this row, then I'll come in and change, and we can talk about what to eat."

An hour later we are at Gray's Beach in Yarmouth Port. We don't frequent this beach much. It's small and tends to have that too-close feeling when overcrowded in the summer. One of its distinctive features is a boardwalk that extends out over a salt marsh. Folks are encouraged to walk on it, and they do. When the weather is nice, like today, it can get busy, but there's hardly a soul here. Where is everybody? One car in the parking lot and that family is on a blanket by the beach. I guess it's the time of year with school ending and many celebrations, parties, graduations, and so forth. Lucky for us. I'm glad we're nearly alone.

We walk along the boardwalk, when I notice a new rhythmic sound, my cane. At the end of the boardwalk, there's a deck-like structure with built-in benches. We sit here enjoying the remains of this perfect sunny day. The sun is beginning to slide down, first behind some clouds so it is not blinding us when we glance at it from time to time, anticipating its setting. There is a light breeze, and it's a warm one. It's too early for bugs. This beach is famous for those nasty no-see-ums. Ugh. I feel itchy just thinking of them. No toes in the sand, but that's OK.

The water is slapping against the pilings under the deck, and as I look over the deck railing I see sand through the clear salt water. It looks and sounds like the tide is coming in.

It's a beautiful evening. Joe takes out two of our crystal wine glasses and a bottle of red wine. We unwrap our dinner. "I brought a bottle of our best wine for our hot meatball subs with melted cheese," says Joe.

I laugh. "A toast!" Joe stares at me quizzically. "To the end of our book, it is finally done!"

"What do you mean? We have much more to say...more to tell."

"Uh-uh," I state emphatically. "The book is over, finished, caput, fini. How many languages do you need?"

"But, but..."

"No more buts," I interrupt.

"But there was..."

"I know, I know." I take a sip of wine. "You definitely came up with good ideas that needed to be included, like the water aerobics, the support group. And I'm glad you pushed me to write more about why I had to give up my practice."

"That was hard for you to write."

"It was. I've said it before, 2008 was a year of grieving." I bite into my sub. "And then when I thought I was finally done, you reminded me of the *thank-you notes.*"

"Those needed to be included."

"Of course."

"But what about…"

"Look," I say, changing the subject. "The sun is almost sinking into the bay. Quick. Grab the camera. I want to capture it." Joe searches for the camera I packed in our large orange beach bag.

"Reminds me of the first sunset you photographed right after we moved here. Wasn't it the end of February?"

"Yes," I say, "and freezing cold. That photograph was beautiful. But the sunset I captured then is different from the photo I will take tonight."

"Just like us," interjects Joe. "We're different people since your brain tumor and its aftermath."

"We've been through a lot."

Joe adds, "I wonder what we will talk about now, and how we will keep our relationship alive."

"There will be something, I'm sure of it. We never run out of things to discuss". I add. "It seems the book gave us a challenge and something to work on together."

"I believe our perspective and expectations in life have changed, too." Joe picks up his glass of wine and turns to me. "Let's finish that toast. To the end of the book."

We clink our glasses. Now that the sun has gone down I'm cold and start to shiver.

"Did you bring a sweater?"

"No, forgot it." Joe moves closer and wraps his arm around me, tilts his head toward mine. He does that when people take pictures of us, too.

"Look," I say. "The sun has sunk below the horizon."

"This the best part, watching the beautiful colors stream across the bottom of the clouds."

Yes, I think to myself, the best part.

IN LOVING MEMORY

Anna Massa

friend, neighbor, "snoop sister"

ABOUT THE AUTHORS

Martie Dumas, a stay-at-home mom while she finished her undergraduate degree in Economics and Computer Science, began a career in the corporate world. Midlife brought a career change when she obtained an MSW, and became a clinical social worker. Martie recently retired as a psychotherapist, and now devotes her time to writing and her granddaughter.

Joe Dumas is enjoying the benefits of a successful career in software development. He has a PhD in Cognitive Psychology and has written three books on the methods used to make computer software easier to use:

Designing User Interfaces for Software, Prentice Hall, 1988.

A Practical Guide to Usability Testing, Intellect Ltd. 1993, revised edition 1999.

Moderating Usability Tests: Principles and Practices for Interacting, Elsevier, 2008.

In 2012, he was awarded the Lifetime Achievement Award by the User Experience Professionals Association and he is Editor in Chief of the *Journal of Usability Studies*.

214

CPSIA information can be obtained at www.ICGtesting.com
Printed in the USA
LVOW10s0252020216

473174LV00010B/821/P